Handbook of Adolescent Gynecology and ARSH

(Adolescent Reproductive and Sexual Health)

Handbook of Adolescent Gynecology and ARSH

(Adolescent Reproductive and Sexual Health)

Editors

Swati Y Bhave (Lele) MD DCH FCPS FIAP FAAP
Senior Visiting Consultant
Indraprastha Apollo Hospitals, New Delhi
Member Technical Steering Committee CAH, WHO Geneva
Member Technical Advisory Group Adolescent Health WHO SEARO
Convener International Pediatric Association (IPA), Adolescent Interest Group
Former Chairperson, IAP Adolescent Chapter
Advisory Consultant "*Expressions*" India

Ashwini Bhalerao-Gandhi MD DGO DFP FCPS DNB MICOG
Consultant Gynecologist
PD Hinduja National Hospital and Medical Research Centre, Mumbai.
Ex-Associate Professor, TN Medical College and BYL Nair Hospital
Chairperson of Adolescent Health Committee, FOGSI

Foreword

Naresh Dayal
Secretary to Government of India
Ministry of Health and Family Welfare
Nirman Bhawan, New Delhi

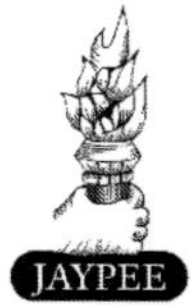

JAYPEE BROTHERS MEDICAL PUBLISHERS
The Health Sciences Publisher
New Delhi | London

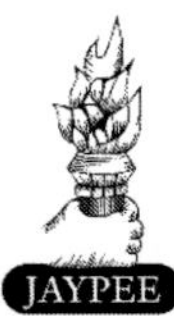

Jaypee Brothers Medical Publishers (P) Ltd

Headquarters
EMCA House, 23/23-B Ansari Road,
Daryaganj New Delhi 110 002, India
Landline: +91-11-23272143,
+91-11-23272703
+91-11-23282021, +91-11-23245672
e-mail: jaypee@jaypeebrothers.com

Corporate Office
4838/24, Ansari Road,
Daryaganj New Delhi 110 002, India
Phone: +91-11-43574357
Fax: +91-11-43574314
e-mail: jaypee@jaypeebrothers.com

Overseas Office
JP Medical Ltd.
83, Victoria Street, London
SW1H 0HW (UK)
Phone: +44-20 3170 8910
e-mail: info@jpmedpub.com

EU GPSR Authorised Representative
Logos Europe, 9 rue Nicolas Poussin
17000, La Rochelle, France
Phone: +33 (0) 6 67 93 73 78
e-mail: contact@logoseurope.eu

Website: www.jaypeebrothers.com
Website: www.jaypeedigital.com

Handbook of Adolescent Gynecology and ARSH
First Edition: 2007
Reprint: 2026
ISBN: 978-81-8448-013-9
Printed at: Samrat Offset Pvt. Ltd.

DEDICATED TO

Our respective spouses

Yashwant Bhave

and

Rajesh Gandhi

for their constant support and cooperation for the effort required for this endeavor Which we hope will benefit the millions of adolescents who require RSH services

Contributors

Kalpana Apte
Assistant Secretary General (Programme Implementation), FPA India
6/B, 701, Alica Nagar
Lokhandwala Township, Kandivali (E)
Mumbai 400 101
Email: kalpanaapte@yahoo.com

L Fahmida Banu
Obstetrician and Gynaecologist
Endoscopic Surgeon
Fehmi Care Hospital
Yousufguda, Hyderabad
Email: dr_lfahmida@yahoo.com

Meenakshi Bharath
Consultant, Infertility Specialist
Director, Centre for Assisted Reproductive Techniques, Bangalore
Email: mandakiniparihar@gmail.com

Swati Y Bhave
Visiting consultant
Indraprastha Apollo Hospitals, New Delhi
Member, Technical Steering Group, WHO Geneva
Convenor, IPA Adol intrest group
Chairperson, IAP Adolescent chapter
Research and training Wing
Email: tambhave@yahoo.co.in

Adarsh Bhargava
Professor and Head
Department of Obstetrics and Gynecology
SMS Medical College, Jaipur 302 004
India

Ashwini Bhalerao-Gandhi
Consultant Gynecologist
PD Hinduja National Hospital and Medical Research Centre, Mumbai.
Ex-Associate Professor,
TN Medical College and BYL Nair Hospital
Chairperson of Adolescent Health Committee, FOGSI
Email: ashwinibgandhi@rediffmail.com

Parag Biniwale
Chairperson Adolescent Committee POGS, Patankar Nursing Home, Pune

PH Chauhan
Consultant Endocrinologist
PD Hinduja National Hospital and Medical Research Centre, Mumbai.
Email: chauhanph@rediffmail.com

Nikhil D Datar
Assistant Honorary
Dr RN Cooper Municipal Hospital, Mumbai
Email: drnikhil70@hotmail.com

Vinay Deshmane
Consultant in Surgical Oncology and Breast Diseases, PD Hinduja National Hospital and Medical Research Centre, Mumbai
Email: deshmanevinay@hotmail.com

Neeta Dhabhai
Consultant, Sunflag Hospital and Research Centre, Sector 16, Faridabad
Email: dr_neeta@yahoo.com

Papia Goswami-Mukherjee
Clinical Assistant, Department of Gynaecology
PD Hinduja National Hospital and Medical Research Centre, Mahim, Mumbai.

Donald E Greydanus
Professor, Pediatrics and Human Development
Michigan State University College of Human Medicine
Pediatrics Program Director
Michigan State University/
Kalamazoo Center for Medical Studies
Kalamazoo, Michigan, USA
Email: greydanus@kcms.msu.edu

Rajiv Joshi
Consultant Dermatologist
PD Hinduja National Hospital and Medical Research Centre, Mumbai
Email: rsjdr@rediffmail.com

Ritu Joshi
Head, Department of Obstetrics and Gynecology
Monilek Hospital and Research Centre
Jaipur 302004; Room 217
E-mail: ritujoshi01@rediffmail.com

Kanchan S Kewalramani

Vijay Kulkarni
Consultant Andrologist and Microsurgeon
Dr. Kulkarni's Clinic
103, Suraj Ventures—A wing,
B. Keer Marg, Mahim,
Mumbai—400 016
E-mail: drvijaykulkarni@rediffmail.com

Murad E Lala
Consultant Cancer Surgeon
PD Hinduja National Hospital and Medical Research Centre, Mumbai
E-mail: muradlala@yahoo.com

Manisha Macha
Family Planning Association of India
E-mail: manisha@fpaindia.org

Neena Madnani
Consultant Dermatologist
PD Hinduja National Hospital and Medical Research Centre, Mumbai
E-mail: ninamadnani@gmail.com

Sheela V Mane
President, Bangalore Society for Obstetrics and Gynaecology, 2004-05
Anugraha Nursing Home
2, Palace Guttahalli Main Road
Bangalore 560 003.
E-mail: sheela_mane@hotmail.com

Jitendra Nagpal
Consultant Psychatrist
VIMHANS, New Delhi
E-mail: Jitendranagpal@rediffmail.com

Roza Olyai
Director, Olyai Hospital, Gwalior, MP
Email: rolyai@hotmail.com

Divya S Prasad
Clinical Child and Adolescent Psychologist
VIMHANS, New Delhi
E-mail: diyasprasad73@rediffmail.com

Mandakini Parihar
Chairperson, Family Welfare Committee, FOGSI
Mandakini IVF Centre,
48, Swastik Park, Chembur, Mumbai 400071
E-mail: map@parihar.com

Harish K Pemde
Associate Professor of Pediatrics
Kalavati Saran Hosptial, New Delhi
E-mail: harishpemde@gmail.com

D Pushpalatha
Lakshmi Nursing Home
3-6-191/1, Hyderguda, Hyderabad—500029
Email: dpushpalata@yahoo.com

Geeta Pandya
Consultant Gynec-Endocrinologist
Jaslok Hospital and Breach Candy Hospital, Mumbai
E-mail: pandya@bom2.vsnl.net.in

Shefali Pandey
Bharatiya Vidya Bhavan's SPA Research Centre,
13th NS Road, Juhu, Mumbai 400 049
E-mail: bhaspa@bom5.vsnl.net.in

Sunil Saini
Research Scholar and Clinical Psychologist
Department of Psychology
Punjab University, Patiala 147 002
E-mail: ssaini@gmail.com

Duru Shah
Consultant Obstetrician and Gynecologist
Breach Candy Hospital, Jaslok Hospital and Research Center
E-mail: durushah@hotmail.com

Anju Seth
Pediatric Endocrinologist
Professoor of Pediatrics
Kalawati Saran Childrens Hospital
New Delhi
E-mail: anju_seth@rediffmail.com

PC Shastri
Former Honorary professor of Psychiatry
TNMC and Nair Hospital, Mumbai
E-mail: Pcshastri@gmail.com

Jay P Shastri
Hon Psychatrist
Srimati Motibai Thackersey Institute of Research in the Field of Mental Retardation
Mumbai
E-mail: Jai31@hotmail.com

Ashok Shukla
Ex-Clinical Assistant
PD Hinduja National Hospital and
Medical Research Centre, Mahim, Mumbai.

Jaydeep Tank

Parikshit Tank

Reena Wani
Consultant Obstetrician and Gynecologist
Breach Candy Hospital, Jaslok Hospital and Research Center, Mumbai

Rama Vaidya
Director: Mother and Child Health
Bhavan's SPARC
E-mail: bhaspa@bom5.vsnl.net.in,
E-mail: avaidya@bom5.vsnl.net.in

Sangeeta Yadav
Professor of Pediatrics
Maualna Azad Medical College
New Delhi
E-mail: sangita_Yadav@hotmail.com

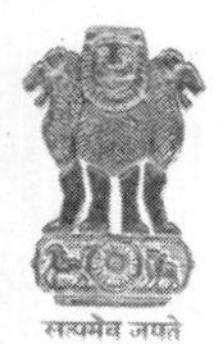

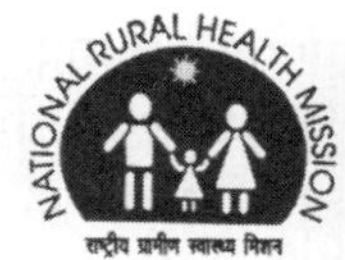

भारत सरकार
स्वास्थ्य एवं परिवार कल्याण मंत्रालय
निर्माण भवन, नई दिल्ली - 110011
Government of India
Ministry of Health & Family Welfare
Nirman Bhavan, New Delhi - 110011

Naresh Dayal
Health & FW Secretary
Tel.: 23061863 Fax : 23061252
e-mail :secyfw@nb.nic.in
ndayal@nic.in

Dated the 23rd November 2006

FOREWORD

India today is a country of a large population of young people, with over 30 percent in the age group of 10-24. Based on the population projections by the Registrar General of India (1996) there are an estimated 300 million young people in the age group 10-24, whose need for sexual and reproductive health information and services remains very high.

In spite of a legal provision against child marriage, almost 50 percent girls remain at a risk of getting married before 18. Also, over 32 percent girls get married by age 15, however, as compared to this only 6 percent adolescent boys get married by that age (IIPS and ORC Macro, 2000).

There is also increasing evidence that the onset of sexual activity before marriage is starting at a younger age amongst men. More young men (ranging from 15-26%) report premarital sexual activity as compared to only (3-6%) young women reporting premarital sexual activity.

Young people are at high risk of negative sexual and reproductive health consequences like unwanted pregnancies, sexually transmitted infections and unsafe abortions. They start sexual activity without adequate knowledge of sexual and reproductive issues and seldom practice safe sex.

The adolescent fertility is very high with 20 percent girls giving births by age 17; 19 percent of the total fertility rates are contributed by girls aged 15-19 years. This early childbearing age contributes to high maternal morbidity and mortality. Many studies have also indicated the risk of closely spaced births in young women.

Between 1 and 10 percent of all abortion seekers are adolescents. 10-30 percent abortion seekers are young women. Most of these are married adolescents, at least 50 percent of unmarried women seeking abortions are adolescent and amongst these there are many below 15 years of age.

The contraceptive use remains low among young married adolescent, 27 percent reporting an unmet need for contraception. Women in the age 15-24 years are more likely to discontinue use of contraceptives because of method failure and due to difficulty in access. The access to services and information depends on their marital status and gender.

The family welfare department, Government of India has introduced a strong adolescent reproductive and sexual service delivery component in the RCH II program. But it is equally important to strengthen the private sector awareness of ARSH has many youngsters will access service in this sector.

I am happy to know that clinicians, pediatricians, gynecologists, psychiatrists, surgeons, clinical psychologists, dermatologists and public health workers have come together to contribute to this Handbook on Adolescent Gynecology and ARSH issues.The topics included take a very holistic view of ARSH and will serve as a good resource material for those who wish to contribute to ARSH services. I congratulate Dr Swati Bhave on her initiative and hardwork.

Naresh Dayal
Secretary to the Govt of India
Ministry of Health and Family Welfare
Nirman Bhawan, New Delhi

Preface

Dear readers,

It has given us a great sense of fulfillment to have come out with this Handbook of Adolescent Gynecology and ARSH (adolescent reproductive and sexual health issues)

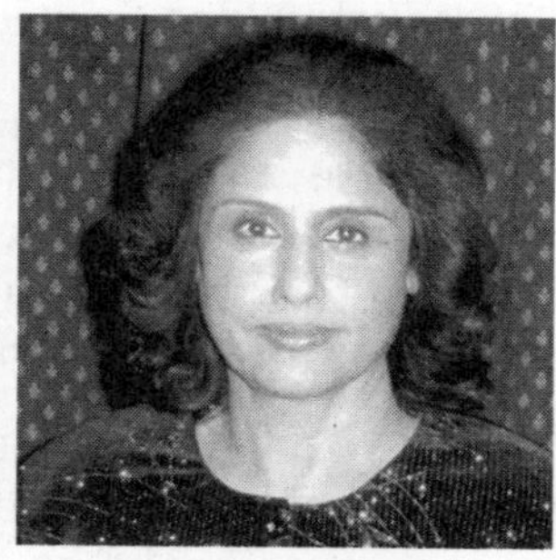

Swati Y Bhave

Adolescent medicine is the field which is overlapped by many specialties. Adolescents are continued to visit to their family physicians and pediatricians for day-to-day problems and immunizations, to adult physicians for diseases, to a gynecologist for menstruation and pregnancy-related problems, to mental health professional, for their anxiety and depression, and so on. Hence, managing an adolescent is a teamwork; and hence this book is aptly contributed by pediatricians, gynecologists, mental health and public health professionals.

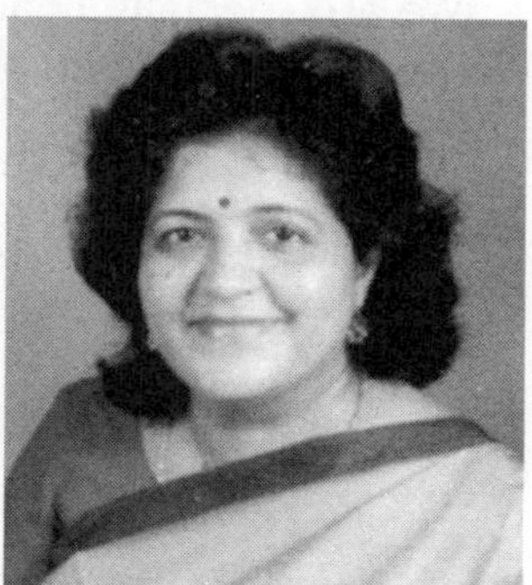

Aswini Bhalerao-Gandhi

Though all aspects of adolescent health are important, the issues related to ARSH are not only vital for affected individual adolescents, but also have a great impact in the public health scenario of the nation. There are trained gynecologists available to look after adolescent girls but very few specialists for dealing with adolescent boys who are often neglected. Andrological problems of the adolescent males should not be forgotten in ARSH services

The national statistics show the importance and need of concentrating on delivering ARSH services in our country. The incidence of premarital sex is rising as shown by the surveys in different parts of the country. Adolescent sexual activity is generally impulsive unplanned; initiated without adequate knowledge of sexual and reproductive issues and seldom with the practices of safe sex. Hence we have a rising incidence of the various negative consequences like sexually transmitted diseases, unwanted teenage pregnancies and unsafe abortions. More than 50% of new cases of HIV/AIDS are in the age group of 15-24 years.

Inspite of a legal provision against child marriage, we have a very high incidence of girls getting married before age of 18 yr. Once married they are pressurized to prove their fertility by producing a child in the very first year of marriage. They are not in a position to neither negotiate the number of births nor ensure good spacing inbetween. It is well proven that teen age pregnancy causes a high incidence of morbidity and mortality in both the mother and neonates. The incidence of abortions is high in both married and unmarried adolescents

Inspite of easy and free access to contraceptives both in the public and private set-up it has been seen that the use of contraceptives in married adolescents continue to be very low. Unmet need for contraception is reported in 27%.Unmarried adolescents cannot freely access ARSH services or supply on contraceptives without parental consent, which ofcourse is unlikely to be easily obtained.

The family welfare dept Government of India has aptly introduced a strong Adolescent Reproductive and Sexual Service delivery component in the RCH II and the NRHM (National Rural Health Mission).

But it is equally important to strengthen the private sector awareness of ARSH as many youngsters will access service in this sector. This book aims at increasing awareness of ARSH issues in the professionals of all the specialties dealing with adolescents, as ARSH is closely related with high risk behavior and mental health problems and substance abuse.

We are happy that this book has been published by M/s Jaypee Brothers Medical Publisher with whom we have had previous publications and we are sure it will reach many readers as our other books have.

We are specially honored that Mr Naresh Dayal, Secretary, Ministry of Health and Family Welfare, Government of India has graciously consented to write the Foreword.

Swati Y Bhave

Aswini Bhalerao-Gandhi

Acknowledgements

- To all our contributors who have added value to this book
- Our families specially our spouses and children for putting up with the long hours dedication to this book, causing deprivation of family time
- God Almighty for giving us motivation when at times we thought the task was impossible.
- Mr Jitendar P Vij, CMD; Mr Tarun Duneja, Manager (Publishing) and all production staff especially Ms Mubeen Bano, Mr DC Gupta, Mr Alok Saxena and Mr Abhinay Kumar Nigam of M/s Jaypee Brothers Medical Publishers for the efforts put by them.
- For photoes: We thank the following for permission to use their photographs for the cover of the book.

  Photo 1: Adolescent girls: Pallavi Sovani, Niyati Sovani Surabhi Gokhale

  Photo 2: Married couple: Prasad and Cresseide Taksal

  Photo 3: Baby: Askshay Sagne

  Photo 4: Joint family: Lata Sagne, Preetam Sagne, Mrs Asavari Sagne, Sharvari Sagne, Akshay Sagne.

Contents

Section 5: Breast Problems

Section 6: Pregnancy, Contraception and Abortion

Section 7: Adolescent Boys

Section 8: Endocrine

Section 9: Infections

Section 10: Skin and Related Issues

Section 11: Sexual Abuse

Section 12: Psychiatric Problems

Section 13: Malignancies

Section 14: Preventive Health

Section 15: Statistical Review

Section 16: Adolescent Friendly Health Services (AFHS)

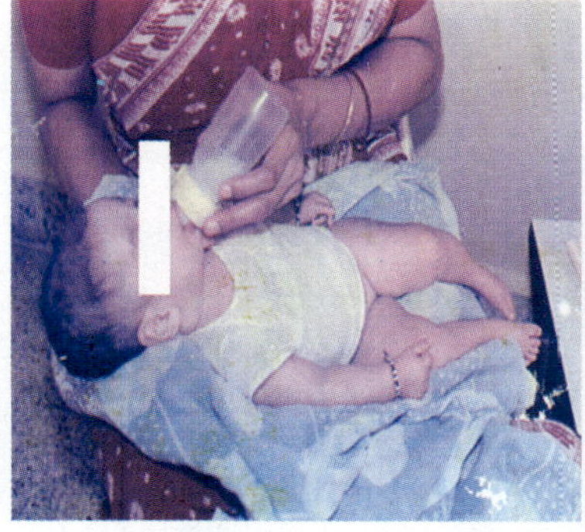

Fig. 10.2A: Progressive weight gain in a case of Prader-Willi syndrome—4 months

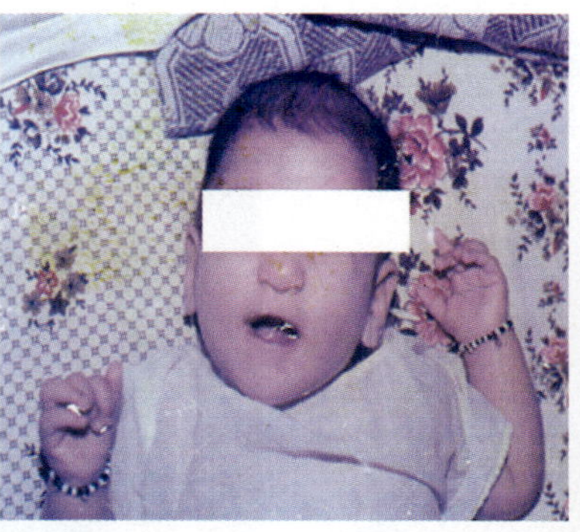

Fig. 10.2B: Progressive weight gain in a case of Prader-Willi syndrome—8 months

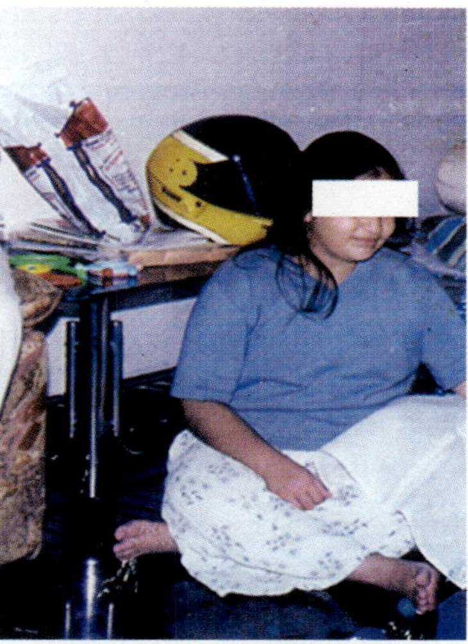

Fig. 10.2C: Progressive weight gain in a case of Prader-Willi syndrome—13 months

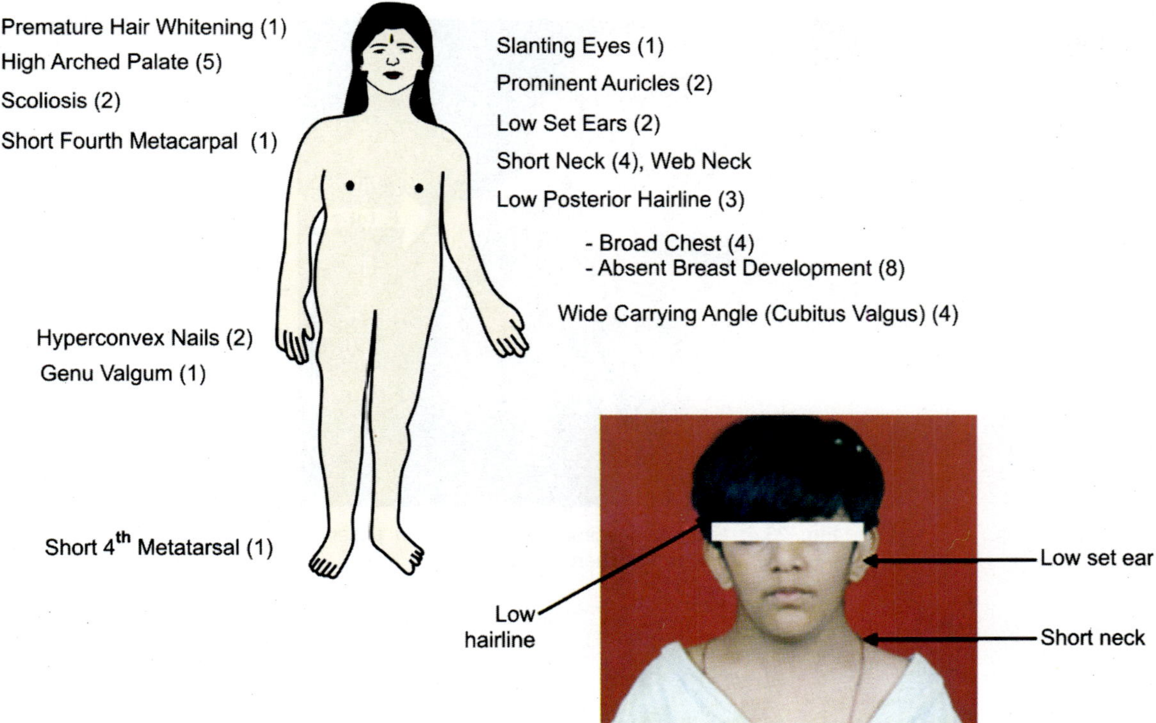

Fig. 10.3: Typical features of Turner syndrome

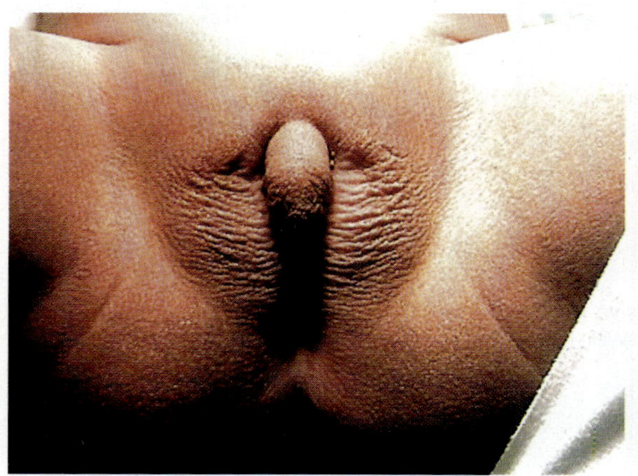

Fig. 23.2: Virilized 46, XX infant with CAH

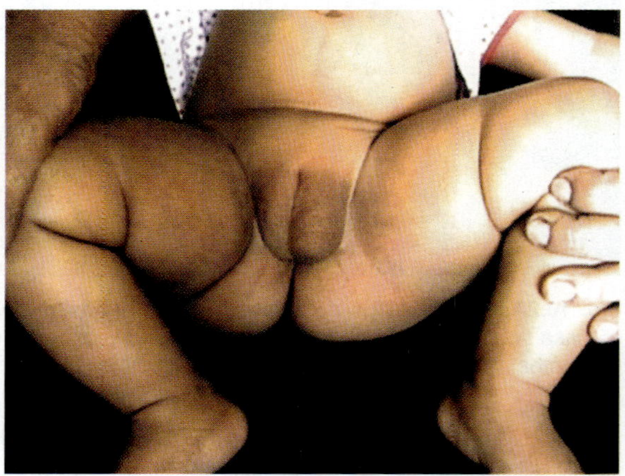

Fig. 23.3: 46, XY infant with complete AIS

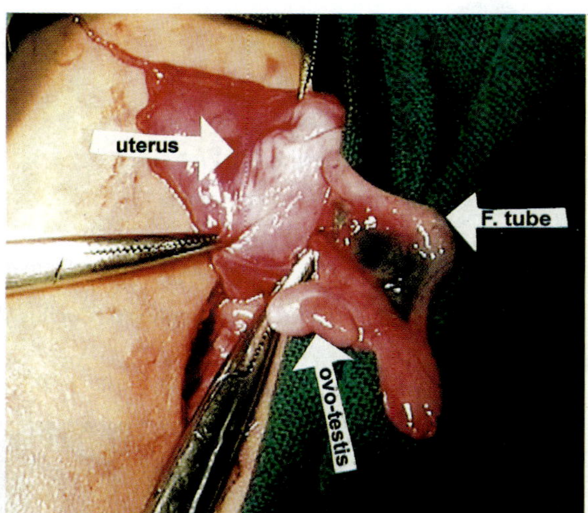

Fig. 23.4: Surgical specimen of ovotestis in patient with true hermaphroditism

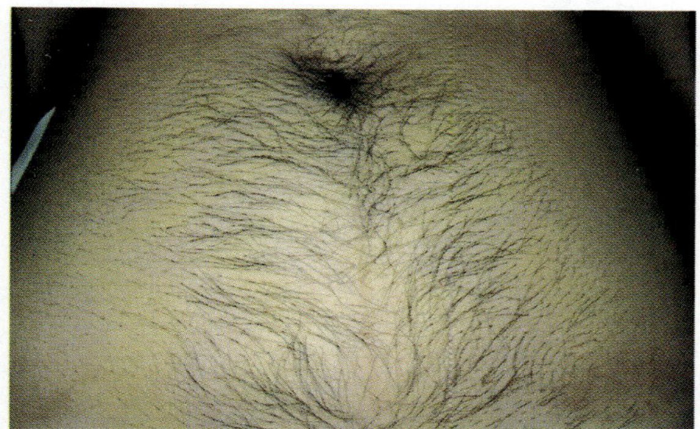

Fig. 30.1: Excessive hair on abdomen in a hirsute woman

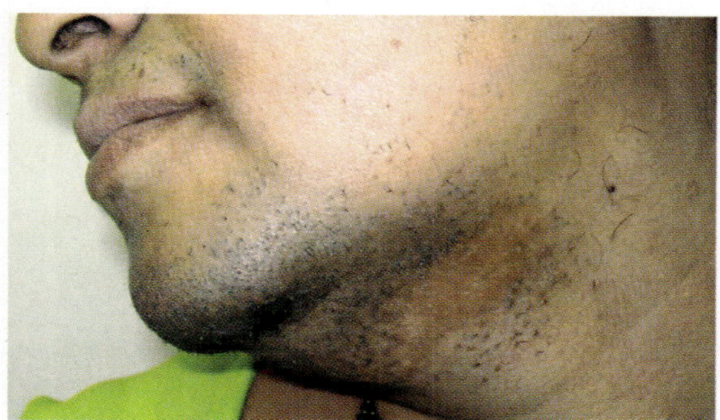

Fig. 30.2: Hirsute chin and neck - Hirsutism

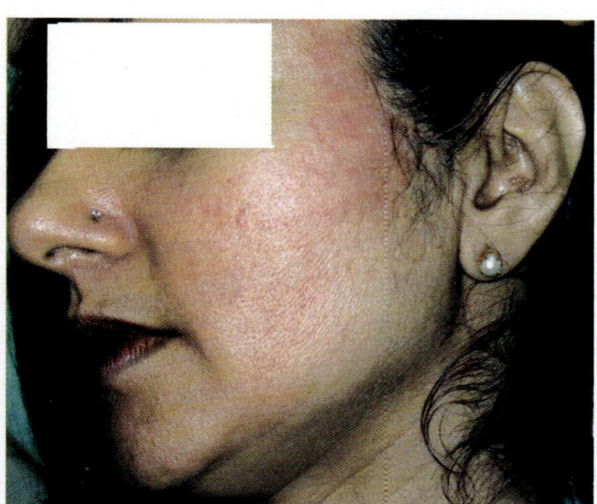

Fig. 31.1: Contact dermatitis to OTC skin-lightening cream (cosmetics)

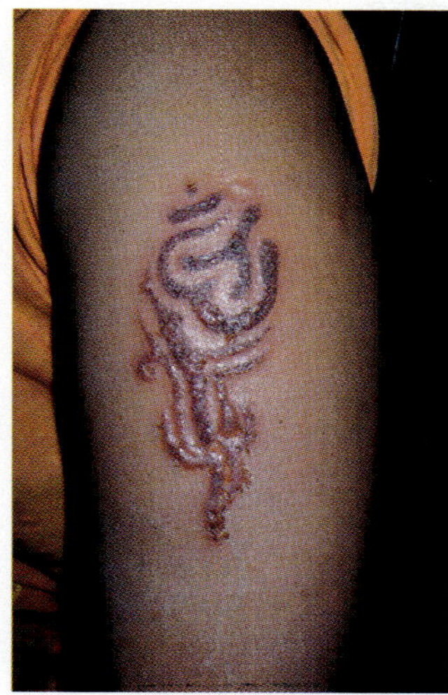

Fig. 31.2: Allergic reaction to henna tattoo (cosmetics)

Section 1: Introduction

1 Importance of ARSH

Swati Y Bhave

INTRODUCTION

Adolescents like to experiment and experience new things, which they enjoy as adventures, this is called risk taking behavior. This applies to sex also. A large number of adolescents enter into sexual activity that is either spontaneous or unplanned or under coercion, without having any knowledge whatsoever of the risk of pregnancy and sexually transmitted diseases. This leads to the increasing number of unwanted pregnancies and increasing incidence of sexually transmitted diseases. Due to lack of information and embarrassment adolescents have poor health seeking behavior on issues of reproductive and sexual health ARSH. To prevent this we have to give sexuality education and make ARSH services available and accessible to both married and unmarried adolescents.

The aim of human sexuality education is to provide accurate and correct knowledge about human sexuality and the hidden dangers involved in reckless experimentation. This will help them to take informed and correct decisions at the appropriate time. Most people oppose programs that teach or discuss ARSH as they believe it will lead to promiscuity, though research by WHO has shown that age appropriate sexuality education delays the age of first intercourse, and increases practice of safe sex, reducing the consequences of early and unsafe sex like unwanted pregnancies and sexually transmitted diseases including HIV /AIDS. As health workers we need to increase awareness in the community that sexuality and HIV education programs do not lead to increase in sexual activity.

Most adult are uncomfortable in discussing sexual matters with adolescents, some have religious taboos. As a result most adolescents lack basic reproductive health information, and skills in negotiating sexual relationships, and access to contraception

The International Conference on Population and Development (ICPD) Program of Action in 1994 called for organizations to initiate or strengthen programs to better meet the reproductive health needs of adolescents.

ARSH concerns have been ignored due to social taboo, related to issues of sexuality. This is true even in case of married adolescents *Focusing on adolescent reproductive health is both a challenge and an opportunity for health care providers.*

EARLY MARRIAGE AND EARLY PREGNANCIES

In India, teenage pregnancies are mainly unintended and unwanted, both in and outside wedlock. Girls are married very early inspite of the law. They cannot take a decision for use of contraception and are dependent on the male partner and a couple is forced to prove fertility by producing a child in the very first year of marriage.

The census 2001 shows that nearly 20% girls under the age of 15 years are already mothers and there is a high incidence of maternal and fetal morbidity and mortality.

According to NFHS 2, 43% of women are married before they attain 18 years of age and TFR amongst 15-19 years old is 19% of the total fertility.

ASSOCIATED RISKS IN TEEN PREGNANCY

Adolescent girls are still growing. Becoming pregnant in this period is like a "child growing in a child". Early marriage pushes the girls into early child bearing and the associated risks include hemorrhage, anemia, delayed or obstructed labor, low birth weight of the baby, miscarriage, damage to the reproductive tract and in some cases, even death of the mother. More than 70% girls in the age group of 10-19 years suffer from severe or moderate anemia (DLHS-RCH 2004). Female mortality rates are higher as compared to males during 15-24 years.

POOR USE OF CONTRACEPTION IN ADOLESCENTS

Among currently married women of 15-19 and 20-24 years age, 5.4 and 16.0 percent respectively ever use a condom. Consistent condom use remains low, only 2.5 in age group 15-19 years and 7.4 percent in age group 20-24 years are currently using condom.

Nearly 27 percent of married female adolescents have reported unmet need for contraception (NFHS-2).

UNSAFE ABORTIONS

Unwanted pregnancies lead to the seeking of abortions. Since parental consent is required for unmarried girls under 18 a large number of them resort to unsafe abortions which account for up to 13% of all maternal deaths and 50% of all maternal deaths in the 15-19 age group. Many married women also resort to unsafe abortions for issue of confidentiality: 38-68% of abortion complications are in women under 20 years of age.

STDs

Adolescents have a higher risk of sexually transmitted diseases and unwanted pregnancy because of many factors: sex is generally impulsive and unplanned hence protection is rarely used. They have lack of knowledge about contraception and STIs, including HIV They think they are invincible and do not perceive themselves to be at risk. Those that have knowledge find it difficult to have easy access to condoms and other contraceptives. They often have high risk sexual behavior involving multiple partners.

Adolescent girls are at a higher risk of contracting HIV and other sexually transmitted infections due to the immaturity of their reproductive system and also because they are often not in a position to say no to the sexual intercourse that may be inflicted upon them.

More than 35-50% of AIDS cases are occurring in the 15-24 years age group mainly through unprotected sex.

POOR EDUCATION STATUS ESPECIALLY IN GIRLS

The age of marriage must be delayed. In early marriages the first conception must be delayed with appropriate use of contraception. To empower women in decision making they have to be literate. Global data has proved that the health statistics improve if women are literate. This is well seen in Kerala state.

But we have a dismal situation of education of adolescents specially of girls in India, 25% of the 15-19 years age group in rural areas and 10% in urban areas are illiterate. Girls account for less than 50% enrollment at all stages of schooling. Enrollment figures are improing but dropout rates are high – 68 percent from class I to X.

Young people not at school join the workforce at an early age – nearly one out of three adolescents in 10-19 years is working.

EXTENDED ADOLESCENCE AND DELAYED MARRIAGES

On one hand we have early marriages and early pregnancies in the rural areas .On the other hand in the urban areas due to higher education there is extended adolescence and very late marriages Majority of girls are getting married after age of 25 years and boys after 30 years due to higher academic persuits .So though the chronological age is higher they still have ongoing adolescent age situation .This long gap between puberty and marriage leads to increasing incidence of premarital sex. Unmarried adolescent boys are far more likely to be sexually active and approve of premarital sexual activity than adolescent girls (Jejeebhoy, 1996). Sexual activity among males was reported at as early as 11 years. For one-third of males, the first sexual partners are sex workers (BSS, 2001, NACO, GOI).

Though we would want them to practice abstinence, it is not possible for many youth to continue doing so and hence we need to empower them to practice safe sex. We need to acknowledge their sexual urges and not remain on high moral grounds. If young couples use effective methods of protection against pregnancy and STIs, and if their decision to enter into a relationship is voluntary, then adverse psychological impact and medical risks are minimized. Adolescents can engage in healthy, fulfilling sexual relationships, and we should not always focus only on the negative outcomes.

SEXUAL ABUSE AND RAPE

Most of the rape victims are in the age group of 14-18 years. In 82 percent of rape cases, the victims knew the offenders. Majority of victims did not understand that they are being sexually abused and had no knowledge or skills to protect themselves.

Most adolescents lack the necessary knowledge of RSH. The information may not be enough to clarify the various doubts they have about sexual activities. Many times information is given without empowering them with skills that help them to take decisions at the proper time and protect themselves.

SUBSTANCE ABUSE IN ADOLESCENTS LEADS TO INCREASE IN SEXUAL EXPERIMENTATION AND ADDS TO THE ARSH BURDEN

Drug abuse rate is low in early adolescence and high during late adolescence.

The estimated number of drug abusers in India is around 3 million and that of drug dependents is 0.5 - 0.6 million, more in the North-Eastern states of the country. Most drug users are in the age group 16-35 years. 21 percent of 40,000 male drug users in a household survey were in the age group 12-18 years.

DIFFICULTIES IN DELIVERING ARSH SERVICES TO UNMARRIED ADOLESCENTS UNDER 18 YEARS IN A CLINICAL PRACTICE

As per the law in our country the parent or guardian consent is required for medical examination and treatment for children under 18 years. While this does not raise any problem in majority of the medical problems, in fact it is essential and desirable to have parental involvement,this leads to a very tricky situation when an adolescent comes with issues of RSH when the adolescents are very reluctant to have the parents involved.

This puts the practicing clinician in a most difficult position. Obviously the law cannot be broken at the same time as a physician the "best interests of the patient" are ethically important. As we start taking care of adolescents patients in our adolescent friendly centers we will be faced with various dilemmas. If an unmarried girl of 16 comes to the gynecologist for an MTP and does not want parental involvement and will go to a quack and undergo a risky unsafe abortion, how does the gynecologists obstetrician help the girl without breaking the law? If an unmarried girl or boy comes for contraception or treatment of STD , how to give these services without informing the parents specially if the parents happen to be your patient as well ! How to ask for a HIV testing without parental consent?

Clinicians need to develop their counseling skills to develop rapport and help the adolescent to confide and seek support and help from the parents, a most difficult situation indeed !In the West in many centers children in chronic disease and terminal illness are allowed to participate in decision making of their treatment protocols. Children from the age of 7 years have cognitive development to understand risk and benefits to be able to make a decision .

As clinicians dealing with adolescents we need to advocate change in laws that will enable us to give RSH services to adolescents without breaking their confidentiality.

SUMMARY

As health care professional dealing with adolescent health issues we need to recognize the importance of RSH and help in spreading awareness and doing advocacy for sexuality education in the community and schools. We also need to strengthen our services to deliver to both married and unmarried adolescents.

SUGGESTED READING

1. Census 2001. Office of the Registrar General India.
2. CSO. 2002. Women and Men in India.
3. DLHS-RCH (District Level Health Survey – Reproductive and Child Health), 2002.
4. DWCD. GOI and UNICEF; NACO and UNICEF, 2001. Knowledge, attitudes and practices of young adults (15-24 years).
5. International Conference on Population and Development (ICPD). Programme of Action. New York: United Nations Population Division, Department for Economic and Social Information and Policy Analysis (1994).
6. MICS (Multiple Indicator Survey). 2001.
7. Ministry of Health and Family Welfare; IIPS and ORC Macro. 2000.
8. Ministry of Home Affairs, GOI; NNMB (National Nutrition Monitoring Bureau) 2001.
9. National Family Health Survey 1998-99; 2002-03.
10. National House Household Survey on Drug Abuse in India.
11. NCRB (National Crime Records Bureau) 2001.
12. NSSO (National Sample Survey Organisation) 2001.
13. 55th Round; SRS (Sample Registration System Statistical Report) 1999. Registrar General, India.
14. UNODC and Ministry of Social Justice and Empowerment, 2004.

2 Changing Trends of Adolescent Gynecology and Various Clinical Problems

Geeta Pandya

INTRODUCTION

Gynec- endocrinology section was started by us at the Jaslok Hospital and Research Centre since its incept in 1973. Similarly it was started, after 2 years at the Breach Candy Hospital too. This has given me a great opportunity for more than 30 years to see the changing trends in clinical practice related to adolescent gynecology.

Initially in early 70's many young girls and even boys with puberty problems were brought for consultations, from all over India and the neighboring countries. Parents were becoming aware of the problems of their adolescent child. Having failed to get proper guidance, and much help from pediatricians, family physicians and even gynecologists, they would bring them to Jaslok Hospital .

THE PROBLEMS SEEN

- Developmental problems of secondary sex organs.
- Growth problems such as height and weight.
- Menstrual problems such as precocious puberty, delayed puberty or secondary amenorrhea, dysmenorrhea.
- Repeated urinary infection, vaginal discharge and vulval itching.
- Breast problems such as underdeveloped, overdeveloped or asymmetrical breast and in boys gynecomastia.

DIAGNOSIS: A BIG DILEMMA

The factors responsible for that were many

- It was difficult to get a proper history. Sometimes parents would not reveal the important history in trying to hide to avoid the problem becoming known to relatives and the world.
- Non-availability of investigating modalities.
- Economic reasons : because even few tests which were available would be beyond their means.
- Time factor required to get full investigations. This is because many patients were coming from out station, and would have difficulty in staying in Bombay.
- Management was even more difficult again due to non-availability of drugs, inability to bear expenses and lack of time to undergo investigations.

CONSERVATIVE THINKING

In those days puberty was shrouded with secrecy.

The classical example being—

1. Appointment would be taken by a woman on her name, but was actually for consultation for her daughter. In the waiting room mother while chatting with other patients would say that she has a gynecological problem, and daughter is just accompanying her. The truth was told to the consultant only after entering the consulting room with the daughter.

2. Many cases of sexual ambiguity at birth were given wrong sex assignment at birth and the child was reared as opposite sex. These cases came with may problems .
3. Delay in bringing adolescent girl, who would hide and lie to parents about the real problem. The girl may complain of pain in abdomen or gaining weight especially on the tummy. This would in fact be due to pregnancy. Even early symptoms of nausea /vomiting may have been treated as GI problem.

UNRECOGNIZED PROBLEMS

The problems of adolescent were not understood well.

This is because the problems were unfortunately not recognized or treated at its onset. Parents were put in a dilemma as to whom they should consult. Children below 9/10 years were treated by pediatrician and above 18 being treated by gynecologist, leaving lacunae of years from age 10-17 where the adolescent problems generally arose. The knowledge regarding Hormones and gynecological endocrinology was insufficient.

Once the awareness of Gynec-Endocrine clinic came up many family physicians and even gynecologists from all over India started referring their patients. We saw many cases of precocious puberty, delayed puberty and unusual cases of missed gender diagnosis. Over the years, media has played a very important role in bringing awareness about various adolescent problems.

DEALING WITH VARIOUS PROBLEMS OVER THE YEARS

Height

In the past, mothers who were short had an anxiety that their child may remain short. The epiphysis fuses when there is well established cyclic estrogen for at least a year. Unfortunately they approached us late when the girl had an already established menstrual cycle for a year, when there was very little that could be done to help them. But now young girls are very conscious and come either on their own or with mother much earlier. When a girl realizes that her parents are short, and she is also likely to remain short, she would like to do almost anything to grow taller.

If tallying the bone age with the chronological age shows that bone age is much lesser than chronological age, then advice regarding stretching exercises was given. But when both ages correspond, decision is based on the time since menarche. If it is less than a year, one can delay her puberty by delaying her periods for a year. We had been giving depot. Provera 75 mg every three weeks. Nowadays monthly GnRH injection can be given. However, one must keep in mind the cost of the drugs. Secondly, one has to emphasize and guide them to do lot of stretching exercises to increase the height. We had an opportunity to delay the puberty in cases of precocious puberty after diagnosing and treating specific cause of precocity.

Weight

Weight in young girls is a much bigger problem now, than in the past. In the past girls were rarely brought in for consultation for weight problems, unless it was associated with known hormonal problems like thyroid, irregular cycles or secondary amenorrhea. We now see a lot more of obese girls with associated PCOS. The changing life style, media, marketing tactic of companies, advertisements and availability of gymnasiums have made young girls very conscious of weight. This has changed the whole out look.

Over and above the young girls after finishing studies get into very demanding jobs where eating habits and balanced diet get the least priority. Obese girls gain weight by eating fast food and doing no exercises, while thin girls do not gain weight due to self imposed discipline to maintain figure by strict diet control, and doing severe exercises.

It is very difficult to maintain balance between the two. One needs to consider many factors and help them.

Development of Secondary Sex Characteristics

Breast problems: Previously development of breast was taken in its stride.

Girls would be very shy to discuss her reaction to her breasts. In fact the girls would wear very tight clothes so that breasts would not look prominent. Now an adolescent girl is conscious of her breast development and wears clothes and brassieres to make them more visible.

The media's role is very important for the change.

- The importance of breast as sex symbol
- The discussions and gossip about how some one has got implants to augment the breasts
- Advertisements of different types of Brassieres and how they give support and give a proper look and shape to the breasts.

In the past a mother often brought the girl with some odd complaints related to periods and then came out with the truth to find out what can be done to make the breasts larger. Occasionally one comes with large breasts and inquire what can be done to make them smaller and not grow further. Some desire to know as to what can be done to the sagging breasts which occurs when a girl who had been obese has lost a lot of weight.

But now the girls come on their own and inquire about beautifying their breasts.

Menstrual problems:

i. *Menarche:* Age of menarche has been changing over decades. In the past it was accepted as normal when it occurred between 12 and 15 years. Nowadays menarche at age 10 or even 9 is acceptable. In some places mothers become very anxious and come running to the doctor for assurance. Mothers always like to compare this with their own age of menarche, and requires reassurance. They need to be guided regarding importance of height and exercises.

ii. *Primary amenorrhea:* It is the absence of onset of periods till age 16 without secondary sexual characters, or 14/15 with the developed secondary sexual characters. The anxiety of the mother increases whenever the periods don't start in a girl above 14 and she is taken to the gynecologist.
In the past when knowledge and availability of investigations were not available she was given hormones usually contraceptive pills.
In mid 70's often we had to resort to Laparoscopy to assess the presence of uterus, tubes and gonads and if present, whether they were normal in size or hypoplastic. But now with the availability of proper investigations, one can find the status and the cause and give necessary treatment or reassure the girls if the cause is genetic/chromosomal.

iii. *DUB (Dysfunctional uterine bleeding):* in adolescent is a challenging problem. It can occur at menarche, or during first 2 to 3 cycles. It can be very severe, sometimes needing hospitalization. It is usually due to hyperplasia of endometrium due to unopposed estrogen. In the past as an absolute emergency means we used to give IV premarin injection to stop bleeding.
One could hardly do any investigations except for hemogram.
The line of treatment was according to hemoglobin levels. If less than 6 gm patient was hospitalized and IV fluids had to be given.
Now the ultrasound has been of great help. It gives measurement of the endometrial thickness and rules out any other pelvic pathology like cyst. One can give medications and get bleeding in control. The availability of low dosage contraceptive pills and other drugs like Mefenemic acid, are able to bring bleeding under control and regulate the cycle. The parents need a lot of explanation and repeated reassurance, especially when the medications have to be continued or repeated for few cycles.

iv. *Hygiene during menstruation:* The past has seen mothers and women using clothes during their periods which were reused after washing, thus maintaining hygiene was always questionable. They were made to live and sleep separately, although in the same house, always from the other members of the family, wash their own clothes and utensils.

Now with the education and understanding of normal physiology, these traditions have gone away. The problem of hygiene has been solved due to easy accessibility of sanitary napkins and tampons available at an affordable rate.

ATTITUDE OF AN ADOLESCENT GIRL TOWARDS FAMILY

The nuclear families have brought parents and child closer. However many times the parents being very busy professionally, child gets lonely and gets into bad company or gets carried away with the peer pressure and starts indulging in smoking, alcohol or even drugs.

In the past the joint family system and having many members in the family had an advantage of getting help from the older siblings, but at the same time there was no openness in discussing many problems.

ATTITUDE TOWARDS SEX

The adolescent age is the age when attraction towards opposite sex is common. Freedom of having a friend of opposite sex is common in today's era. They get involved into sex and sometimes get confused as when to draw a line. In the past, by and large, premarital sex was unheard. But now the knowledge and use of birth control pills or an emergency contraception has changed the attitude towards sex.

SEXUAL IDENTITY CRISIS

In the past one hardly got cases of adolescents wanting to change their sex. It used to be called sex perversions. Homosexuality did exist but it was hush hush. But now with new laws, liberal attitude of government and people, adolescent are becoming aware of their inner feelings and do come forward to seek help from a specialist.

Then the same sex perversions were given names as transsexuals. But now they are called as having gender dysphoria - Where a child feels that God has made a mistake and given him or her a wrong sex identity and they would like to change the sex. They start taking hormones of opposite sex, and go through all the sex change pre-requisite check ups and go through the operations.They require to take hormones for life.

ATTITUDE TOWARDS ONE'S BODY

The media and available internet knowledge has made most adolescents conscious of their body and want to have a body that can be admired. They do not hesitate to get surgeries done or going to beauty clinics to improve or correct whatever they think will make them more beautiful or give them confidence. Sometimes to keep their body slim, they put in too much effort and may end up as anorexia nervosa.

HAIR, SKIN AND BEAUTY

In these days of youth oriented society, media has played a very important role. Young adolescents are very much beauty conscious. Now they know that without formal education also, beauty and a good body can give them many opportunities to come up in life, become popular and become economically sound.

Knowledge through media and internet, and availability of cheap cosmetic products have changed the outlook of adolescents who go for various creams and surgeries like electro-cautery, laser, and skin peels to enhance their beauty. Such treatments have in fact done more harm and started a vicious cycle.

Acne and unwanted hair (hirsutism) make them very anxious. They keep on worrying and end up doing various treatments advertised by media. The mushrooming of beauty clinics and advertisements of the laser and skin care clinics attract many teenagers. Many times they end up having infection and it becomes a factor for end-organ sensitivity leading to acne.

PCOS

Some have definite problem like PCOS. Unfortunately PCOS is a poorly understood and an over diagnosed condition. They end up going to different specialists – dermatologists, gynecologist, endocrinologist, plastic surgeons, beauticians, homeopaths and ayurvedic doctors. They get all kinds of advise, treatments and find themselves completely confused.

MATERIALISTIC ATTITUDE

Another very important factor is wanting to have latest fashions and its accessories, for which they want to have more money. Thus many young adolescents have indulged in prostitution to meet their needs. This has led them to being exposed to various sexually transmitted diseases, vaginal discharge, AIDS and unplanned pregnancies.

GENERATION GAP

Having modern ideas, an adolescent finds older family members including parents 'DESI'; far behind their way of thinking. Thus generation Gap keeps on increasing. This leads to improper communication between children and adults and adolescents get influenced by friends. The peer pressure increases and attitude towards family is disturbed. Parents find it difficult to guide them. Another factor also comes into picture - The nuclear family with working mother puts an adolescent at a loss, as to where to turn to; this results into feeling of loneliness. Broken families and divorces also increase adolescent's fear and anxiety. This increases many psychological problems, and increase identity crisis. In the past with the joint family system, children grew up together and could share their anxiety, knowledge and problems with each other and older siblings.

PSYCHOLOGICAL PROBLEMS AND STRESS

The rapidly growing Indian population has led to increased competition in every field. To achieve higher education, jobs and luxurious life style, an adolescent goes through a lot of stress. This in turn results in psychological and psychiatric problems. An adolescent thus indulges in various bad habits of smoking, alcohol and drugs. Stress is one of the major factors responsible in going in for bad company and bad habits. And of course stress is known to cause Hormonal imbalance leading to many medical and psychological problems.

INVESTIGATIONS

Availability of specialized investigations has completely changed the trends of adolescent management. These lead to a proper diagnosis in a large number of cases.

However the drawbacks of these investigations are:

- Economics
- The expense of installing such expensive equipments
- The cost of the tests
- Experts to conduct the test and interpret them correctly.

ULTRASONOGRAPHY

Ultrasonography has absolutely revolutionarized the management of adolescent problems. In this age group per vaginal examination is difficult and we had to do per rectal examination to judge the presence of uterus and adenexae.

Now with USG, we can properly judge pelvic pathology:

- *Presence or absence of uterus:* If present, Normal, hypoplastic or enlarged
- *The thickness of endometrium:* Very important to know for the cases of puberty menorrhagia (DUB)
- *Presence and size of ovaries:* Enlarged or very small, streak ovaries. Presence of follicles, their number and size.
- Appearance of ovaries to rule out PCOS
- Presence of fibroids or ovarian cyst or any other pelvic mass
- If pregnant, the duration of pregnancy and whether intrauterine or extrauterine.

It is important to know what day of the cycle (if cycle is present) USG should be done.

Evaluation and interpretation of the USG findings with its clinical application is a must.

CT SCAN

In the past diagnosis of pituitary Microadenoma was difficult. RIA was not available to give levels of serum Prolactin. Whenever galactorrhea–amenorrhea complex was associated with headaches we used to get X-ray of skull done and looked for pituitary fossa, which had its limitation. With the advent of CT scan and availability of RIA (serum prolactin), the diagnosis of pituitary adenoma has become easier. Now with MRI, results are more informative. For all these investigation, cost is the limiting factor. So one needs to consider all the symptoms and signs before subjecting the patient for these tests. Fortunately availability of drugs like Bromocryptin has made it easier to treat the micro-adenomas conservatively.

MRI

By and large one does not need to resort to MRI investigations, unless the USG findings are inconclusive. However the cost of MRI is beyond reach of an average person. Sometimes it may be better to subject the girl to diagnostic laparoscopy, which can actually visualize the pelvic organs.

HORMONAL ASSAYS (RIA)

This modality is important in diagnosing many of the adolescent problems which occur due to Hormonal imbalance or abnormality. In the past just to judge the presence of estrogen, we used to do vaginal smear and in some cases even buccal smear to see the pyknotic nuclei in the cells. As chromosomal evaluation was not available, even to confirm gonadal dysgenesis, we had to depend on buccal smear for pyknotic nuclei and laparoscopy. For hyperandrogenism, only clinical signs of acne and Hirsutism were considered of value.

Now with RIA, it has become easy to get the values of necessary hormones and monitoring the progress of the treatment.

SPECIAL TESTS: ANTIBODIES, CA 125

We used to see many adolescents who had Tuberculosis affecting different organs and its sequelae on the genital organ affecting either normal pubertal growth or affecting menstrual cycles. We have seen cases of tuberculous meningitis occurring in childhood ending up as hyopituitarism, or having precautious puberty, delayed puberty or secondary amenorrhea.

Tuberculosis was and is still rampant in our country. The family physicians, and doctors of practically every specialty face the diagnostic dilemma. In 70's we used to send menstrual blood for guinea pig inoculations and confirm diagnosis of TB.

Few years ago, antibodies IgG and IgM for Kochs were started but unfortunately it is not of absolute 100% diagnostic value. Nowadays nucleic acid amplification test is more than 90% accurate. But its availability is only in few selected labs.

However the laparoscopy is much more valuable for diagnosis of pelvic tuberculosis, and we have been using it for a long time especially in adolescent girls.

CA125 is most useful for ovarian cancer. Fortunately it is not common in adolescent girls. But it is also elevated to some extend in cases of Endometriosis. Frequently we use it to monitor the response of the drug therapy in already diagnosed cases of endometriosis.

LAPAROSCOPY

Laparoscopy has been a great boon. We had started diagnostic laparoscopy at the Jaslok Hospital as early as 1974/75 in young adolescents with delayed puberty / primary amenorrhea. With no other investigating modalities like ultrasonography or karyotyping available, we had to undertake diagnostic laparoscopy to visualize pelvic organs.

In cases of streak ovaries we would undertake gonadal biopsies to judge whether the gonad is ovary or it had an element of testes. Unfortunately the biopsy would only say 'basic gonadal tissue'. This did not help much. In few cases when we would suspect that gonads are not purely female looking (mainly due to the look of the tube and fimbria), we would want chromosomal evaluation which unfortunately was not available in mid 70's. We used to send blood to Banglore where Dr Manorama Thomas had started chromosome evaluation on research basis under WHO grant. We had found gonadal dysgenesis with mosaics having Y chromosome. These cases were then subjected for gonadectomy. But now with the availability of karyotyping facilities, diagnosis has become easier.

Laparoscopy has become so valuable, that over a period of time it has not only become important diagnostic tool, but also has become a minimally invasive surgical treatment procedure.

KARYOTYPING OR CHROMOSOMAL EVALUATION

In the past, when karyotyping was not available, we had to take help of various means like vaginal smear or buccal smear to judge presence of estrogen. Buccal smear for chromatin was also done for cases to see presence of barr body. Unfortunately it was not always conclusive. Initially as mentioned earlier we used to send blood to Banglore for the chromosomal evaluation. But now many centers have come up with advanced techniques.

We use this modality a lot and judge the reproductive growth of an adolescent. Once the diagnosis is made of gonadal dysgenesis, or testicular feminization or Klinefelter's and many more, one can plan the line of management, treatment and conseling the adolescent and the family about life style, and reproductive function of an adolescent.

I would like to narret an incidence:
I still remember the day in early 70's when I had diagnosed a Turner, some colleague had mentioned to me - "What is a big deal, you cant help her in anyway" and my answer was, "Yes, I know I can't help her much, but I can stop her going from doctor to doctor and spend money and get frustrated. I can also advice and guide her to be independent and get into a field where she can stand on her feet". In fact earlier I have helped 5 girls with genetic abnormality and got them admission in nursing school.

SUMMARY

following are the important factors which have changed and evolved over last few years.

1. Genetic tendencies
2. The knowledge - Internet and media plays a very important role
3. The environment
4. Life style, socioeconomical status, nutrition
5. Chronic illnesses
6. Economic independence of older adolescents
7. Availability and knowledge of clinics
8. The diagnostic modalities
9. Availability of required drugs.
10. The changing attitude towards sex;
11. Availability of contraception including emergency contraception, abortion.
12. Liberalization and acceptance of gender dysphoria.

The number of adolescent girls coming for consultation in private clinic has increased ten folds in recent years. What could be more confirming than this, as the changing trend in adolescent gynecology?

3 Sexuality Education in Schools and Community

Swati Y Bhave, Diya S Prasad

INTRODUCTION

Research world over has shown that educational interventions focused on life skills development have proved very effective in empowering adolescents to manage their ARSH issues and concerns including avoidance of risky behaviors. Sex education given in a scientific manner in the early stage for adolescence before they start sexual experimentation has a positive effect on their practicing abstinence and delaying the first sexual activity.

WHAT IS THE NEED FOR SEXUAL EDUCATION FOR ADOLESCENTS?

Indian society is conservative and with high moral standards but in reality many things are happening that are behind a garb of mortality. The TV serials, movies all depict explicit sexuality and extramarital and premarital affairs. This hypocrisy is very confusing to growing adolescents. Easy access to internet and CDs and DVDs exposes to pornography that distort the perception of human sexuality.

Many adults suffer a great deal of anxiety because of the lack of knowledge of sexuality, and also from myths and misconceptions. This tracks from adolescence when information was not given at the right time.

Masturbation leads to tremendous guilt and anxiety in young boys. They need guidance about first seminal emission and sexual fantasies.

Not only young girls, but many adult woman also remember their menarche as one of the most negative experiences of growing up. A teenage girl needs information and an adult to guide her when she gets her first menstrual period.

Both boys and girls need information about body changes of puberty, masturbation, boy-girl relationships and sexual attraction, and to guidance to cope with newly emerging sexual urges.

Children get information about sex from wrong sources such as domestic servants, friends, and media. This information may be incorrect and could have damaging effects.

A study conducted by expressions India showed that though most adolescents would like information on sexuality by parents teachers and professionals and least by friends, ultimately they get it from their friends as it is most easily available (Figs 3.1 and 3.2).

WHAT ARE THE ADVANTAGES?

Adolescents understand what is sexual abuse, which will enable them to protect themselves. Most sexual abuse takes place because the victim does not understand he or she is being sexually abused and also lacks the skill to resist.

Adolescents develop positive attitudes towards human sexuality, if they are given honest answers to queries at any age.

Delhi HSE schools 2003

Boys 349, Girls 354 **12-18 yrs**

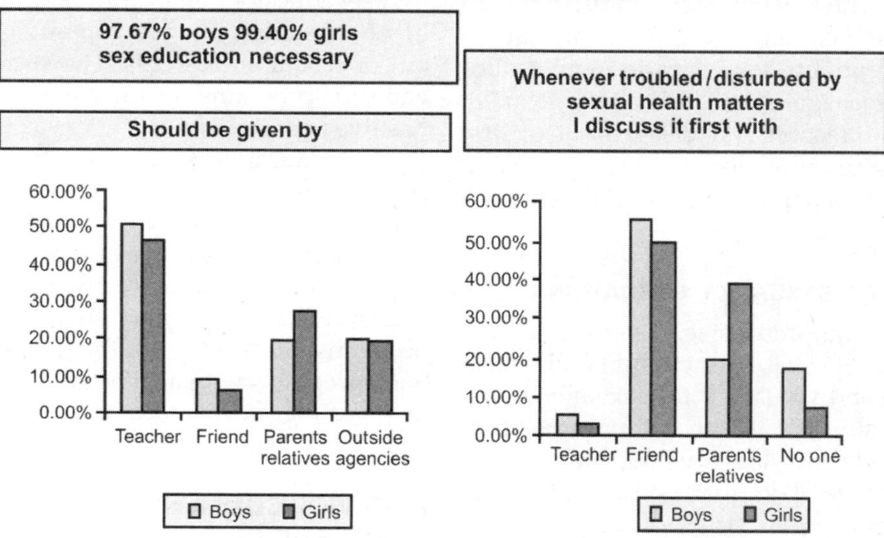

Fig. 3.1: Analysis of 703 adolescents in regarding sexuality education Delhi-2003

Dr J Nagpal, SY Bhave, Prasad D (n=1200 ado 13-18 yrs)

Expressions Delhi, 2004

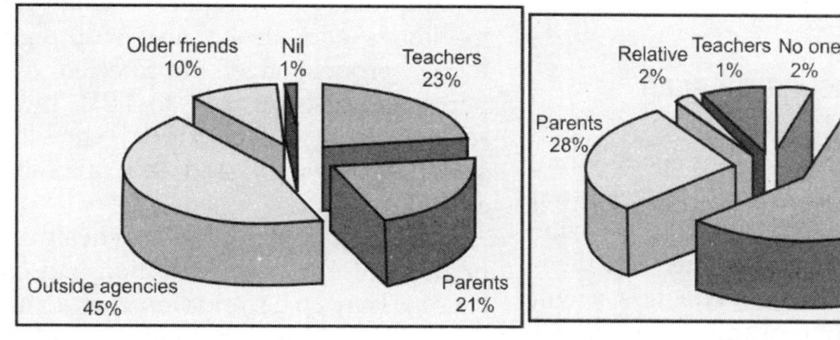

Preferred source of information for adolescent reproductive and sexual health issues

First contact person for the adolescent whenever in trouble for sexual issues

Fig. 3.2: Analysis of 1200 adolescents in Delhi regarding source of sexual information 2004

Adolescents, who are comfortable with their own sexuality and have an understanding of their body and their feelings, would develop self-confidence and self-esteem. It has been seen that adolescents with low self esteem indulge in high risk behavior including sexual experimentation.

Age appropriate sex education will reduce unwanted teenage pregnancies and sexually transmitted infection and delay onset of first sexual act. It certainly does not lead to promiscuity as wrongly perceived by most parents and teachers.

ESSENTIAL OF SEXUALITY EDUCATION

It should be comprehensive, covering the biological, psychological, sociocultural and ethical aspects. An individual's total sexuality is the interrelationship of all these four aspects. It should provide knowledge, values and attitudes and appropriate skills that will help them in dealing with complex issues of sexuality non-judgmental and nondiscriminatory attitude towards other people's sexual preferences, religious beliefs, etc.

Sexuality education is more than just sexual intercourse and prevention of HIV/AIDS with condom use. It is understanding what it means to be a man or woman and acquiring the capacity to experience fulfilling love and affection through a relationship.

POSITIVE PEER PRESSURE BY PEER EDUCATORS

Sexual behavior of friends influences young people's own sexual behavior. If a peer group thinks that unprotected sex is not risky, then they are more likely to have unprotected sex themselves. Many adolescent girls equate sex with love and/or peer acceptance and suffer undesirable consequences as a result of their actions such as HIV-infection, other sexually transmitted diseases and pregnancy, about which they have no knoweldge and hence they are not empowered to prevent them. Lack of maturity, sexual experimentation, alcohol and drug abuse put adolescents at increased rate of unwanted pregnancy and disease transmission.All these negative factors can be effectively combated with peer educator programs.

Peer educator training can be school based for in school adolescents and community based for out of school adolescents. The success of peer educator programs lies in the effectiveness of positive peer pressure.

Peer education gives children and adolescents an environment and opportunity to ask questions to someone who is not an authority figure and they don't have to appear for an exam. It also has the advantage of avoiding embarrassment which prevents them from asking questions to a teacher or other authority figure. Such programs with a "life skill approach" also help young people acquire skills of sexual negotiation and assertiveness.

BEHAVIOR COMMUNICATION AND CHANGE (BCC)

WHAT CAUSES RISK TAKING BEHAVIOR?

Impulsive personality trait, that has poor self-control can lead a person to indulge in many risk-taking behaviors. Sexual desire and its expression is a natural part of healthy living. Highly impulsive adolescents in a "last three month analysis" reported more frequent marijuana and alcohol use with significantly higher proportion of unprotected sex, higher perceived susceptibility to HIV, more AIDS-related anxiety, greater HIV knowledge, less sexual self-efficacy, and less favorable sexual attitudes.

BCC is quite different from health education or IEC (information, education and communication). They go beyond simple dissemination of information. They aim to give people the skills and support they need to protect them and their partners and create a supportive social environment that helps people adopt and maintain safer sexual behavior.

Helping people move from unsafe to safer behaviors is a complex task that can only be accomplished through concerted efforts to master both the science and the art of behavior change communication.

AFRICAN EXPERIENCE

In Tanzania, the AIDSCAP-supported program emphasizes preventing STDs rather than HIV because key informants advised program planners, that members of the target audience would be more receptive to such a message. STDs are common and familiar in the areas served by the project, but most people are afraid to admit that they might be at risk of HIV infection.

Nigerian students expressed discomfort asking their peers certain questions about HIV, so the Nigerian Youth AIDS Program developed a radio call-in show to complement peer education efforts.

Audience research in Uganda determined that although sexually active young women wanted their partners to use condoms, they did not dare suggest it because of popular attitudes that associate condoms with commercial sex. To counteract this perception, the National AIDS Control Program designed BCC materials depicting savvy, popular young women buying and carrying condoms.

MEDIA CAMPAIGN USED FOR POSITIVE IMPACT

Most of the programs shown on TV and movies have the effect of promoting unsafe attitudes and behavior and portraying sex in ways that encourage risk-taking. Research in Zimbabwe showed that young people reached by a communication campaign to encourage "saying no" to sex were 2.5 times more likely than those whom the campaign did not reach to change their sexual behavior for the better.

JAMAICAN EXPERIENCE

Performances of "Vibes," a musical revue by the ASHE Caribbean Arts Ensemble in Jamaica, have delighted and informed thousands of young people and their parents about HIV/AIDS.

BANGKOK

A "Love and Sex Fair," in Bangkok on Valentine's Day drew more than 2,500 people to compete in quizzes testing their knowledge of STDs, watch condom demonstrations, and participate in frank discussions about sex, sexuality and reproductive health.

INDIAN EXPERIENCE

Studies showing that Indian film stars were the most influential spokespeople in Madras led to the use of their voices in the voice-response system for an HIV/AIDS hot line.

YOUNG PEOPLES SEXUAL AND REPRODUCTIVE HEALTH AND RIGHTS (YPSRHR)

The India Population and Reproductive Health (PRH) program focus on two thematic areas over the next few years. These are: reducing maternal mortality and morbidity (MMM), increasing young people's sexual and reproductive health and rights. In India, the two themes are closely inter-connected as fertility begins early for almost 50 percent of young girls, who get married well before the legal age of 18 years and are exposed to high risks of MMM.

The word sexuality or sex education gets a negative reactions from parents and school authorities. It is better to call it family life education (FLE) or adolescent education for better receptivity

ADOLESCENCE EDUCATION PROGRAM (AEP) IN INDIA

The government of India has taken a decision to upscale National School AIDS Education Program (SAEP) and implement Adolescence Education Program (AEP) as a component of National Population Education Program, Adolescent Reproductive and Sexual Health (ARSH) project in schools in all secondary and higher secondary schools.

AEP is an educational intervention to help students acquire authentic knowledge about adolescent reproductive and sexual health (ARSH) including HIV/AIDS and substance (drug) abuse. And inculcate essential life skills to develop healthy attitude and responsible behavior towards these issues AEP program in schools has three *modules: (1) Process of growing up, (2) HIV/AIDS (3) Substance abuse.*

The AEP has been accepted as a Curricular Approach by Council of Board of School Education (COBSE). There will be integration in syllabi at secondary and higher secondary stages through State Boards. It may be subject specific inclusion of content or unit based separate module within the subject. There will be Continuous and Comprehensive Evaluation (CCE).

National Institute of Open Schooling (NIOS) will have integration of AEP in open schooling and distance learning system via the strategy of Interactive Voice Response System (IVRS).

Coverage of AEP (MHRD-NACO) will be through the State Education Department.

(UNICEF supported) in Govt. Secondary Schools.

National Organizations (UNFPA supported) will be through COBSE,(41 State Boards 11 for curriculum integration), CBSE (5000 schools) KVS(837 schools), NVS(470 schools) and NIOS (2750 Study Centers).

The authors are actively involved in the implementation of this program as a core group of " Expressions " A *school based program on holistic health through a life school approach* from VIMHANS New Delhi who have been given the charge of developing training modules and conducting TOT's across the nation.

The program is being implemented in most states/UTs across the country through the state/ UT Departments of Education (DoE) in collaboration with the State AIDS Control Societies (SACS).

The program will be conducted for a minimum of 16 hours per academic year (more than 16 hours, wherever feasible) At least 2 Nodal Teachers per school will undergo training between the period : March to June 2006.

State level action plans are prepared incorporating curricular and co-curricular approaches. While the curriculum change is a lengthy process and will take time, co-curricular activities are to be conducted in all secondary and higher secondary schools using interactive methods facilitating experiential learning with a special focus on life skills development.

There is an Intersectoral linkage for adolescent health services through various ministries.

Ministry of health and family welfare: Adolescent friendly health services (AFHS) and delivery of adolescent reproductive and sexual health (ARSH) is a very important component added to the RCH **2** services, reorganized at primary health centers on dedicated days and timings for adolescents: It gives great focus on counseling and services for RTI/STI prevention education and management. NACO has school based programs on HIV/AIDS that will increase awareness and utilization of these services.

Ministry of Human Resource Development through the education department and NSS is implementing AEP program for schools.

Ministry of Youth Affairs and Sports is working on adolescents outside schools through the NYKD (Nehru Yuvak Kendra) and Bharat scouts and guides.

The 1994 International Conference on Population and Development (ICPD) program of Action called for organizations to initiate or strengthen programs to better meet the reproductive health needs of adolescents.

SUMMARY

As doctors we need to increase the awareness of need of sexuality education in schools.

If professional organizations like IAP, FOGSI, IMA, FPA join hands we will not duplicate efforts and achieve better impact.

SUGGESTED READING

1. AEP program, MHRD – NCRT Module 1 - *Advocacy module for principals* 2006;1-8.
2. DiClemente R. Preventing HIV/AIDS among adolescents. Schools as agents of behavior

change. [Editorial]. Journal of the American Medical Association 1993;270(6):760-62.
3. Devieux J, Malow R, Stein JA, Jennings TE, Lucenko BA, Averhat C, Kalichman S. Impulsivity and HIV risk among Adjudicated Alcohol- and Other Drug-Abusing Adolescent Offenders. Supplement HIV/AIDS in Correctional Settings 2002;5:24-35.
4. Expressions India. *A school based program of holistic health through life skill approach and peer educators* Training modules III for adolescent age group, VIMHANS, New Delhi, 2004.
5. Horizons Project. Peer education and HIV/AIDS: Past experience, future directions. Washington DC, Population Council, 2000;53.
6. Kirby D, Short, L, Collins J. School-based program's to reduce sexual risk behaviors: A review of effectiveness. Public Health Reports 2006;09:339-60.
7. National Youth Policy of India, 2003.
8. Nair MKC. How to introduce sexuality in schools in Bhave's Textbook of Adolescent Medicine 1st (ed) Jaypee Publishers New Delhi 2006;8:6307-16.
9. International Conference on Population and Development (ICPD). Programme of Action. New York: United Nations Population Division, Department for Economic and Social Information and Policy Analysis 1994.

4 Psychosocial-sexual Development Related to RSH Issues

Swati Y Bhave

INTRODUCTION

Adolescence is a period of transition where a child metamorphosis into an adult. Only human species have the period of adolescence.

Some adolescents sail through this period pretty easily especially if they have a stable family life and are well settled in school and community. Most adolescents pass through the phase with a lot of confusion, and some may through an identity crisis.

Most parents make an effort to study the development milestones of children and can remember when their child cut his first tooth, when the first step was taken, when the first word was spoken and so on. But very few parents make an effort to understand the normal psychosocial and physical development of early (10-13) middle (14-16) and late (17-19) adolescence.

Failure to understand the normal milestones that adolescents pass through, like daydreaming, moodiness, wanting to be more with friends and family leads makes them feel their adolescents are abnormal and rebellious and they are subjected to unnecessary criticisms, and comparisons. Parents must learn to develop skills in communicating with their adolescents, as this will reduce the adolescent- parent conflicts, improve interpersonal relationships problems. It has been well documented that connectedness between parents and adolescents is a protective factor against risk taking in sexual reproductive health.

ONSET OF PUBERTY, RELATION TO CHRONOLOGICAL AGE AND IMPACT ON SEXUAL BEHAVIOR

There is a wide range in normal pubertal development adolescents. Most want to look like their peers. Adolescents who have who have early puberty, i.e. ***early bloomers*** or late puberty, i.e. ***late bloomers*** look and feel different from their peers and this can cause stress which can make them indulge in risky sexual behavior.

Early puberty in boys is a matter of pride as they can boss over their peers but also can lead to early sexual experimentation. Early puberty in girls makes them awkward and shy due to early breast development. They are at risk of being subject to sexual abuse and exploitation as they are mentally still not mature enough to understand and withstand sexual advances specially from older males.

Boys who are "late bloomers" can be ridiculed as being puny and can be unwilling victims of bullying or homosexuality by more powerful boys. Girls who are late bloomers can feel inadequate and not sexually attractive to peers, which can lead to low self esteem and indulgence in sexually risky behavior to prove that they are attractive.

Parents, teachers and society treats them as per their physical maturity and not chronological age. This can lead to lot of conflict as the early bloomers are given more responsibility and more maturity is expected from them whereas late bloomers are treated as infantile.

DEVELOPMENTAL MILESTONES OF EARLY, MIDDLE AND LATE ADOLESCENCE

EARLY ADOLESCENCE 10-14 YEARS (CAN BE EARLIER DEPENDING ON WHEN PUBERTY OCCURS)

This falls in Tanners stage 1 and 2. There is development of secondary sexual characteristics. There is peaking of height velocity in girls, making them look older that the boys in their class. Boys start feeling their growth is delayed,. This is the time when they may become victims of sexual abuse especially by older adolescents and adults hence there is need to give sexuality education in schools They are emotionally very labile.

Regarding friendships there is predominance of the same age. They ignore members of opposite sex. Girls may often say "I hate boys" and boys may hate girls. Same sex groups predominate. They like to discuss body changes with peers. They are concerned with body image. They can start self exploration.

They are unable to think and plan about future and understand the implications and long term impact of current decisions They appear to be move away from family towards friends. They do not like to participate in family functions.

This is the time when parents should continue to remain connected with them and use every opportunity to openly discuss bodily changes of puberty, onset of menarche and other age appropriate sexual issues.

MIDDLE ADOLESCENCE 14-17 YEARS

This falls in Tanners stage 3 to 5. The secondary sexual characteristics are well-defined. And they now accept the body changes as norm. Menarche and spermarche take place.

This is the time to discuss about night falls and wet dreams with boys. If the girl has any problems with menstruation like irregularity, menorrhagia or dysmenorrhea they should be shown to a doctor.

The peak height velocity (PHV) declines in girls whereas it. PHV peaks in boys. So now suddenly the boys become taller than the class girls.

Emotionally they are very argumentative, like to rebel and anger outbursts take place. They question authority and demonstrate need for privacy and confidentiality and struggle for independence in all activities This leads to major interpersonal conflicts with parents This is the time when adults have to understand that this is a development phase and not take it personally and spoil the relationship by reacting in the same manner.

There is heightened preoccupation with sexual organs. There is increase in thinking skills and fantasy life. In the event of opportunities sexual experimentation begins. It is mainly heterosexual in most. Self-stimulation increases. Masturbation should be discussed in a scientific manner so that they do not have guilt and do not get infections due to unhygienic practices.

Preventive counseling and anticipatory guidance regarding health and sexual matters is very important to be give at this state because they are now able to understand consequences of actions. They are also able to understand that a person's emotions are influenced by their previous experiences.

Parents have to understand that peers are respected more than parents and the peer group approval considered as foremost. Hence, the codes of conduct and dressing follow the peer group's recommendations. Group counseling and sexuality education by peer educators has a great role to play at this stage. Strategies for reducing high risk sexual behavior has to be tackled with group based interventions rather than individual parental pressures. If parents pressurize too much, or the adolescents do not feel connected they are pushed into adverse peer influences. Peer influences are not always negative. Belonging to a good group will motivate them to excel in studies and other activities and also keep them away from high risk sexual behavior. Parents and treating physicians should make an effort to have some understanding about the peer group to which the adolescent interacts.

There is disparity between biological maturity and responsible adulthood. They are sexually mature and are capable of producing a child. But most adolescents who are sexually active do not realize the dangers of unprotected sex, i.e. unwanted pregnancy and sexually transmitted diseases. They feel invincible at this age thinking such bad things cannot happen to them.

LATE ADOLESCENCE 17-19 YEARS

This falls in Tanners stage 5. Final changes in secondary sexual characteristics happen. The height stabilizes and boys gain muscle bulk and power. They are now emotionally more composed and mature and able to show empathy.

They now come back to the family norms with a broader outlook and perceive rights and responsibilities as an adult. Peer group influence wanes. This is replace by individual intimate friendships with either sex, which may last over a long time, sometimes lifelong.

Commitment in the relationship develops and adult pattern of sexual intimacy evolves. Now nonsexual intimacy is also given importance for a stable mutually satisfying relationship in future.

If they have been given proper sexuality education and preventive counseling during early and middle adolescence they are unlikely to indulge in high risk sexual or drug abuse behavior because by now they are able to understand the consequences and strong enough to face peer pressure.

ISSUES OF BODY IMAGE AND BODY DISSATISFACTION

Body image has been defined as the way we picture our body. Body dissatisfaction is "negative evaluation of one figure and body parts." Poor body image means a person focuses on the negative or the imaginary negative aspects related to the body. This is a emerging problem in today's adolescents. It is associated with preoccupation with appearance and many times can lead to unnecessary cosmetic surgery in affluent adolescents. The emotional distress gives rise to many problems liked depression, irritability, anger, aggression, and eating disorders.

Adolescents are self-conscious and are worried about external appearances. They have a feeling that they are continuously 'On Stage' and every one else is staring at them. Body image is well established by 10 years of age. This feeling is accentuated at puberty and the related body changes. Disproportionate growth of arms and legs during adolescence can gives an awkward, gawky look. Early maturing girls and late maturing boys need special support. Once somatic growth is completed there is a change in body image perception by the adolescents.

Body dissatisfaction is a common problem of adolescents. There are a number of factors associated with the development of such negative image of their body. These are negative peer pressure and impact of media. Unhappy family life and low self esteem. We have to help them overcome the media effect of giving undue and false impression of physical beauty.

We must foster the importance of developing personality and moral qualities which are far more important than physical attributes alone and more longer lasting. As the old saying goes beauty is only skin deep. Adolescents may feel self conscious and consider even positive aspects like a good height as negative. It is human nature to want what we don't have, so it is with physical attributes also.

Poor body image leads to poor self esteem and this can lead to depressive disorders and substance abuse. Poor self esteem leads to failure in other fields of life: academics, sports social interactions, interpersonal relationships. When body dissatisfaction is extreme it leads to eating disorders either anorexia nervosa or binge eating and bulimia. These are discussed in detail in chapter 40.

Protective factors for positive body image are connectedness with family and parents, positive peer group, fostering security and good self esteem.

Adolescents often obsess about their complexion, lack or excess of hair, facial features or size and shape of sexual organs. Research has shown that boy have less body image problems as compared with girls as they are developing muscles and height and generally receive a positive feedback. However, with the "metro sexual man culture" this may no longer hold true. The impact of media the body image on boys is more healthy than the effect on girls as it leads them to eat better and exercise and go to the gym for better development of muscle mass. How ever some of them may want short cuts and this leads to the abuse of anabolic steroids. Boys are troubled with issues of acne, body hair, and majority with the size of their genitalia.

Girls are also concerned with acne but far more important is a fair complexion. Breast size too big or too small is another important consideration. Most Indian figures are not suitable for western clothes which are the norm today and this leads to lot of anxiety in girls. Majority of girls suffer from "Perceived obesity, as opposed to actual obesity". The normal fat increase in puberty can play havoc in their mind.

As clinicians dealing with adolescents we need to spend time and effort in advocacy and awareness to change improve adolescent distorted ideas of body image and encourage healthy life style. They must understand the importance of not skipping meals and accepting healthy curves as a fact of life. Boys should be made aware of the adverse effects anabolic steroids Girls must be discouraged from following the present trend of being excessively slim bordering on malnutrition. The recent press report of not allowing models of BMI < 18 not to walk the ramp is certainly a step in the right direction.

SUMMARY

If an adolescent has body dissatisfaction he or she suffers from low self esteem and also can have depression. Such adolescents are more likely to indulge in tobacco, alcohol and substance abuse. They may also be vulnerable to sexual exploitation. They may succumb to pressure of sexual relationships as this makes them feel they are attractive and wanted by the opposite sex leading to high risk sexual behavior and its consequences of unwanted pregnancy and sexually transmitted diseases.

SUGGESTED READING

1. Byely L, Archibald AB, Graber J, Brooks-Gunn J. A prospective study of familial and social influences on girls' body image and dieting. International Journal of Eating Disorders 2000;28:155-64.
2. Chorgade SW, Bhave Swati Y. Identity crisis in adolescents, ITPAH Course. Manual for Adolescent Health, Part II published by the IAP adolescent Task Force and IAP Adolescent Chapter Ed Swati Bhave et al 2002;237-48.
3. Culbertson JL, et al. Childhood and Adolescent Psychological Development. Pediatrics Clinics of North America 2003;50:741-64.
4. Cusamano DL, Thompson JK. Media influence and body image in 8 to 11-year-old boys and girls: A preliminary report on the multidimensional media influence scale. International Journal of Eating Disorder 2000;29:37-44.
5. Field AE, Carmargo CA, Taylor CB, Berkey CS, Roberts SB, Colditz GA. Peer, parent, and media influences on the development of weight concerns and frequent dieting among preadolescent and adolescent girls and boys. Pediatrics 2001;107:54-60.
6. Flannery Schroeder EC, Chrisler JC. Body esteem, eating attitudes, and gender-role orientation in three age groups of children. Current Psychology 1996;15:235-48.
7. Gardner RM, Sorter RG, Friedman BN. Development changes in children's body images. Journal of Social Behavior and Personality, 1997;12:1019-36.
8. Gerner B, Wilson PH. The relationship between friendship factors and adolescent girls' body

image concern, body dissatisfaction, and restrained eating. Int J Eat Disord 2005;37(4):313-20.
9. Hargreaves, D. Idealized Women in TV Ads Make Girls Feel Bad. Journal of Social and Clinical Psychology 2002;21:287-308.
10. Hill AJ, Silver EK. Fat, friendless and unhealthy: 9-year-old children's perception of body shape and stereotypes. International Journal of Obesity 1995;19:423-30.
11. Hoffman JM, Brownell KD. Sex differences in the relationship of body fat distribution with psychosocial variables. International Journal of Eating Disorders 1997;22:139-45.
12. Hofman AD. Adolescent Growth and Development. In: Adolescent Medicine, Hofman AD, Greydanus DE,(Eds), 3rd ed. Appleton and Lange, Stamford, CT, USA, 1997:10-22.
13. Hofschire LJ, Greenberg BS. Media's impact on adolescents' body dissatisfaction. In Brown JD, Steele JR, Walsh-Childers K (Eds) Sexual Teens, Sexual Media. NJ: Lawrence Erlbaum Associates, Inc. 2000.
14. Holt K, Ricciardelli LA Social comparisons and negative affect as indicators of problem eating and muscle preoccupation among children. Applied Developmental Psychology 2002;23:285-304.
15. Irving LM, Wall M, Neumark-Sztainer D, Story M. Steroid use among adolescents: Findings from Project EAT. Journal of Adolescent Health 2002;30, 243-52.
16. McCabe MP, Ricciardelli LA, Finemore J. The role of puberty, media, and popularity with peers on strategies to increase weight, decrease weight, and increase muscle tone among adolescent boys and girls. Journal of Psychosomatic Research, 2002;52: 145-53.
17. Mundell EJ. Sitcoms, Videos Make Even Fifth-Graders Feel Fat. Reuters Health 26,2002. (last visited 9/16/02.
18. Nayar PD. Body image in adolescents. In Bhave's Textbook of Adolescent Medicine 1st ed. Jaypee Brothers Medical Publishers, New Delhi 2006;6,2,166-73.
19. Neumark-Sztainer, D, Story, M, Flakner, NH, Beuhring T, Resnick MD. Sociodemographic and personal characteristics of adolescents engaged in weight loss and weight/muscle gain behaviors: Who is doing what? Preventive Medicine, 1999;28:40-50.
20. Newman DL, Moffitt TE, Caspi A, Magdol L, Silva PA, Stanton WR. Psychiatric disorder in a birth cohort of young adults: Prevalence, comorbidity, clinical signifi-cance, and new case incidence from ages 11 to 21. Journal of Consulting and Clinical Psychology 1996;64:552-62.
21. Olgetree SM, Williams SW, Raffeld P, et al. Female attractiveness and eating disorders: Do children's television commercials play a role? Sex Roles 1990; 22: 791-97.
22. Ricciardelli LA, McCabe MP, Banfield S. Body image and body change methods in adolescent boys: Role of parents, friends, and the media. Journal of Psychosomatic Research, 2000;48:189-97.
23. Ricciardelli LA, McCabe MP. Sociocultural and individual influences on muscle gain and weight loss strategies among adolescent boys and girls. Psychology in the Schools, 2003;40:209-24.
24. Saini S. Body dissatisfaction among adolescents in Asian Journal of Pediatric Practice 2006.
25. Sigel EJ. "Adolescent Growth and Development" In: Essential Adolescent Medicine : DE Greydanus, DR Patel, HD Pratt. Eds: New York: McGraw-Hill Medical Publishers, 2006;1:11-15.
26. Stice E, Whitenton K. Risk factors for body dissatisfaction in adolescent girls: A longitudinal investigation. Developmental Psychology, 2002; 38,669-78.
27. Thompson JK, Heinberg LJ, Altabe M, Tantleff-Dunn S. Exacting beauty: Theory, assessment, and treatment of body image disturbance. Washington, DC: American Psychological Association 1999.
28. Tiggemann M, Pickering AS. Role of television in adolescent women's body dissatisfaction and drive for thinness. Int J Eat Disord 1996;20:199-203.
29. Tiggemann M, Wilson-Barrett E. Children's figure ratings: Relationships to self-esteem and negative stereotyping. International Journal of Eating Disorders 1998;23,83-8.
30. Wiseman CV, Gray JJ, Mosimann JE, Ahrens AH. Cultural expectations of thinness in women: An update. International Journal of Eating Disorders 1992;11:86-9.
31. Worell J (Eds). Beyond appearance: A new look at adolescent girls. Washington, DC: American Psychological Association 85–108.
32. Yamuna S. Psychosexual development in adolescents in Bhave's Textbook of Adolescent Medicine 1st ed. Jaypee Brothers Medical Publishers, New Delhi 2006,3.3,78-84.

have concluded that more adolescents in the present are involved in behavior that threatens their health than in the past generations.

UNHEALTHY EATING HABITS

In India, school based data has demonstrated an incidence of overweight and obesity ranging from 5.6 to 24% among adolescents. Recent epidemiological trends in obesity indicate that the present day generation of adolescents because of their lifestyles is markedly sedentary and indulges in energy dense foods. There are major shifts in diet which includes increased consumption of vegetable oils, refined grains and more meat and eggs. There is decline in physical activities in school, increased use of transportation less physically demanding activities, more technology and leisure activities at home. Obesity among adolescents compounds their problems like depression, poor self image, and medical conditions like Type 2 diabetes mellitus, dyslipidemia, hypertension, etc.

An adolescent who engages in unhealthy weight control practices or an obsessive behavior towards food, weight, body shape and exercise is considered to be having an eating disorder. This disorder begins most commonly in adolescent years and more often 90-95% in females. There is a failure to attain and maintain a healthy weight. The prevalence both in Western and non-Western literature ranges from 0.5 to 3.7 percent for anorexia nervosa and 1.1 to 4.2 percent for bulimia nervosa.

SUBSTANCE ABUSE

Adolescence and young adulthood are the period most associated with the onset of illicit drug use all over the world. Adolescents, who are without healthy family and peer support or attachment, drift towards social settings of drug using crowd. Smoking and alcohol use lead to drug use/abuse. They often progress from one drug to next which is usually more potent and hazardous than the previous one. Children of parents using and abusing drugs are at increased risk of use and dependence of drugs. The children of these families develop a variety of problems, including school underachievement, abusive, defiant and disruptive behaviors .

SEXUAL BEHAVIORS

Among adolescents sexual behavior is in a state of flux under the influence of media, breakdown of traditional family structures, widespread availability of information on sexual activity. There is a consistent high level of premarital sexual activity across all socioeconomic backgrounds which makes them vulnerable to sexual abuses, STI's and unwanted teenage pregnancies.

SEXUAL ABUSE AND EXPLOITATION

The magnitude of adolescent sexual abuse and exploitation cannot be judged truly because the abuse takes place more often within the four walls of a supposedly secure home by close family, members and relatives. In the article, written and compiled by Rao mentions that 88% of girls are subjected to eve teasing, 13% visually and vocally harassed, 47% molested, and 15% of boys are abused. The system of silence, social, cultural and religious attitudes allow the abuse to thrive. It has a wide range of varied symptoms. The adolescent experiences emotional trauma, or socially withdraws, have self destructive behavior, develop eating disorders or becomes aggressive. The adolescent sexual abuse is to be tackled by counseling and support services and strengthening communications.

ACCIDENTS AND INJURIES

Adolescents by nature are adventurous and rash. They indulge in vehicular driving before the age of 18 years without proper training and documents. They may be involved in many life-threatening accidents especially if they are under the influence of alcohol. Youth under the age of 19 are at greatest risk of motor vehicle fatalities.

5 Risk Taking Behaviors and Protective Factors

Swati Y Bhave, Sangeeta Yadav

INTRODUCTION

Clinicians dealing with adolescents need to know that many problems of adolescent reproductive and sexual health is associated with the risk taking behavior inherent to this age group coupled with lack of protective factors. Medical management alone will not produce optimal results unless the psychosocial issues are also simultaneously looked into. *Risk behaviors are defined as actions that can jeopardize physical, psychological and emotional health.*

Adolescence is a time for natural experimentation, because in this phase of development they are curious and adventurous. Risky behaviors also result from lack of knowledge and understanding of consequences. This can lead to unprotected and often unwanted sexual activity, accidental injuries, addictions and substance abuse, and violence. The health problems are closely inter-related, e.g. drug abuse and depression, alcohol use and accidents and violence, poor nutrition and pregnancy and childbirth. There are several common determinants which underlie these health problems. The factors which influence these behaviors are family relations, abuse and neglect, abuse of alcohol and drugs, school failures, poor skills development and low self esteem. The circumstances which lead to risk are poverty, lack of family support system, mental and physical disabilities, sexual abuse and exploitation, addiction, poor access to education and health services, unemployment, ethnic and gender discrimination, war and emergency situations.

MORBIDITY AND MORTALITY IN ADOLESCENT AGE GROUP

Review of adolescent health data has revealed that there has been a major shift in the cause of adolescent morbidity and mortality. Among school aged youths the major causes of morbidity are related to substance abuse, sexual abuse, teenage pregnancies, sexually transmitted diseases and HIV, intentional and unintentional injuries, homicide and suicide. A large number of deaths are due to accidents, homicide and suicide which may be related to alcohol and drug use.

All segments of adolescent populations are at risk for involvement in behaviors that adversely affect their health. The adolescents from affluent families are more at risk for problems such as eating disorders, substance abuse, motor vehicular accidents, suicide and homicide whereas those who live in poverty are more at risk for intentional injury STI's, pregnancy, school drop out, unemployment. The risk profiles cannot be determined by demographic data alone but has to be ascertained through direct assessment. Many studies over the past decade

VIOLENCE AND AGGRESSION

Adolescents are known to be aggressive and violent. They are not only violent but are also subjected to violence and aggression. Violence is observed in various forms like physical, non-physical, sexual and non-sexual. The phenomena is seen as intimidation and stalking, bullying, physical fighting and abuse, kicking, hitting, violent crimes with weapons, homicides, sexual abuse and assault, self-mutilation, suicidal ideation and attempts. In some parts of the world adolescents are forced into war and other terror activities.

Other risky behaviors leading to HIV AIDS, Tobacco, alcohol, adolescent suicide and depression are discussed in chapters 25, 35, 36 and 37.

MANAGEMENT

Adolescents need places and environment that offer nurturing, guidance, rules, structures, clear expectations and consistent limits. A safe and supportive environment motivates them to make healthy choices. Safe means absence of trauma, violence, excessive stress and abuse. Supportive means an environment that provides a positive and close relationship with family, other adults and peers. A healthy environment provides both support and opportunities for their healthy developments.

It is important to understand the adolescents' physical, emotional and social development to decide what type of guidance to be imparted and facilitate development of healthy lifestyle choices. They often have little understanding of their own maturation, are unprepared for new relationships and are unaware of health services available to them. They need guidance to set limits when needed and to accept challenges of life. Health enhancing behavior is primarily the responsibility of young people themselves and therefore, they must learn to make decisions related to major health consequences for their own present and future.

ROLE OF CLINICIAN

When dealing with adolescent patient the clinician should pay careful attention for a comprehensive risk assessment because these behaviors are associated with prediction and intervention of risky behaviors and essential in promoting healthy sexual and reproductive health. They can help in spotting risk factors, assessing and referring or managing problems. They can focus on health and safety while assisting with healthy lifestyle choices.

PREVENTIVE AND PROMOTIVE COUNSELING

In dealing with adolescents preventive and promoting counseling has a great role to play in reducing many associated problems. Preventive Psychiatry is an emerging field that looks at risk factors and protective factors for psychiatric problems and illnesses. Prevention by only reduction of risk is not adequate.

PROTECTIVE FACTORS

That can enhance an adolescents resilience can be from individual factors and family and school environment. An adolescent must feel connected to the family and have a sense of belonging and closeness. Giving "quality time" is not enough but parental presence at crucial events and timing in the adolescents life is what creates a greater impact. Parents being at home when the adolescent goes and returns from school and mealtime sharing is the most effective. The ability to communicate and confide problems with parents is a great protective factor. *An adolescent who is happy with the school environment and has satisfactory relationship with peers and teachers is less likely to go astray. Also the adolescent who has good self esteem and good coping skills that are nurtured by the parents, not being overprotective are able to resist peer pressure and other temptations that can cause risk taking.*

Excessive stress of academics and not enough leisure time to spend in sports and cultural activities leads to lot of emotional stresses in adolescents and makes them vulnerable to seek relief by various other methods that can be injurious to health. Involvement in religion or religious activity helps against emotional disorders, as long as it does not turn into fanaticism.

SUMMARY

As clinicians we need to be aware of the risk taking behavior that leads to negative consequencies in ARSH.

Increasing the awarness of protective factors in parents and community is an important preventive strategy.

SUGGESTED READING

1. Bhave Swati Y, Yadav S. Risk taking behavior in adolescents in Bhave's Textbook of Adolescent Medicine. 1st ed Chief Ed Swati Y Bhave Jaypee Brothers Medical Publications, New Delhi 2006;25.2:887-93
2. Bernard B, Marshall K. Protective Factors in Individuals, Families, and Schools: National Longitudinal Study on Adolescent Health Findings. www.cpc.unc.edu/projects addhealth /files/refer.pdf
3. Bezbaruah S. Adolescents in India. A profile, UNFPA, New Delhi 2000, 3-25.
4. Blum, R Rinehart P. Reducing the risk: Connections that Make a Difference in the Lives of Youth. Division of General Pediatrics, University of Minnesota, Minneapolis 1997.
5. Major interventions In: Programming for Adolescent Health and Development, WHO Technical Report Series 886, Geneva 1999:28-66.
6. Mohan Raj. Protective factors in adolescent risk taking behaviors in "Bhave's Textbook of Adolescent Medicine 1st ed Swati Y Bhave Chief Ed. Jaypee Brothers Medical Publishers, New Delhi 2006;25.3 893-97
7. Programming for adolescent health and development, Report of WHO/UNFPA/ UNICEF Study group. WHO Technical Report Series 886, Geneva 1999:9-15.
8. Rao M I S. Adolescent Sexual abuse. In: Course Manual for Adolescent Health Part II. Indian Perspective. Bhave SY, Gupta PK, Jain TS, Nair MKC (Eds); IAP ITPAH. Cambridge Press, Delhi 2002;225-28.
9. Resnick M, et al. Protecting adolescents from harm: Findings from the National Longitudinal Study on Adolescent Health. Journal of the American Medical Association 1997: 278, 823-32.
10. Report of the working group on Adolescents. TFYP working group Sr. No. 1/2000 GOI, New Delhi 1001; 3-11.
11. Strasburger VC, Greydanus DE. The high risk adolescent: Problems and Solutions. State of the Art Review. Adolescent Medicine 2000, 11:1-100.
12. Yadav S, Walyat N. Adolescent risk taking behaviors: In: Course Manual for Adolescent Health Part II. Indian Perspective. Bhave SY, Gupta PK, Jain TS, Nair MKC, (Eds): IAP ITPAH. Cambridge Press Delhi 2002; 385-91.

6 Alternate Sexual Orientation

Donald E Greydanus, Swati Y Bhave

INTRODUCTION

Clinicians dealing with sexual and reproductive (SRH) issues of adolescents need to upgrade their knowledge about human sexual orientation.[1-7] *Sexual orientation* is a reflection of a person's sexual and emotional feelings toward persons of the same or opposite gender and is expressed by individual sexual fantasies, actions, attitudes, and behavior. Sexual orientation emerges over time through various stages of adolescence. By middle adolescence the majority of adolescent boys and girls begin to feel romantically and sexually attracted to the opposite sex (i.e. heterosexual orientation).

Some young adolescents may have a transient attraction to the same sex which may not result in sexual experimentation. Other girls and boys may go through a passing phase of intense emotional dependence on a friend of the same sex and at some stage the attraction can turn physical or sexual. They can indulge in kissing, serious petting, oral sex or genital stimulation. As clinicians we have to remember that such situations have a risk of transmission of disease by contact with body fluids. In the long run most of these youth develop lasting heterosexual relationships. However, some adolescents may have an alternative orientation that reflect being homosexual (gay), lesbian, bisexual, transgender, or simply questioning their sexuality (GLBTQ).

HOW SHOULD A CLINICIAN SENSITIVE TO RSH ISSUES DEAL WITH SUCH ADOLESCENTS?

Sexual orientation is a personal matter and clinicians should remember that even if we do not approve or feel comfortable regarding the orientation, we need to avoid having hatred or negative feeling towards a person with such alternative orientations. As clinicians we need to treat them as adolescents that have high risk behavior and resultant consequences that need preventive counseling as well as medical treatment if sexually transmitted diseases arise. We also need to empower them with the knowledge to resist sexual exploitation, sexual abuse and violence.

In 1973 The American Psychiatric Association concluded that homosexuality is not a mental disorder and removed it from the list of psychiatric illnesses in the third of their Diagnostic and Statistical Manual (DSM-III). The International Statistical Classification of Diseases and Related Health Problems (9th revision)[9] also agrees with this same concept of removing mental illness labels from someone just because they are homosexual or lesbian. However, in our country, this is a very tricky issue for clinicians, as unlike the West, homosexuality is considered abnormal in our society and punishable by the law of our country.

DEFINITIONS OF TERMS IN SEXUALITY

1. *Anatomic sex:* Phenotypic appearance (male, female, intersex) and includes variations such as the adrenogenital syndrome and the incomplete masculinization syndrome.
2. *Anti-homosexualism:* The pervasive and often institutionalized attitudes denigrating homosexuality.
3. *Asexuality:* The absence of erotic response or motivation.
4. *Bisexuality:* The capacity to sexually respond to both sexes to a significant but not necessarily equal degree.
5. *Core gender identity:* Self-identification as either male or female, typically occurring by age 3 years of age.
6. *Cross dressing:* Dressing in clothing of the opposite sex with the intention of expressing identification with or caricaturing the opposite sex role identity; does not generally involve erotic stimulation; often seen in males.
7. *Genetic sex:* Chromosomally determined sex (i.e. XX, XY, XXY, XYY, others).
8. *Gender role identity:* The summation of actions that indicate to self and society the degree to which one is male, female, or ambivalent. It is influenced by familial, cultural, and social role expectations, and includes but is not limited to sexual arousal and response. It may also be referred to as one's "sex role."
9. *Heterosexuality:* An erotic preference, including fantasies and experiences, for persons of the opposite sex, with minimal erotic interest in the same sex.
10. *Homosexuality:* An erotic preference, including fantasies and experiences, for persons of the same sex, with minimal erotic interest in the opposite sex.
11. *Hyposexuality:* The paucity of erotic response or motivation.
12. *Homophobia:* The condition in which those whose love and lust are attached to others of the same sex are dreaded or feared.
13. *Sexual dimorphism:* The structural, physiologic, and behavioral differences between the sexes.
14. *Sexual (erotic) orientation:* Defined by one's prevailing, unrepressed sexual longings and fantasies.
15. *Transvestitism:* The expression or belief that one's gender identity does not match one's anatomic sex ("woman trapped in a man's body, or the reverse").
16. *Deviant sexual behaviors:*
    i. *Exhibitionism:* Obtaining sexual arousal by exposing genitals to an unsuspecting stranger.
    ii. *Fetishism:* Obtaining sexual arousal using or thinking about an inanimate object or part of the body.
    iii. *Frotteurism:* Obtaining sexual arousal and gratification by rubbing one's genitals against others in public places.
    iv. *Masochism:* Sexual arousal by having pain and/or humiliation inflicted upon oneself.
    v. *Pedophilia:* Sex or sexual activity with children who have not reached puberty.
    vi. *Sadism:* Sexual arousal through inflicting pain on another person.
    vii. *Transvestitism:* Dressing in clothing of the opposite sex, predominantly by males, for the purpose of erotic stimulation (i.e. sexual arousal from dressing in the clothes of the opposite sex).
    viii. *Voyeurism:* Sexual arousal by observing nude individuals without their knowledge.

CAUSES OF DIFFERENT SEXUAL ORIENTATION

A small percentage of people in every culture are homosexual or lesbian. Sexual orientation cannot be changed by therapy or medicines, though some individuals may be confused about their sexual orientation until finally arriving at what they conclude is their true sexual orientation. There is no accepted psychological or psychiatric explanation for homosexuality.[1,4,5] The biological cause of homosexuality is not clear, with a large number of un proven theories to explain why it occurs. Genetic factors, prenatal hormonal influences, psychosocial and socio-cultural factors and various combinations of these determine sexual orientation.

There are three theories that are presented to explain homosexuality: *Biological / genetic, psychological*, and *behavioral*. All of these theories have supporting but non-conclusive evidence, however, scientists lean towards genetic factors. Most social scientists do not support the idea that people simply decide to become gay because it is a latest fad, or because they want to rebel, or because they are misinformed in sex education class. The biological theory is that the hypothalamus is affected *in utero* that combines with social factors in childhood and results in a homosexual orientation. [11] Though there is no identified genetic marker for homosexuality, genetic studies note an increased incidence of homosexuality among monozygotic twins versus dizygotic twins. [1,5,8,11] Female fetuses with some types of congenital adrenal hyperplasia are exposed to increased amounts of male hormones, leading to later exhibition of male-like traits in childhood, such as being involved in aggressive playing.[1] Some research has identified differences in the anterior commissure size as well as differences in the size and structure of the hypothalamus in homosexual men versus heterosexual men; however, the meaning of such findings is unclear.[10,11]

PREVALENCE PERSPECTIVES ON HOMOSEXUALITY

A largest and classic study in USA is by Kinsey et al[12,13] which lead to the Kinsey Scale of Sexual Orientation dividing human sexual orientation into a range of 7 points, from 0 to 6.[1,2,6] This Sexual Orientation Scale is identified as:

0 Exclusive heterosexual (in sexual behavior and fantasy).
1 Essentially heterosexual with incidental or limited homosexual history.
2 Largely heterosexual with distinct homosexual history.
3 Equal heterosexual and homosexual orientation (ambisexuality).
4 Largely homosexual with distinct heterosexual history.
5 Essentially homosexual with limited heterosexual history.
6 Exclusive homosexual in sexual behavior and fantasy.

A survey of medical students in 1979 showed that 60% were aware of homosexual feelings as adolescents and 40% still had these feelings.[14]A survey of 34,706 students in the United States grades 7 through 12 noted that 88.2% were heterosexual, 10.7% were not sure of their sexual orientation, and 1.1% were bisexual or predominately homosexual.[1,4] 17 Additional research concludes that 2% of adult males are homosexual, 3% of males are bisexual, and 3 to 7% of adult females are lesbian since the adolescent years.[1,4] In India, since homosexuality is punishable by the Indian penal code, statistics are difficult to find.

PERSPECTIVES ON THE DEVELOPMENT OF A GAY OR LESBIAN IDENTITY

The understanding of how an individual becomes aware of and accepts a gay or lesbian identity in a world that remains extremely hostile to a homosexual lifestyle is well brought out by the research of Green in 1974[15] and Troiden in 1979. [16,17] Green identifies three stages of "coming out" phase as the teenager seeks to reveal this "secret" to others, family, peers or a health care professional: [15]

Stage 1: Feeling "different."

Stage 2: Develop a crush on a same sex individual

Stage 3: Overt awareness of personal gay/lesbian identity.

The process of acceptance of a homosexual identity is described by Troiden (1979) who identifies four stages of development: [16,17]

Stage 1: Sensitization: Gains homosexual experiences in childhood and adolescence while learning of society's homophobic views on homosexuality.

Stage 2: *Dissociation and signification*: Struggles to refute the idea that society's negative opinions on being gay or lesbian refers to oneself.

Stage 3: Coming out: Self-identification as gay or lesbian and seeks to find others of similar orientation; reflects on this pathway as a worthwhile direction.

Stage 4: Acceptance: Total acceptance of this pathway.

All gay or lesbian persons will not go though all the stages. Some are "arrested" at Stage Three while others eventually reach Stage Four. Sometimes, the denial of one's sexual orientation persists for a lifetime or may slowly progress over many decades.

When a adolescent gets the self-awareness that she/he does not share the same feelings as heterosexual peers, the first realization is that the she/he will face anger and rejection from mainstream society. This itself is very painful to accept. Then comes the struggle to understand what a homosexual identify is and how to become part of the gay or lesbian culture in one's surroundings and how to let others know about this sexual orientation. Some adolescents will have the courage to develop a gay or lesbian lifestyle, while others acquire a bisexual identity, allowing them to function better in society by projecting the heterosexual orientation and keeping the homosexual orientation a secret.

Other bisexuals state they are truly orientated to both sexes in a process not understood by medicine.

Sexual orientation begins in middle childhood but may not be accepted or understood until some time in adolescence or adulthood—sometimes never. Some adolescents will remain confused regarding their sexual identify, and "question" who they are for a variable amount of time. Thus, the clinician will be faced with some adolescents with different sexual orientations identified as GLBTQ (gay, lesbian, bisexual, transgender, or questioning).

CARING FOR ADOLESCENTS WITH ALTERNATIVE SEXUAL ORIENTATIONS

CLINICIAN'S ATTITUDE

In the West where homosexuality is not punishable by law. The unbiased clinician often works with such adolescents who can come openly for health care. It then becomes necessary for the clinician to identify his/her personal feelings regarding homosexuality as these feelings may interfere with the creation of a trusting doctor-patient relationship. The clinician should review his or her personal views and experiences and become aware of any negative feelings which may make the adolescent patient feel uncomfortable or even rejected. If the personal negative feelings are too strong to overcome, referral to unbiased clinicians is recommended. If one decides to care for homosexual adolescents, the issue of confidentiality becomes important, in which the clinician defines what issues cannot stay strictly between patient and clinician—such as the adolescent expressing active desires of suicide or homicide. The sexual orientation should not be disclosed to others (as parents, for example) unless the adolescent gives permission to do so.

HISTORY TAKING AND MEDICAL EXAMINATION OF GLBTQ ADOLESCENTS [1,4,5]

History should cover in detail all aspects of the following: Social, School, Family Employment, Substance use, Psychosocial problems, and Suicidal ideations and attempts.

The sexual history should include the number of partners and sexual practices.

PHYSICAL EXAMINATION[1,4,5]

This should include a general physical examination and specifically, an evalution for signs of for sexually transmitted diseases or infections (STDs/STIs). Procedures such as pelvic examination and anoscopy will be useful for the appropriate patient.

LABORATORY EVALUATION[1,4,5]

This should include testing for *Neisseria gonorrhoeae, Chlamydia trachomatis, Treponema pallidum,* Human immumodeficiency virus (HIV), Herpes simplex virus (HSV) and Human papillomavirus (HPV); other STD microbes may be looked for depending on the specific circumstances.

TREATMENT PLANS[1,4,5]

Appropriate management of any identified medical problems is necessary. STDs, if present, should be treated with emphasis on the importance of getting the partner (s) also treated.

REFERRAL AND FOLLOW-UP [1,4,5]

The adolescent should be given appropriate referral including to mental health professionals if necessary. A good rapport should be established so that the adolescent will come for regular follow-up. The family also should be included if supportive and with the permission of the adolescent.

PREVENTIVE ASPECTS[1,4,5]

This includes Hepatitis B immunization and preventive counseling for risk reduction that cover the importance of abstinence, contraception, and condoms.

SEXUALITY EVALUATION

In adolescents with different sexual orientation, the clinician also needs to do a sexuality evaluation which will include the various factors:[1,4,5]

SEXUAL IDENTITY EVALUATION

Sexual identity is based on the genetic make-up as a male (XY) or female (XX) and requires a careful physical examination with accurate sexually maturity rating or Tanner staging. This should include a complete physical examination especially for genital abnormalities, including ambiguous genitalia. Genetic testing, if needed, should also be done. If a genital anomaly is noted, referral to another clinician may be necessary, such as an endocrinologist, gynecologist, and/or urologist. [1,5]

GENDER IDENTITY EVALUATION

Gender identity involves the youth's sense of masculinity or femininity. The gender behavior of the adolescents has to be noted. A good history should be taken to elicit the following: history of persistent cross-dressing (*transvestism*), persistent feelings of being "trapped in the body of the opposite sex" (*transsexualism*) with a persistent desire to be the opposite sex (i.e. seeking to actually be the opposite sex because of intense discomfort with one's anatomic sex):[1,4,5] A psychiatric evaluation is very important for these patients.

SEXUAL ORIENTATION EVALUATION[1,4,5]

It is important to ask if there is sexual attraction to the opposite sex (*heterosexual*), same sex (*homosexual* or *lesbian*), or both (*bisexual*) to determine the youth's sexual orientation; some youth are unsure and can be labeled as *questioning*.

Take a Good History to Elicit the Following Points

- Predominant sexual fantasy and attraction towards the opposite sex, same sex, both sexes
- Knowledge and awareness of variations of sexual orientations
- Psychological adjustment, substance abuse
- Depression, suicidal ideation and plan
- Familial knowledge and support/family unaware/family unsupportive
- Social knowledge and support/school/friends
- Sexual relationships
- Religious conflicts/legal problems/special problems/prostitution/bullying, other forms of violence.

They should be given accurate information regarding human sexuality and if needed, help in obtaining appropriate Gay and Lesbian resources; they can be referred to mental health professionals if necessary.

SEXUAL BEHAVIOR EVALUATION[1,4,5]

The clinician should also ask about the range of sexual activity to determine the actual sexual behavior of the patient. If the youth is sexually active, further questions include the type of sexual behavior, number of sex partners, and if there is use of condoms, sex toys, and pornography. Once such basic information is obtained, the clinician is in a better position to identify if medical or psychiatric problems are present and what advice is needed by the patient.

They Need to be Given Advice Regarding

- A therapist may be necessary for those disturbed by cross-dressing behaviors or having transsexualism
- The antagonism that s/he may encounter from the general and religious community may be extremely negative and difficult to handle
- It is also very difficult for the homosexual or lesbian youth to explain to parents, peers, and the general society that they are different than their heterosexual family members and peers
- Options for safe sex and condom use/advise on risk for STDs/STIs
- Family planning
- Hepatitis B and other immunizations
- Necessary medical tests.

When and why will Adolescents with Different Sexual Orientation Seek Medical Help?

- They may come simply to get more information about homosexuality or other aspects of human sexuality
- They may come because they have fear of infection like HIV or STDs, or because they already have symptoms of such infections
- They may come for other medical disorders
- They may come for various psychosocial issues and problems
- There may be Family, School, Personal problems, Vocational concerns, Religious conflicts, Substance abuse problems or overdose, and legal issues like Theft or Prostitution
- RTI's and STI's may be present. In addition to the usual STD's, there can also be enteritis/proctocolitis due to *Giardia lamblia, Salmonella enteritidis, Entamoeba histolytica, Cryptosporidium, Campylobacter, Shigella species,* and *Ectoparasites.*
- Psychological problems may be present. These adolescents may undergo a lot of psychological problems because of guilt and, need to keep secrecy. In general because of lack of support and understanding from the family and environment, they suffer from anxiety and depression, and have a higher incidence of suicide than their heterosexual peers.[1,4,5,18-26] Homophobia from peers can lead to mental abuse and physical beatings. Rejection by parents and society can lead them into sexual exploitation and prostitution. Internet abuse is also occurring.

REACTIONS OF PARENTS

In general, the world rejects this lifestyle on various grounds of religion, ethical, moral, and legal arguments.

How the parents react to the news of their son or daughter emerging as a gay or lesbian has a great impact and consequences for this adolescent.[1,4,5]

- Some parents perceive this as a rejection of their ancestral, cultural, and religious background and blame themselves for not given the children a "proper: upbringing.
- Parents brought up in a culture that is hostile to alternate sexual orientations can become as confused as their son or daughter about this development.
- Parents may feel isolated form their own friends and find it difficult to discuss this issue with anyone and go through a severe emotional turmoil; if they do not seek help, they may develop a variety of psychological sequelae, such as like anger, anxiety, and depression.
- Parents may reject their child—sometimes even asking their child to leave the home as

they would like to separate him or her from siblings, fearing negative influence on the "healthy" siblings.

- Parents who are looking forward to having grand children may feel an acute sense of deprivation and loss.

MANAGEMENT APPROACH

MANAGEMENT PRINCIPLES

Therapy may be necessary for those who are finding it difficult to cope up with rejection of family and community. There are various behavioral therapy approaches, including counseling for social skills training, individual therapy, family therapy, and group therapy.

If the adolescents are sexually active, they need advice regarding the value of both abstinence (if accepted) as well as condoms for STD protection (if coital behavior continues). They have to be empowered with the knowledge of prevention of sexually transmitted diseases and also made aware of sexual exploitation and sexual violence that they are likely to encounter. They also need to understand the impact of drug and alcohol use before and after sexual behavior.

Parents and their youth need to understand that there is no scientific evidence that therapy, often called reparative therapy or conversion therapy, will change the sexual orientation of a youth or adult committed to a specific orientation.[1,4,26] Counseling is necessary for them to develop coping skills to face all the above mentioned problems they have to face in the family, peers and society. Finally, clinicians must be prepared to evaluate and manage these youth in a confidential manner. [3,27]

SUMMARY

Clinicians had to be aware of alternate sexual orientation and update themselves on the various issues in their management.

REFERENCES

1. Greydanus DE, Sison AC. Focus on Adolescents with Same Sex Attraction and Sexual Behavior AJPP accepted for publication Jan-March 2007.
2. Rowlett JD and Greydanus DE: Homosexuality in adolescence. Adolescent Medicine 1994; 5(3):509-26.
3. Sigel EJ: "Adolescent growth and development" In: Essential Adolescent Medicine Greydanus DE (Eds): New York: McGraw-Hill Medical Publishers 2006;1:11-15.
4. Greydanus DE, Sison AC. "Homosexual attraction and sexual behavior in adolescents." In: Behavioral Pediatrics, 2nd Edition. Lincoln, Nebraska, USA Universe Publishers 2006;13: 444-76.
5. Rowlett J, Greydanus DE. "Gender Identity" In: Behavioral Pediatrics. Greydanus DE, Wolraich M (Eds): NY: Springer-Verlag 1991;3: 40-65.
6. Greydanus DE, Dewdney D. Homosexuality in adolescence. Sem Adol Med 1985; 1:117-30.
7. Sadock, Benjamin J Sadock, Virginia A. Kaplan and Sadock's Synopsis of Psychiatry. Lippincott Williams and Wilkins 2003.
8. American Psychiatric Association. Diagnostic and Statistical Manual of Mental Disorders, DSM-IV, 4th ed., (text revision) (DSM-IV-TR). Washington, DC: American Psychiatric Association 2000.
9. International Classification of Diseases and Related Health Problems, 10th Revision. (ICD-10), 2004.
10. Dalton R. "Homosexuality" In: Nelson Textbook of Pediatrics, 17th edn. Behrman RE, Kliegman RM, Jenson HB, (Eds): Philadelphia: WB Saunders Co 2004;26.2: 91-2.
11. Allen L, Gorski R: Sexual orientation and the size of the anterior commissure in the human brain. Proc Natl Acad Sci 1992; 89:7199.
12. Kinsey A, Pomeroy W, Martin C. Sexual Behavior in the Human Male. Philadelphia: WB Saunders 1948.
13. Kinsey A, Pomeroy W, Martin C, Gebbard P. Sexual Behavior in the Human Female. Philadelphia: WB Saunders 1953.
14. McConaghy N, Armstrong B, Birrell P, et al, The incidence of bisexual feelings and opposite sex behavior in medical students. J Nerv Ment Dis 1979;167:685-88.
15. Green R (Ed). Sexual Identity Conflict in Children and Adults: New York: Basic Books 1974.
16. Troiden RT. Becoming homosexual: A model of gay identity acquisition. Psychiatry 1979; 42:362-73.

17. Troiden R. Homosexual identify development. J Adoles Health Care 1989; 9:105.
18. Allen LB, Glicken AD. Depression and suicide in gay and lesbian adolescents. Phys Assist 1996; 20:44-60.
19. Shaffer D, Fisher P, Hicks RH, et al. Sexual orientation in adolescents who commit suicide. Suicide Life Threat Behav 1995; 25 (Suppl):64-71.
20. Remafedi G. Sexual orientation and youth suicide. JAMA 1999; 282:1291.
21. Nicholas J, Howard J. Better dead than gay: Depression, suicide ideation, and attempt among a sample of gay and straight-identified males 18 to 24. Youth Stud Aust 1998; 17:28-33.
22. Harrison AE, Silenzio VMB: Comprehensive care of lesbian and gay patients and their families. Prim Care 1996; 23(1):31-45.
23. Garofalo R, Harper GW. Not all adolescents are the same: Addressing the unique needs of gay and bisexual male youth. Adolesc Med 2003; 14:595-611.
24. Federal Bureau of Investigation. Hate Crime Statistics, 2003. U.S. Department of Justice, Washington, DC 20535, 2004; 9-12, (November).
25. Garofalo R, Wolf RC, Kessel S, et al. The association between health risks behaviors and sexual orientation among a school-based sample of adolescents. Pediatrics 1998; 101: 895-902.
26. American Academy of Pediatrics. Homosexuality and Adolescence. Committee on Adolescence. Pediatrics 1993; 92: 631-34.
27. Ford C, English A, Sigman G: Confidential health care for adolescents: Position paper of the Society for Adolescent Medicine. J Adolesc Health 2004; 35: 160-67.

7 Internet and Sexual Activity

Sunil Saini, Swati Y Bhave

INTRODUCTION

Internet has become an important part of daily life among adolescents. Internet abuse is emerging as a great threat to society and affecting human beings physically, psychologically, socially and culturally.

Researches have shown that using computer displaces time spent on athletics and other physical activity; extensive computer use may contribute to a sedentary lifestyle that puts children at risk for obesity and associated health problems (Hill and Peter, 1998; Attewell et al, 2003) social isolation (Kraut et al, 1998; Sanders et al, 2000) and the potential for violent games to cause increases in hostility and aggression (Irwin 1995, Kirsh 1998). Adolescents are unable to complete homework or get enough sleep due to misuse of Internet, which result in poor academic results.

INTERNET USE RELATED TO ARSH

The Internet is also a medium that exposes or provides access for some young people to several kinds of inappropriate material. This may include pornography and inappropriate advertising (Shields and Behrman, 2000; Thornburgh and Lin 2002; Mitchell et al, 2003), online sexual solicitation (Mitchell et al, 2003), and the means to acquire cigarettes (Ribisl et al, 2003) or materials to facilitate cheating on school assignments (Lathrop and Foss, 2000).

Internet offers uncensored access to online sex, pornographic images and results in addictive sexual behaviors, eating disorders, job loss, isolation and financial problems. It encourages sexual fantasy, which makes a person vulnerable to many physical and psychological health problems. Most importantly, sexuality on internet is easily accessible and affordable. Sexuality is one of the common topics in all most every commercial, serial, movie, Internet and other media programs are messaging sexuality and justifying teenage sexuality.

All commercials on media including television, radio, magazines, newspaper, internet, etc. promoting perfect body figure, skinny, tall, beautiful girls or well developed muscular men which makes adolescents to seek sexual pleasure with opposite sex.

Studies have shown that individuals who log on to Internet with intention of finding sex partners are at greater risk for sexually transmitted diseases (STDs), including HIV infection than those who do not seek sex partners online (McFarlene et al, 2000).

Research with college students suggests that conversations with friends during the high school years was an important source of sex-related information (Kallen et al, 1983); conversations with best friends has been found to be related to sexual attitudes and behaviors (Lefkowitz et al, 2004). Other conversation topics with peers during the adolescent years include appearance (Giblin, 2004).

Internet is most frequently used as sexual medium than any other medium. Adolescents are curious about sexuality and frequently search for sexual stimulation. We know little about the extent to which adolescents expose themselves to sexuality on internet.

A study conducted in Taiwan in 2001 found that 38% of adolescents had surfed the Internet for sexually explicit material (Lo and Wei, 2005), whereas a US study carried out in 1999 and 2000 reported that 8% of the 10- to 17-year-old surveyed looked intentionally for sexually explicit material on the Internet (Ybarra and Mitchell, 2005). Steele and Brown (1995) link adolescents' selection of (sexual) media content to at least three groups of variables: (a) demographics (e.g. gender, ethnicity) as proxies for underlying sociocultural variables, (b) developmental characteristics (e.g. pubertal status, sexual experience), and (c) social context variables (e.g. parental control, religiosity, peer culture).

Other researches (e.g. Greenberg et al, 1992, Vanwesenbeeck, 2001; Collins et al, 2004, Ybarra and Mitchell, 2005) suggest that adolescents' exposure to online sexually explicit material may be associated with two more groups of variables: (d) personality characteristics, such as sensation seeking, and (e) media use characteristics, such as exposure to sexual content in media other than the Internet.

People are becoming addicted to internet in the same way as others became addicted to drugs, alcohol and gambling which resulted in academic failure (Brady, 1996), reduced work performance (Robert Half International, 1996), marital discord and separation (Quittner, 1997) and other social and occupational impairment.

There are many ways of interaction on internet, e.g. email, chat rooms, instant messaging and blogs. Research suggests that adolescents mostly use instant messaging to communicate with friends from school mostly about friends and gossip (Gross, 2004).

Chat rooms are another most important online venue among adolescents. A chat room is a "room" in cyberspace where people congregate for online conversations, writing, reading messages and exchanging porn materials. Adolescents spend most of their time talking about sex, exchanging sexual jokes, and sex-oriented literature as well as using sex slang (Rice, 2001). Students pass their time on dirty chat and in exchanging porn pictures. The more pornography these individuals access, the higher the risk of their acting out what they see, including sexual assault, rape, and child molestation.

The habitual consumption of pornography can result in a diminished satisfaction with mild forms of pornography and a correspondingly strong desire for more deviant and violent material (Eysneck, 1984). Adolescents express their feeling in chat rooms and on webcams. Bremer and Rauch (1998) observed AOL Teen chat rooms for 321 weekend and after-school minutes and found that one sexual comment was made every four minutes in the chat spaces.

Cyber sex can transform sex from a personal, face-to-face to encounter to an anonymous relationship. Cyber sex is introducing new health risks such as romantic fantasy, sexual addictions, compulsive sexual behavior, obsession, isolation, broken relationships, financial problems, etc. As there is no physical contact in a net relationship, therefore adolescents freely communicate with one another free from parental and social pressure in expressing sexuality. Young children talk with their partners, which they cannot talk in real situation.

Webcam has reached to the bedrooms of adolescents where they expose themselves freely. They do sexual flirt doing indecent acts online on webcam. Newspapers have reported many cases of raids on cyber cafes where young children were caught watching porn movies and doing sexual acts.

Mobile phones are emerging as a new choice for bullies. Mobile pornography is one of the serious problems nowadays. A study conducted by researchers at the University of Oslo is raising concerns after it found that teenagers who use mobile phones are more likely to have had sex. They found that 60 percent of teenagers who use mobiles a lot had sex, whereas, only nine percent of the children who seldom or never used mobile phones had sex. Researchers also found that children with mobile phones often started having sex at the young age of 13. They are attributing this disturbing behavior to the fact that children often flirt on SMS and can also make "speedy contact" with their phones (YIN, 2004).

Transfer of porn images from mobile to mobile has become common among school/ college-going children. Mobile use among school children is also increasing day by day posing a great threat for parents. Mobile with camera and Internet facility has threatened the parents of school going children. According to Professor Willy Pederson "The use of mobile phones is directly responsible for the early sexual encounters directly; they are as harmful as porn sites and adult magazines" (YIN, 2004).

CONSEQUENCES

Although the Internet has consistent positive impacts on modern society, it has also caused various societal concerns about privacy, security, pornography, Internet crime, and virtual community (Greenfield and Yan, 2006).

There is a growing concern about early sexual activities among adolescents and its potential effects on their sexual attitudes, beliefs, moral values, and behaviors. According to a National Attitudinal Poll by Common Sense Media (2006), 85% of parents reported that among all forms of media, the Internet posed the greatest risk to their children. Parental concerns are valid, especially considering that teens are essentially free to view and post whatever they choose and communicate with whomever they want. Boys and girls both are engaging in such activities. According to a survey performed by the London School of Economics (2002), 90% of children between ages 8 and 16 have viewed pornography on the Internet.

Findings indicate that adolescent girls choose network programs with sexual content more often than do adolescent boys (Greenberg and Linsangan, 1993) and spend more time watching it, often in the company of parents. This is the most serious problem of almost every society around the world.

New trends of sexual activities are also emerging among adolescents. There are many sexual practices other than intercourse that predispose young people to negative health outcomes.

Research suggests that teenagers who have not experienced vaginal intercourse, substantial numbers engage in other intimate sexual behaviors that carry health risks (Schuster et al, 1996). According to Rosenthal (2000), a professor of pediatrics and a pediatric psychologist at Cincinnati Children's Hospital Medical Center, "girls are clearly talking about oral sex and masturbation (of their partners or by their partners) more frequently than I used to hear about, but whether this is because they talk more openly about it or are doing it more is unclear. The article published in The New York Times (Lewin, 1997) asserted that high school students who had come of age with AIDS education considered oral sex to be a far less dangerous alternative, in both physical and emotional terms, than vaginal intercourse.

In 2000, an article published in Talk magazine reported that students of 12-16 years old set seventh grade as the starting point for oral sex, which they claimed begins considerably earlier than intercourse. By 10th grade, according to the reporter, "well over half of their classmates were involved (Frank, 2000). Many STDs can be transmitted by either fellatio or cunnilingus, although some are more easily passed than others. Other viral STDs that can be transmitted orally include human papillomavirus, herpes simplex virus and hepatitis B while gonorrhea, syphilis, chlamydia and chancroid are among the bacterial infections that can be passed through oral sex (Edwards and Carne, 1998).

Excessive use of internet result in many physiological, psychological, social, economic problems such as body ache, disturbed digestive system, time sink, substance abuse, sleep disorder, depression, frustration, anger, separation, loneliness, social isolation, financial problems, job loss, disturbed marital relationships, etc.

Research has shown that "males who are exposed to a great deal of erotica before the age of 14 are more sexually active and engage in more varied sexual behaviors as adults than is true for males not so exposed" (Davis and Braucht, 1970). Marshall (1988) found that early exposure (under fourteen years of age) to pornography is related to greater involvement in deviant sexual practice, particularly rape.

Pornography encourages adolescents to have sex before they are ready for it. It is likely that early exposure to pornography is related to greater involvement of deviant sexual practices such as rape, sexual illness, unplanned pregnancies, sexual addictions and child molestation.

Pornography encourages sexual expression without responsibility, which endangers children's health. Slightly more than one-third of the child molesters and rapists found to have at least occasionally been incited by exposure to pornography. The habitual consumption of pornography can result in a diminished satisfaction with mild forms of pornography and a correspondingly strong desire for more deviant and violent material (Eysenck, 1984).

Researchers have found that entertainment application of internet is related with heightened levels of depression, deficient self-regulation, and habitual tendencies (LaRose et al, 2003).

Other serious consequences may include early sexual maturity, unwanted pregnancies, early parenting, abortions, multiple sex partners, homosexuality/lesbianism, lack of education, anxiety, depression, anger, aggression, guilt and shame, masturbation, sexual dysfunction, sexual violence, decline of moral values, drinking, drug abuse suicidal ideation, and other physical and mental health consequences. Studies have shown that among adolescent girls in the United States aged between 15 and 17 years, 75 per 1,000 become pregnant each year (Fleming, 1996).

INTERVENTION

Some important tips for safeguarding adolescents from the negative impacts of cyber age have been suggested here

Parental supervision of their adolescents is extremely important

- They should strictly limit the amount of time spent on internet
- They should be aware of the programs seen
- They should become the primary source of information regarding sex
- They should know their adolescent's friends and their families
- Restrict the use of mobile phones by monitoring the bill and restricting use
- Discourage early and frequent dating
- Talk with them about suitable and unsuitable dating activities and appropriate ways for interacting with the opposite sex
- Talk about the results of irresponsible sexual behavior and why it is important to delay sex.

PARENTS SHOULD EDUCATE AND WARN THEIR ADOLESCENTS TO FOLLOW THE FOLLOWING PRECAUTIONS

- Never to give out any personal identifying information to another individual or website online
- Never agree to actually meet someone they have met online. If they insist it should be under parental supervision
- In a chat not everything they see or read online is true
- Not to disclose personal information to strangers
- Not to give out phone number or address to others

- Not to make phone calls to people that they meet online
- Not to reveal their password to anyone except parents
- Not to send their pictures over the Internet or through the mail to an online acquaintance.

OTHER INTERVENTIONS IN THE COMMUNITY

- Sex education
- Peer education.

FOR ADOLESCENT AFFECTED ADVERSELY

- School counseling
- Family therapy may be beneficial.
- Professional help.

SUGGESTED READING

1. Attewell P, Suazo-Garcia B, Battle J. Computers and Young Children: Social Benefit or Social Problem? Social Forces 2003; 82, 277-97.
2. Brady K. Dropouts raise a net result of computers. The Buffalo Evening News, April 21, 1996; 1.
3. Bremer J, Rauch P. Children and computers: Risks and benefits. Journal of the American Academy of Child and Adolescent Psychiatry 1998; 37, 559.
4. Collins RL, Elliott MN, Berry SH, Kanouse D E, Kunkel D, and Hunter, SB. Watching sex on television predicts adolescent initiation of sexual behavior. Pediatrics, 2004;114, E280-E89.
5. Common Sense Media www.commonsense.com/>
6. Davis KE, Braucht GN. Exposure to Pornography, Character and Sexual Deviance. Technical Reports of the Commission on Obscenity and Pornography 1970;7.
7. Edwards S, Carne C. Oral sex and the transmission of non-viral STIs. Sexually Transmitted Infections 1998;74(2), 95-100.
8. Eysenck HJ. Robustness of experimental support for the general theory of desensitization. In Neil M. Malamuth Edward Donnerstein, (Eds.), Pornography and Sexual Aggression (P, 314). Orlando, Florida: Academic Press 1984.
9. Fleming, M. Healthy youth 2000: A mid-decade review. Chicago (Ill): American Medical Association, Dept of Adolescent Health 1996.
10. Franks L. The sex lives of your children, Talk Magazine 2000; 102-07 and 157.
11. Giblin AA. Adolescent girls' appearance conversations: Evaluation, pressure, and coping. Dissertation Abstracts International 2004;0419-4209.
12. Greenberg BS, Linsangan R, Soderman A, Heeter C, Lin C, Stanley C. Adolescents' exposure to television and movie sex. In Greenberg BS, Brown JD, Buerkel-Rothfuss N: (Eds.): Media, sex, and the adolescent. Creskill, NJ: Hampton 1992;61-98
13. Greenfield P, Yan Z. Children, adolescents, and the Internet: A new field of inquiry in developmental psychology. Journal of Applied Developmental Psychology 2006;42 (3), 391-4
14. Gross EF. Adolescent Internet use: What we expect, what teens report. Journal of Applied Developmental Psychology 2004;24, 633-49.
15. Hill JO, Peter JC Environmental Contributions to the Obesity Epidemic. Science 1998;280, 1371-74.
16. Irwin AR. Cognitive Tempo, Violent Video Games, and Aggressive Behavior in Young Boys. Journal of Family Violence 1995;10, 337-50.
17. Kallen, DJ, Stephenson. JJ, Doughty, A. The need to know: Recalled adolescent sources of sexual and contraceptive information and sexual behavior. Journal of Sex Research 1983; 19, 137-59.
18. Kirsh SJ. Seeing the World through Mortal-Kombat-Colored Glasses: Violent Video Games and the Development of a Short-Term Hostile Attribution Bias. Childhood: A Global Journal of Child Research 1998;5:177-84.
19. Kraut R, Patterson J, Lundmark, V, Kiesler S, Mukopadhyay T, Scherlis, W Internet Paradox: A Social Technology that Reduces Social Involvement and Psychological Well-Being? American Psychologist 1998;53(9), 1017-31.
20. LaRose R, Lin C, Eastin, MS. Unregulated Internet usage: Addiction, habit, or deficient self-regulation? Media Psychology 2003;5:225–53.
21. Lathrop A and Foss KE. Student Cheating and Plagiarism in the Internet Era: A Wake-up Call. Englewood, CO: Libraries Unlimited 2000.
22. Lefkowitz ES, BooneTL, Shearer CL. Communication with best friends about sex-related topics during emerging adulthood. Journal of Youth and Adolescence 2004;33, 339-51.

23. Lewin, T. Teen-agers alter sexual practices, thinking risks will be avoided, New York Times 1997.
24. Lo VH, Wei R. Exposure to Internet pornography and Taiwanese adolescents' sexual attitudes and behavior. Journal of Broadcasting and Electronic Media 2005;49,221-37.
25. Marshall WL. The use of sexually explicit stimuli by rapists, child molesters, and nonoffenders. The Journal of Sex Research 1988;25,2267-88.
26. McFarlane M, Bull SS, Rietmeijer CA The Internet as a newly emerging risk environment for sexually transmitted diseases. JAMA 2000; 284,443-46.
27. Mitchell KJ, Finkelhor D, Wolak J. The Exposure of Youth to Unwanted Sexual Material on the Internet: A National Survey of Risk, Impact, and Prevention. Youth and Society 2003;34,330-58.
28. Quittner J. Divorce Internet style. Time, 1997:72.
29. Ribisl K, Williams RS, Kim AE. Internet Sales of Cigarettes to Minors. Journal of the American Medical Association 2003;290,1356-59.
30. Robert Half International, Inc. (October 20, 1996). Misuse of the Internet may hamper productivity. Report from an internal study conducted by a private marketing research group 1996.
31. Rosenthal S. Children's Hospital Medical Center, Cincinnati, OH, personal communication 2000.
32. Saini S, Trama S. Cyber age and adolescents. AJPP 2006;9(3);30-4
33. Sanders CE, Field TM, Diego M, Kaplan M. The relationship of internet use to depression and social isolation among adolescents. Adolescence 2000;35(138):237-42.
34. Schuster MA, Bell RM, Kanouse DE. The sexual practices of adolescent virgins: genital sexual activities of high school students who have never had vaginal intercourse. American Journal of Public Health 1995;86,1570-6.
35. Shields MK, Behrman RE. Children and Computer Technology: Analysis and Recommendation. Future of Children 2000;10(2),4-30. Available at http://www.futureofchildren.org/
36. Steele JR, Brown JD. Adolescent room culture: Studying media in the context of everyday life. Journal of Youth and Adolescence 1995;24, 551-76.
37. Thornburgh D, Lin HS, (Eds): Youth, Pornography, and the Internet. Washington DC: National Academy Press 2002.
38. Vanwesenbeeck I. Psychosexual correlates of viewing sexually explicit sex on television among women in the Netherlands. Journal of Sex Research 2001;38, 361-8.
39. Yahoo India News: Technology. Cell phone boosts teen sex 2004.
40. Ybarra ML, Mitchell KJ. Exposure to Internet pornography among children and adolescents: A national survey. Cyber Psychology and Behavior 2005;8, 473-86.

8 Normal, Precocious and Delayed Puberty

Sangeeta Yadav

INTRODUCTION

Puberty is a biological process in the continuum of life which is characterized by the appearance of secondary sex characteristics and the achievement of reproductive capacity. Puberty is a gradual process culminating in ovulatory menstrual cycling in the female and fully mature spermatogenesis in the male. It is temporally linked to the onset of breast or genital development in the majority of individuals.

a. There is reactivation of the hypothalamic-pituitary gonadal axis.
b. There is pulsatile release of the gonadotropins i.e. increased amplitude and frequency in production of LH and FSH.
c. There is decreased sensitivity of the CNS gonadostat to negative feedback by sex steroids.
d. There is increase in the levels of sex steroids.

The following are important to note:

At the onset of puberty, accentuated periodic release of LH first occurs during sleep because of increased amplitude of pulsatile secretion every 60 to 90 minutes.

As puberty progresses the peak of gonadotropin increases in amplitude and extends throughout the 24 hours period with no diurnal variation as in the adults.

FSH stimulates ovarian follicle formation and estrogen secretion in girls and estradiol exerts negative feed back inhibition on FSH secretion.

LH stimulates the Leydig cells of the testes to secrete testosterone in boys and this testosterone exerts negative feedback inhibition of LH secretion.

LH has little effect in girls until after ovulation occurs, when it supports the corpus luteum.

FSH has little effect in boys until spermarche, when it supports the development of sperm Inhibin, a protein, is produced by seminiferous tubules in males and ovarian follicles in females that exerts negative feedback inhibition on FSH secretion.

The theca cells of the ovaries secrete progesterone after ovulation and its measurement in serum may be used as a reflection of ovulation.

With the onset of puberty, mean unstimulated LH and FSH levels increase. Stimulation testing with GnRH increases the LH and FSH levels.

The LH to FSH ratios, either baseline or stimulated, may be useful as an indicator of pubertal status. A ratio of less than 1 is typical during childhood and a ratio of more than 1 is characteristic of pubertal secretion.

These parameters may be useful but not always adequate to differentiate especially for precocious puberty (progressive) from the early onset normal variant (non-progressive) puberty.

Sex steroid secretion is more constant throughout the day than it is with the gonadotropin secretion, but definite variation is found, so that the concentrations may vary from less than 10 pg/ml to 40 to 50 pg/ml within a 24 hour period. Sensitive testosterone and estradiol assays are available for accurate analysis in the diagnosis of endocrine conditions.

AGE OF ONSET OF PUBERTY

The normal age at onset of puberty is 9 to 14 years in boys and 8 to 13 years in girls and this has not changed appreciably in the last several decades. The average age of onset of puberty in girls is 10 years and is complete in 1.5 to 6 years with a mean of 4.2 years. The secular trends occurring over the last century towards earlier puberty is continuing but at a very reduced rate.

CHANGES IN PUBERTY

a. Gonadal changes
b. Adolescent growth spurt
c. Secondary sexual character
d. Changes in body composition
e. Skeletal maturity and growth of internal organs.

GONADAL CHANGES

In girls accelerated growth rate is the usual first evidence of puberty, but thelarche is usually the first evidence to be noted.

The mean age of breast development (Tanner stage 2) among girls, not considering race, is between 9.5 and 10 years of age with 5% girls having breast development by their eighth birthday with full maturity at 14 years. The interval between pubertal onset and menarche is variable, the average interval is 2 years.

Ovulation may occur before menarche or later. There is considerable variation in the tempo of puberty, with earlier onset, the tempo is slower.

There is increase in the size of the genitalia i.e. uterus, vagina, clitoris, ovaries. Menarche occurs around stage 3-4.

There is activation of the Bartholin glands.

Adolescent Growth Spurt is Characterized by Increased Peak Height Velocity

The average growth spurt lasts 2.5- 3 years.

In girls it is 9 cm/year (around stage 2-3)i.e. before menarche. In girls total height gain is 24-26 cm. It is important to assess the growth in relation to sexual development rather than age. Most of the spurt is due to an increase in the trunk length than the leg length.

The mean gain in sitting height in boys is 15.4 cm and girls is 13.5 and 11.5 cm and the leg length is 12.5 cm for boys and 11.5 cm for girls. Initially the foot and hand grows, then the calf i.e. the legs followed by trunk.

BODY COMPOSITION

The peak weight velocity is preceded by peak height velocity.

The females have higher fat content whereas males have more muscular growth.

The girls have a pear shaped body and wider pelvis. Whereas boys have an apple shaped body and have broader shoulders.

There is accelerated growth of the maxilla and mandible and the jaw becomes prominent.

In the eyes, there is change in axial dimension, resulting in myopia.

The skeletal maturity is characterized by ossification and fusion of epiphysis.

The bone mineral density increases under the influence of sex steroids.

SEXUAL MATURITY RATING

The physical changes of puberty are widely known as Sex Maturity Rating (SMR). The development in girls are shown in Table 8.1.

The adolescents are very often brought by parents seeking consultation regarding growth and development. The major issues bothering them are height, timing of puberty and development of secondary characters.

In clinical practice the common concerns are Short stature and early or delayed puberty. Therefore, these issues will be primarily focused upon in this article.

Table 8.1: Sexual maturity rating

Breast development	
B1	Prepubertal: elevation of papilla only
B2	Breast buds with enlargement of areola.
B3	Further enlargement of breast tissue and areola, without separation of contours.
B4	Breast contour is separate from chest wall, areola and papilla form a secondary mound.
B5	Mature breast with projection of papilla.
Female pubic hair	
P1	Prepubertal: No pubic hair
P2	Sparse long, straight, slightly curly, minimally pigmented hair.
P3	Darker and coarser hair on mons pubis
P4	Adult type hair, not yet spreading to thighs.
P5	Adult type distribution of hair.

SHORT STATURE

Short stature is defined as height below the third centile of the reference range or height below 2.5 S.D. below the mean for age.

Mid Parental Height (MPH) or Predicted Adult Height (PAH) is the height the child is expected to have at the age of 18 years.

In males it is calculated as (Father's Height + Mother's Height)\2 + 6.5 cm and

In Females as (Father's Height + Mother's Height)\2 - 6.5 cm.

The other way to assess the growth is the height gained over a period of time i.e.1 year-*annual growth velocity.*

A child is said to be having growth failure when the growth velocity is > 2.5 SD below the mean or, 25th centile of the mean height velocity for age.

As a rule, any growth rate < 4.5 cm/year between 2 and 12 years in either sex is pathological.

The growth velocity falls to a nadir just before the pubertal growth spurt.

EPIDEMIOLOGY OF SHORT STATURE

In the majority of cases, short stature (SS) is due to normal physiologic variations in growth and maturation. The most common cause of short stature is: Normal variant short stature i.e. familial and/or constitutional.

The etiological causes of short stature in the various studies available show that growth hormone deficiency and other endocrine causes are observed more often especially in a pediatric referral center, chronic systemic illnesses, nutritional causes, etc. are also commonly seen.

ETIOLOGY OF SHORT STATURE

Classification of short stature on the basis of etiology is given in Table 8.2.

Table 8.2: Etiological classification of short stature

A. Normal
- Constitutional growth delay
- Genetic/familial
- Idiopathic

B. Pathological
- Psychosocial growth retardation
- Nutritional
- Hypocaloric
- Rickets
- Gastrointestinal:
  - Malabsorption
  - Chronic inflammatory bowel
  - Hepatic-chronic hepatitis
  - Glycogen storage disease.
  - Cardiac (Congenital heart disease/ rheumatic.
  - Pulmonary chronic lung diseases
- Renal:
  - Chronic pyelonephritis
  - Renal tubular acidosis
  - Chronic renal insufficiency

  Rheumatoid disease
- Endocrine:
  - GH deficiency- congenital/acquired
  - Hypothyroidism
  - Pseudohypoparathyroidism
  - Hypercortisolemia
  - Precocious puberty
  - Poorly controlled IDDM
  - Skeletal dysplasias and chondrodystrophies
  - Low birth weight
  - Sporadic
  - Characteristic appearance
  - Chromosomal defects
  - Turner's syndrome
  - Down syndrome
  - Others

Familial/Genetic Short Stature

It is the most common cause of short stature.

In this parents and/or close relatives are short but child's projected adult height falls within 2 SD of the MPH.

This 2 SD for boys is 7.5 cm and for girls 6 cm at 18 years.

Growth velocity is normal.

Results of physical examination including signs of sexual maturation are normal.

The child passes puberty at normal time.

The bone age is equal to chronological age which may be slightly greater than the height age.

No treatment is required, parents and child need to be reassured.

Final height is in consonant with the parental height and likely to be shorter than the peers.

Constitutional Growth Delay

These are also called late maturers. It is more common in boys with a Male: Female ratio of 10:1.

Periods of slow growth occurs in the first 3 to 4 years of life, so their height falls below the 3rd centile, after which the growth velocity is normal for age, such that their growth pattern runs parallel to the normal growth but below the 3rd centile.

Height and bone age are usually delayed by 2 to 4 years.

History of delayed growth and sexual development is present in parents and other family members.

Puberty and pubertal growth spurt is delayed by 2 or more years

Bone age is equal to height age, both are in turn less than chronological age. Final adult height is reached around 18-20 years, and is within low normal range.

Sexual development and fertility is normal.

Growth hormone levels, if measured, are normal.

Parents and the child must be explained that the child would continue to grow for a longer period than usual and ultimately will reach normal adult height.

Growth Hormone Deficiency

GHD may be congenital or acquired.

1. Congenital or genetic GHD may be due to defects in pituitary transcription factors, mutations in growth hormone gene, receptor defects or GH biosynthesis or there may be structural defects.
2. Acquired defects may be the result of hypothalamic-pituitary damage due to infections, neoplasias, trauma, irradiation or surgery.

Growth hormone deficiency presents with

- Extreme short stature and delayed puberty.
- The body proportions are normal with a prominent forehead and depressed mid face development.
- There is truncal obesity with decreased muscle bulk.
- The extremities and hands and feet are small.
- It may be associated with features of hypoadrenalism and hypothyroidism if multiple pituitary hormones are affected.
- The dentition is delayed
- Both height and growth velocity are less than 3rd centile.
- Bone age is < 2 SD below chronological age

Growth hormone estimation in serum after stimulation test if > 7 ng/ml rules out GH deficiency.

Nutritional Insufficiency

The single most important cause of growth failure and short stature globally is poverty related. The bone age is significantly retarded.

The GH levels are normal to increased but IGF–I levels are reduced.

Zinc deficiency has been particularly implicated in growth retardation. Vitamin D deficiency rickets can result in impaired growth. Eating disorders can present with linear growth retardation.

Hypothyroidism

Thyroxin is an important regulator of GH secretion and low thyroxin leads to decreased GH pulsatility.

In short statute due to hypothyroidism, the US:LS ratio is infantile and the bone age is markedly reduced.

Other clinical features of hypothyroidism would be present.

All patients should have assessment of thyroid function as part of initial work-up of short stature.

Replacement therapy with thyroxin results in rapid catch up growth but also causes early bone maturation and epiphyseal fusion.

CLINICAL ASSESSMENT OF SHORT STATURE

The work up consists of a detailed history including details of birth and development history, mental retardation, headache, vomiting, diplopic, feeding problems and anorexia, edema feet and hand at birth, chronic diarrhea or constipation, fever, breathlessness, cyanosis, polyuria, polydypsia, parental height, details of parental puberty and detailed nutritional review.

Physical Examination

It includes interaction with parents and detailed head to toe examination and search for abnormalities related to systemic illnesses.

Each abnormal finding can indicate etiology of short stature. The flow diagram delineates the evaluation (Fig. 8.1)

Anthropometric evaluation is the most important parameter for assessment of growth.

The following measurements should be taken with most accuracy. It is also important to plot the growth measurements on the available charts.

Growth velocity should be assessed and plotted on the growth velocity curves. Special growth charts have been developed for various conditions.

The adolescent's stature should be assessed in relation to parents and siblings.

Standing Height

Lower Segment – Length from top of pubic symphysis to the ground

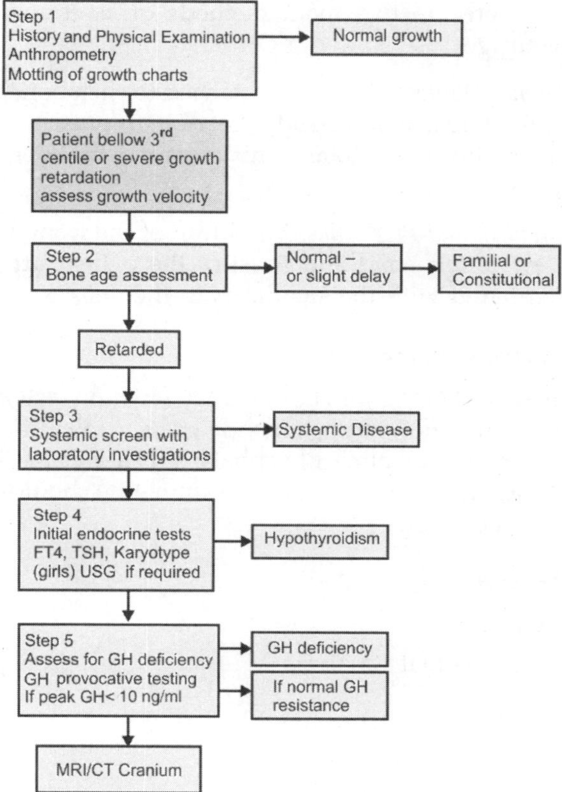

Fig. 8.1: Evaluation of short stature

Upper segment –Total Height – Lower Segment

US : LS ratios are useful to decide whether the SS is proportionate or disproportionate.

INVESTIGATIONS

Bone Age

It refers to the skeletal maturation attained by the subject at that chronological age.

A short child with delayed bone age carries a better prognosis for attainment of ultimate height than a short child where bone age is consistent with chronological age.

When bone age is less than 2 SD or < 2 years of chronological age, it is considered delayed. Bone age of 17 years in males and 15 years in females means full maturation, i.e. no more increase in height is likely to be possible.

There are two main methods of assessing bone age:

Tanner-WhiteHouse Score: Attached to each bone of the forearm and hand according to presence and maturity. The total score determines the bone age

Greulich and Pyle Atlas: X-ray film of the frontal view of left hand and wrist of the patient are compared with the standards in the atlas.

Systemic Screening

Includes hemogram, ESR, kidney function tests, liver function tests, blood gases, calcium, phosphate, alkaline phosphatase, celiac panel, chest X-ray, Mantoux, urine examination should be done.

Thyroid Function Tests

Karyotyping

Chromosomal analysis—Turner's and Gene defects.

GH Stimulation Test

Since GH has pulsatile secretion, single reading of serum GH are not useful. The serum GH > 7 ng/ml after stimulation test, rules out GH deficiency. Clonidine test is done in early morning fasting state. 150 gm/kg orally clonidine is given and samples collected at 0, 30, 60, 90 and 120 minutes. In Insulin Tolerance test plain insulin 0.1 unit/kg IV is given. A 50% fall in blood sugar is necessary for adequate test. Nadir in blood sugar occurs around 20-30 min. Samples are collected at 0, 30, 60, 90, 120 min.

Other agents used for stimulation are arginine, L-dopa, propranolol, glucagon.

CT Scan/MRI

Evaluation of the hypothalamic pituitary area is essential if GH deficiency is apparent.

Insulin like Growth factors

The growth promoting action of growth hormone is mediated by insulin like growth factors (IGF-1) and IGF binding proteins(IGF BP). They are commonly being used as screening tests.

The interpretation of serum IGF-1assays must be done with caution since it is influenced by nutritional status, skeletal age, puberty and liver functions.

IGF BP3 is GH dependent and low levels along with IGF-1 add accuracy to the diagnosis of GH deficiency.

TREATMENT OF SHORT STATURE

The physician must balance the needs of the adolescent and family, the severity of growth retardation, the expected adult height while chalking out the treatment plan.

The normal variant short stature requires reassurance and support alongwith close follow-up for growth velocity.

Patients with Pathological cause need Specific Medical Therapy

Growth Hormone Therapy

Administration of GH increases growth velocity in most children with GHD . They respond very well to exogenous GH treatment.

The dose of GH may be increased if necessary while maintaining IGF-I levels within the normal range.

Higher doses may be needed during puberty, a time of increased physiologic GH production.

When children with GHD who are receiving GH enter puberty, additional treatment modalities may be considered to optimize growth and adult height attainment.

One option is to combine GH with a GnRH agonist to delay puberty. Issues with this treatment option include the psychological aspect of halting puberty and potential effects on bone mineral density.

Sex Steroids and Anabolic Steroids

Oxandrolone is useful in short stature secondary to pubertal delay as well as in Turner's syndrome. It is an anabolic steroid with minimal androgenic affects. Dose is 1.25 -2.5 mg /day x 3 months orally. It is useful in constitutional delay.

Long acting LHRH agonist are shown to delay puberty. A delayed puberty leads to delayed epiphysial fusion which causes longer bones. It increases adult height in LHRH dependent precocious puberty. A randomized controlled trial on effect of LHRH agonist in girls with short stature with normally timed puberty has shown an increase by 0.6 SD in adult height but a significantly reduced bone mineral density.

VARIANTS OF NORMAL PUBERTY

They include premature thelarche i.e. isolated early breast development or premature adrenarche i.e. mild androgen effect leading to sexual hair growth.

Occasionally premature menarche may be observed due to transient ovarian overactivity but puberty occurs at usual time.There is no evidence of maturation of the hypothalamic-pituitary gonadal axis. There are no other signs of estrogen effect and no linear growth. Serum estradiol values and LH are pre-pubertal, FSH may be slightly higher when compared with normal age matched children. Ovarian follicular cysts may be present which regress spontaneously. The condition requires reassurance but continued follow-up and observation at 3 to 6 months interval is necessary. The child may remain in the same category or may progress to precocious puberty.

PRECOCIOUS PUBERTY

Puberty occuring before the age of 8 years in girls and 9 years in boys is termed precocious.

Puberty can occur prematurely because of the early stimulation of the hormonal axis or disturbance outside the axis. The former is complete or true and isosexual with the accelerated somatic growth, development of secondary sexual characters and fertility. The latter is incomplete or pseudoprecocious with only one type of sexual characteristic developing i.e. androgenization or estrogenization e.g. premature adrenarche or premature thelarche.

Table 8.3 shows the etiology of sexual precocity.

Table 8.3: Etiology of sexual precocity

Complete and isosexual	
Hypothalamic – Pituitary – Idiopathic	
• Neurogenic	
• Hypothalamic hamartomas	
• CNS tumors	
• Neural tube defects	
• Infections	
• Irradiation	
• Advanced somatic maturation	
Incomplete + Heterosexual	
Neuroendocrine-premature thelarche	
• Hypothyroidism	
• Isolated LH excess-testotoxicosis	
Adrenal	• Premature adrenarche
	• Congenital adrenal hyperplasia
	• Adrenal tumors
Gonadal	• Tumors-germcell tumors
	• Teratomas
	• Chorioepitheliomas
Ectopic	• Hepatomas
	• Hepatoblastomas
Exogenous	• Anabolic/contraceptive steroids
	• McCune Albright syndrome

TRUE PRECOCIOUS PUBERTY

Is idiopathic in more than 70% girls and there is a CNS lesion in 70% boys. Hypothalamic hamartomas are now frequently identified on imaging techniques and there may be other diverse CNS disorders.

Gonadal tumors and congenital adrenal hyperplasia must be looked for esppecially if incongruity between physical appearance or chronologic age is observed. McCune Albright syndrome is an intriguing cause of sexual precocity, with polyostotic fibrous dysplasia and café-au-lait nevi and endocrine overactivity syndrome.

Testotoxicosis is a familial form of precocious puberty affecting males with marked elevation of testosterone and Leydig-cell activity.

THE EVALUATION: OF A CHILD WITH PRECOCIOUS PUBERTY

Requires a complete clinical history with emphasis on rate of pubertal progression and growth, previous infection, neurological events, hypothyroidism, exposure to gonadal steroids, family history.

The physical examination should assess sexual maturity rating, secondary sexual characters, abdominal, gonadal, CNS examination with visual and fundus exam.

The investigation commences with a bone age and an assessment for estrogenization (plasma estradiol and vaginal hormonal cytology) or androgenization (plasma testosterone and DHEAS measurements).

Besides basal hormonal functions, should be evaluated for FSH, LH, hCG, GnRH stimulation test, thyroid function, etc.

Imaging techniques like USG, CT abdomen, CT/MRI of CNS as and when required.

TREATMENT

Premature thelarche, adrenarche and menarche require reassurance and a close follow-up. Central precocious puberty is treated with GnRH analogues. Medroxy progesterone acetate is effective in diminishing symptoms but has no effect on advancement.

Testolactone is useful in McCune-Albright syndrome and ketoconazole and spironolactone are useful in testotoxicosis.

In case, there is an underlying abnormality, surgical excision of CNS lesions, adrenal or gonadal tumors is advocated.

Hypothalamic hamartomas are to be left alone.

Radiosensitive germ cell pineal tumors and hCG producing tumors are treated by radiotherapy.

The adolescent and the family are stressed due to dyssynchrony in age and body appearance therefore, a psychosocial support is essential especially for social reasons.

DELAYED PUBERTY

Pubertal delay is defined as lack of any evidence of pubertal maturation by the age of 13 years in girls and 14 years in boys and needs to be evaluated. It is of common concern both among boys and girls.

A careful examination, i.e. assessment of breast development in girls very often allay the anxiety and avoid further work-up.

However, subsequent follow-up for progression is necessary.

The delay is not only in sexual maturation but also in relation to stature, i.e. constitutional delay in growth and puberty is the most frequent reason for the delay.

The causes of delayed puberty are outlined in the Table 8.4.

Table 8.4: Causes of delayed puberty

A. Delay of H-P-G-axis reactivation
   1. Constitutional delay of growth and puberty
   2. Chronic systemic illness
   3. Endocrinological disorders
      - IDDM (poorly managed)
      - Cushing's syndrome
      - GH deficiency
      - Hypothyroidism
   4. Malnutrition
   5. Stress/Depression
   6. Anorexia nervosa girls

B. Hypogonadotrophic hypogonadism
   1. Hypothalamic tumors
   2. Craniopharyngioma
   3. Hypopituitarism
   4. CNS
      - Surgical intervention
      - Radiation therapy
   5. Kallmann's syndrome

C. Hypergonadotropic hypogonadism
   1. Genital tract aplasia } Females
   2. Oophorectomy/irradiation } Females
   3. Turner's syndrome } Females
   4. Anorexia } Females
   5. Cryptorchidism
   6. Testicular insufficiency/insensitivity
   7. Testicular-surgical/radiation therapy

Syndromes-Klinefelter's, Noonan's Prader-Willi, Laurence Moon-Biedle

HYPERGONADOTROPIC HYPOGONADISM

Primary gonadal failure resulting from a range of chromosomal and syndromic causes, disorders of steroid and androgen synthesis or any insult to gonads can result in impaired pubertal development.

Girls will present with lack of feminization and amenorrhea.

Serum gonadotropins are elevated because of lack of feedback inhibition from the gonads.

TURNER'S SYNDROME (TS)

It Turner's syndrome is the most common form of primary gonadal failure in females and Klinefelter's syndrome (KS) and its variants in males. The clinical features of TS and KS are shown in the Tables 8.5 and 8.6.

Table 8.5: Features of Klinefelter's syndrome

- Tall stature
- Poor school performance
- Decreased testicular volume and azoospermia
- Decreased body hair
- Decreased sexual function
- Gynecomastia
- Increased gonadotropins
- Decreased testosterone

This has been discussed at length in the chapter of primary amenorrhea.

NOONAN'S SYNDROME

Noonan syndrome is a dominantly inherited condition with some features similar to Turner's and some different from Turner (normal karyotype) triangular shaped face, pectus excavatum, right sided heart disease, mental retardation, affected boys may have undescended testes.

MIXED GONADAL DYSGENESIS

Results from 46XY/45X mosaicism and usually presents with ambiguous genitalia at birth or as pubertal failure later. The streak gonads should be removed.

EVALUATION

During initial evaluation, pertinent history related to nutritional status/linear growth, chronic illnesses, malignancies, CNS lesions and age of onset of puberty of parents or siblings is important.

The physical examination includes anthropometry, pubertal assessment, genital examination, neurological and ophthalmological examination and specific features in relation to syndromes.

Assessment of skeletal maturity can further guide. In girls if bone age is < 11 years it suggests primary hypogonadism, in CDGP—it is 11-13 years and if it is > 13 years it is due to gonadotropin deficiency.

THE LABORATORY EVALUATION

consists of screening for chronic diseases, other endocrine disorders, chromosomal analysis and pelvic ultrasound.

The gonadotropins - FSH and LH are

- elevated in primary hypogonadism and low in secondary hypogonadism, i.e. in pituitary/hypothalamic defects.
- In constitutional delay they are normal for age.

Table 8.6: Features of Turner's syndrome

Infancy	*Childhood*	*Adulthood*
Lymph edema	Short stature	Pubertal failure
Shield chest	Short neck	Amenorrhea
Widely spaced nipples	Cubitus valgus	Hypertension
Web neck	Hypoplastic nails	Obesity
Low-set hairline	Short fourth meta-carpals	Dyslipidemia
Cardiac defects	Scoliosis	Insulin resistance
Coarctation of the aorta	Ptosis/amblyopia	Increased:Cardiovascular disease-
Horse-shoe kidney	Otitis media/hearing loss -	Osteoporosis
	Multiple nevi	Colon cancer
Urinary tract malformations	Autoimmune thyroid disease -	Inflammatory bowel disease
	Visuospatial learning difficulties -	Gonadoblastoma

If the estradiol level > 70 pg/ml indicates some ovarian function.

Similarly hCG testing and DHEAS levels help with further differentiation.

A CT/MRI of CNS/ abdomen are accordingly required for further work-up.

TREATMENT

The goal of treatment is to achieve a normal progression of physical changes of puberty to physical maturity and the normal potential for sexual function.

The treatment involves both psychological counseling and support and endocrinologic treatment.

Patients with constitutional delay need reassurance but occasionally may require a brief course of sex steroids for promoting pubertal growth and development and in improving psychosocial parameters.

Those with hypogonadism require hormone replacement therapy.

Later, especially in secondary hypogonadism hCG and GnRH analogues have to be added.

SUGGESTED READING

1. American Association of Clinical Endocrino-logists medical guidelines for clinical practice for growth hormone use in adults and children-2003 update. Endocr Pract 2003;9:64-76.
2. Ora H, Prescovitz, Erica A, Eugster. Pediatric Endocrinology Lippincott Williams and Wilkins; Philadelphia; 2004:316-48.
3. Pediatric Endocrinology. Dennis M. Styne. Lippincott Williams and Wilkins, Philadelphia: 2004:159-95.
4. Reiter EO, D'Ercole AJ. Disorders of the anterior pituitary gland, hypothalamus, and growth. In: Rudolph CD, Rudolph AM (Eds). Rudolph's pediatrics. New York: McGraw-Hill, 2002:2011-24.
5. Reiter EO, Rosenfeld RG. Normal and abnormal growth. In: Larsen PR, Kronenberg HM, Melmed S, et al. (Eds). Williams textbook of endocrinology. Philadelphia: WB Saunders, 2003:1003-114.
6. Styne DM. Constitutional delay in growth and adolescence. In: Finberg L, Kleinman RE, (Eds). Saunders manual of pediatric practice. Philadelphia: WB Saunders, 2002:838-39.
7. Styne DM. Evaluation of short stature. In: Finberg L, Kleinman RE, eds.Saunders manual of pediatric practice. Philadelphia: WB Saunders, 2002:946-49.
8. Wilson TA, Rose SR, Cohen P, et al. Update of guidelines for the use of growth hormone in children: The Lawson Wilkins Pediatric Endocrino-logy Drug and Therapeutics Committee J Pediatr 2003; 143: 415-21.

9 Obesity Related to Reproductive and Sexual Health

Anju Seth

INTRODUCTION

Prevalence of obesity has increased globally across all age-groups in the last few decades and is now emerging as an important public health problem. Obesity during childhood and adolescence is an issue of major concern since it is a well recognized fore-runner for adult obesity, which in turn, may be the basis of various chronic disorders including hypertension, hyperlipidemia, respiratory diseases, diabetes, orthopedic conditions, etc.

In India too, obesity has made its presence felt among the urban affluent. A study from Ludhiana, Punjab has reported an overall prevalence of obesity and over weight as 11.1% and 14.2% respectively among 9-15 years old children, the difference among children belonging to higher and lower socioeconomic state being statistically significant.[1] Another study from Chennai has reported 9.7% adolescent public school girls to be over weight and 6.2% obese.[2]

SIMPLE OBESITY

Vast majority of obese adolescents suffer from 'simple obesity', which is the result of excessive calorie intake, decreased energy expenditure or a combination of the two. In <1% of cases, obesity may be the result of an underlying pathological process.

PATHOLOGICAL OBESITY

Important disorders associated with 'pathological obesity' that may present during adolescence are presented in Table 9.1.

- ***Endocrine disorders*** like hypothyroidism, GH deficiency and hypercortisolism cause decreased energy expenditure and decreased growth resulting in mild obesity. Enhanced fluid retention is an additional contributing factor in hypothyroidism. In all these disorders obesity is invariably associated with poor linear growth.
- ***Prader-Willi*** syndrome is the commonest genetic syndrome associated with obesity. It is an autosomal dominant disorder characterized by short stature, mental delay, hypotonia and genital hypoplasia along with obesity.
- ***Lawrence-Moon-Beidl syndrome,*** another autosomal recessive disorder associated with

Table 9.1: Causes of pathological obesity

- Endocrine disorders: Hypothyroidism, hypercortisolism, Hyperangrogenism (PCOS)
- GH deficiency (uncommon)
- Genetic syndromes: Prader-Willi, Laurence-Moon-Beidl, Cohen or Alstrom Syndromes
- Specific genetic mutations: Leptin gene, Leptin receptor gene, POMC gene, MC4R gene.
- CNS causes: Trauma, tumor (e.g. craniopharyngioma), post infections (encephalitis, TB).
- Others: Immobilization, drugs

obesity have retinitis pigmentosa, polydactyly, mental retardation, hypogenitalism and short stature.

These disorders generally get identified during childhood, but it is not unusual for the diagnosis to be delayed till adolescence when lack of pubertal development may be the reason for seeking medical consultation.

Hypothalamic and pituitary dysfunction secondary to CNS tumor-craniopharyngioma being the most common or inflammatory process like encephalitis, TB, trauma, etc. may lead to alteration in appetite center leading to hyperphagia and obesity.

OBESITY: IMPACT UPON THE REPRODUCTIVE HEALTH

Obesity leads to increased insulin secretion, insulin resistance, and alterations at the level of hypothalamo-pituitary-adrenal and hypothalamo-pituitary-gonadal axis.

Menarche tends to occur earlier in obese girls, and these girls often have symptoms suggestive of abnormal ovarian function such as irregular menses, oligomenorrhea, amenrrhoea, hirsutism and infertility.[3]

There is evidence to suggest that insulin mediates a regulatory influence on ovarian function, including ovarian androgen synthesis. A positive correlation has been found between the degree of hyperinsulinemia and hyperandrogenism in obese women.[4]

This regulatory effect of insulin is mediated via LH. Some obese girls have been shown to have elevated LH, low FSH and elevated free testosterone levels.[4]

Adolescent hyperandrogenemia is a forerunner of adult polycystic ovaries syndrome (PCOS) which may subsequently develop in some of these girls[5] and has been extensively discussed in the chapter of PCOS.

COMPLICATIONS RELATED TO SEXUAL AND REPRODUCTIVE HEALTH

Obesity leads to many psychosocial problems too.

An obese adolescent often gets discriminated against by family and friends. They may be teased or ridiculed as being clumsy, unattractive and over-indulgent.

This leads to a lowered self-image and withdrawal from social contact.

To overcome these and to prove their worth, they indulge in various risk taking behaviors, they indulge in sexual activity, substance abuse, binging followed by purging behaviors leading to bulimia nervosa.

They are easily blackmailed into having sex with its attendant risks.

The pregnancy may go unrecognized due to obesity or irregular cycles.

The patient may go into depression or anxiety and mood disorders.

OTHER COMPLICATIONS OF OBESITY

Obesity can affect many organ systems. These in turn have an effect upon the overall health including the reproductive health of the adolescent. Table 9.2 lists the various complications of obesity.

Table 9.2: Complications of obesity

1. Cardiovascular diseases, hypertension, deranged lipid profile
2. Steatohepatitis, gallstones
3. Endocrine consequences: Insulin resistance, Type 2 DM, and hyper-androgenism
4. Menstrual abnormalities, polycystic ovaries
5. Orthopedic sequelae: Genes varum, valgus deformity, slipped capital femoral epiphysis, tibia vara
6. Pseudotumor cerebri
7. Psychosocial consequences: Poor self-esteem, depression, poor scholastic performance
   Increased sexual activity, substance abuse, bulimia nervosa

Obesity is a major risk factor for *cardiovascular diseases* in the adolescent age group, the other risk factors being decreased physical activity, dyslipidemia, hypertension and tobacco use.

Since obesity predisposes to all of these except tobacco use, obese adolescents are at a substantial risk of suffering from cardiovascular disease.

They are found to have a 2.4 fold risk for increased blood pressure and up to 10 fold risk for adult hypertension, a greater increase being noted in children with abdominal adiposity. In a study from Ludhiana 15.33% of overweight and 93.1% of obese school going children were found to have *hypertension*.[6]

The prevalence of diabetes mellitus is also high in obese children and adolescents. A global increase in prevalence of *type II DM* is noted parallel to increase in the prevalence of obesity. Thus, Japan has reported a 30 fold increase in its prevalence over the last 20 years.

A high prevalence of *insulin resistance and hyper-insulinemia* has also been reported from post-pubertal urban Indian children in association with abdominal obesity and excess body fat.[7] Most obese adolescents with diabetes tend to be asymptomatic, being picked up on routine blood glucose testing.

Presence of *acanthosis nigricans* (velvety, hyper keratotic, dark skin found at the nape of the neck, axilla and the groin folds) indicates possible presence of hyper-insulinemia and impaired glucose tolerance.

EVALUATION

An adolescent with obesity needs a comprehensive medical and nutritional evaluation. The purpose is to:

1. Ascertain the etiology: whether the obesity is 'simple' or 'pathological'
2. Screen for the complications related to obesity.

Table 9.3 summarizes the clinical evaluation of the obese adolescent.

- As a general rule, an adolescent with simple obesity is usually tall for age/genetic potential, though weight for height is disproportionately higher.
- On the other hand, most individuals with pathological obesity are short.
- Look for thyroid enlargement, clinical features of Cushing syndrome and other genetic syndromes associated with obesity.

Table 9.3: Clinical evaluation of an obese adolescent

History

1. Dietary details
2. Activity pattern
3. Mental development
4. School performance
5. Drug intake
6. H/o CNS injury / infection
7. Snoring, day time sleep
8. Psychosocial concerns- Life styles
9. Prevalence of obesity and body fat distribution in other family members
10. Prevalence of obesity related morbidity in family
11. Review of past weight and height records, if available

Examination

1. Height, weight:BMI calculation
2. Parental height
3. Blood pressure
4. Acanthosis nigricans
5. Pubertal staging
6. Dysmorphic features

- Most of the pathological conditions will present with short stature, features of hypothyroidism or cushing's and hypogonadism and dysmorphism.
- A child with normal cognitive function and good linear growth is very unlikely to have syndromic obesity.
- Patients with hypothyroidism and GH deficiency have increased weight for height though they are seldom grossly obese.
- Some patients with simple obesity may have a fat distribution suggestive of Cushing Syndrome. However, Cushing syndrome is a rare cause of obesity.
- Long-term use of corticosteroids may lead to obesity along with growth retardation. The obesity tends to be transient and resolves once the drug is stopped. History of prolonged intake of certain drugs like sodium valproate and anti-psychotic drugs have also been associated with weight gain.[8]

All adolescents with BMI > 85th centile should be investigated as per Table 9.4. Bone age should be assessed in all of them. It is mildly advanced, but appropriate for height age in subjects with simple obesity, while those with hypothyroidism and GH deficiency would have a retarded bone age.

Table 9.4: Investigations of an obese adolescent

Suspected pathological obesity:
Condition suspected tests:
- Hypothyroidism—FT4, TSH.
- Cushing syndrome—Urine free cortisol or morning and evening plasma cortisol.
- GH deficiency—GH provocative testing
- Pradar-Willi syndrome—Karyotyping; deletion of chromosome 15.
- CNS disorder—MRI brain.
- **Consequences of obesity:**
  - Fasting lipid profile
  - Fasting and PP Blood sugar
  - AST, ALT – If elevated : consider USG for steato-hepatitis
  - Suspected PCOS: Serum free testosterone, USG abdomen for ovaries

MANAGEMENT

Obesity is a notoriously difficult and frustrating to treat disorder especially among adolescents.

Physicians tend to avoid taking care of the obese. Dieticians may hand out meal plans which probably have been unsuccessful on previous many occasions.

Most interventions prescribed half-heartedly by the physician and followed even more casually by the individual result in small short term weight loss with a relapse soon thereafter.

Thus the teenager has to be highly motivated and has to balance the management protocol handed to them.

The objective of obesity management is life long weight control and not merely shedding of a few kilograms. The energy intake is to be restrained while allowing normal growth to take place.

This is crucial since adolescent growth spurt contributes significantly to the final stature and bone mass too builds up rapidly during this phase. Nutritional deprivation at this time can have long lasting sequelae.

It is imperative that weight cycling is avoided since it makes subsequent weight loss even more difficult.

If a weight reduction is planned, it has to be done with a serious commitment of all involved: the adolescent, his/her family and the physician in-charge. Care has to be taken such that the teenager is not indulging into bingeing and purging behaviors.

For every person an individualized plan needs to be charted out according to the current eating pattern, intellect and degree of motivation. Treatment of underlying cause is indicated where applicable and possible.

For simple obesity, the corner stones of management are dietary management, a regular exercise programme and life style/behaviour modification.

Pharmacological interventions have limited role in management of adolescent obesity.

CHALLENGE AHEAD: ROLE OF PHYSICIANS

Physicians need to:

a. Identify overweight adolescents by recording height and weight at visits. Many parents do not recognize the weight problem of their child.
b. Screen obese adolescents for obesity related complications.
c. Promote a healthy life style and be a role model for the same for the patients under their care and their families.

KEY MESSAGES

1. Most obesity during adolescence is "simple". However, it can have impact on various organ systems including endocrine, cardiac and orthopedic. These directly influence the quality of life of an adolescent.
2. Few endocrine disorders presenting during adolescence can also lead to obesity. These include hypothyroidism, GH deficiency and Cushing syndrome. These are invariably associated with growth failure.
3. All obese adolescents should be screened for obesity related complications.

4. The cornerstones of management include dietary modification, regular physical exercise and behavioral modification. The objective is life-time weight control.

REFERENCES

1. Chhatwal J, Verma M, Riar SK. Obesity among pre-adolescents and adolescents of a developing country (India). Asia Pac J Clin Nutr 2004; 13(3): 231-35.
2. Subramanyam V, Jayashree R, Rafi M. Prevalence of overweight and obesity in affluent adolescent girls in Chennai in 1981 and 1998. Indian Pediatr 2003; 40(8): 775-79.
3. Glass AR. Endocrine aspects of obesity. Med Clin North Am 1989;73: 139
4. Singh KB, Mahajan DK, WortsmanJ. Effects of obesity on the clinical and hormonal characteristics of the poly-cystic ovary syndrome.J Reprod Med 1994;39: 805-08
5. McCartney CR, Prendergast KA, Chhabra S, Eagleson CA, Yoo R, Chang RJ, Foster CM, Marshall JC. The association of obesity and hyperandrogenemia during the pubertal transition in girls: Obesity as a potential factor in the genesis of post-pubertal hyperandrogenism. J Clin Endocrinol Metab 2006; 91 (5): 1714 –22.
6. Mohan B, Kumar N, Aslam N, et al. Prevalence of sustained hypertension and obesity in urban and rural school going children in Ludhiana. Indian Heart J 2004; 56(4): 310-14.
7. Misra A, Vikram NK, Arya S, et al. High prevalence of insulin resistance in post-pubertal Asian Indian children is associated with adverse truncal body fat patterning, abdominal adiposity and excess body fat. Int J Obes Relat Metab Disord 2004, 28(10): 1217-26
8. Keck PE, McElroy SL. Bipolar Disorder, Obesity, and Pharmacotherapy-Associated Weight Gain. J Clin Psychiatry 2003; 64:1426-35.

Section 4: Problems Related to Menstruation

10 Primary Amenorrhea

Rama Vaidya, Shefali Pandey

INTRODUCTION

Amenorrhea or absence of menstruation is a symptom and not a disease. Normal menstruation is the end result of coordinated cyclic events in the hypothalamo-pituitary-ovarian-axis and appropriate responses by the uterine endometrium, the target organ for ovarian hormones. Amenorrhea is a reflection of an interruption in the function of this chain or may be due to aberrations in the genital tract.

The causes of amenorrhea are diverse and many. Amenorrhea could be one of the clinical manifestations of a serious underlying disease like space occupying lesion of the central nervous system (CNS) or simply a constitutional delay of growth and/or pubertal development. Hence, a thorough history taking, meticulous examination and appropriate investigations are mandatory in order to establish a correct diagnosis.

PRIMARY AMENORRHEA—DEFINITION

Primary amenorrhea is a condition where menarche has never occurred by the age of 16 years. The amenorrhea can be physiological or pathological. However, primary amenorrhea defined as absence of menses by 16 years of age is a restrictive term and conveys only the absence of one of the aspects of pubertal development namely, menstruation.

Instead, term *delayed puberty* includes some or all aspects of the physiological process of pubertal development, development of breast (thelarche), axillary and pubic hair (Pubarche), pubertal growth spurt and skeletal maturation. There is loose inter-relationship in time of sequence of these events.

However, in the majority of girls, development of breast along with the onset of growth spurt precede pubic and axillary hair development. The menarche usually appears with stage 4 of breast development (Tanner's classification) and after peak height velocity has occurred. The majority of girls have a skeletal age between 13 and 14 years at the menarche. Therefore absence of thelarche/pubarche by the age of 14 years demand appropriate evaluation. On the other hand if mecharche does not occur by the age of 16 years in presence of normal growth and development of secondary sex characteristics there is a need for proper work-up.

ETIOLOGICAL FACTORS

Primary amenorrhea is a multifactorial condition with diverse etiological factors (Fig. 10.1).

HISTORY TAKING FOR A PATIENT WITH PRIMARY AMENORRHEA

History of Headache, Visual Disturbances

Patient presenting with a history of headaches and/or visual disturbances should point

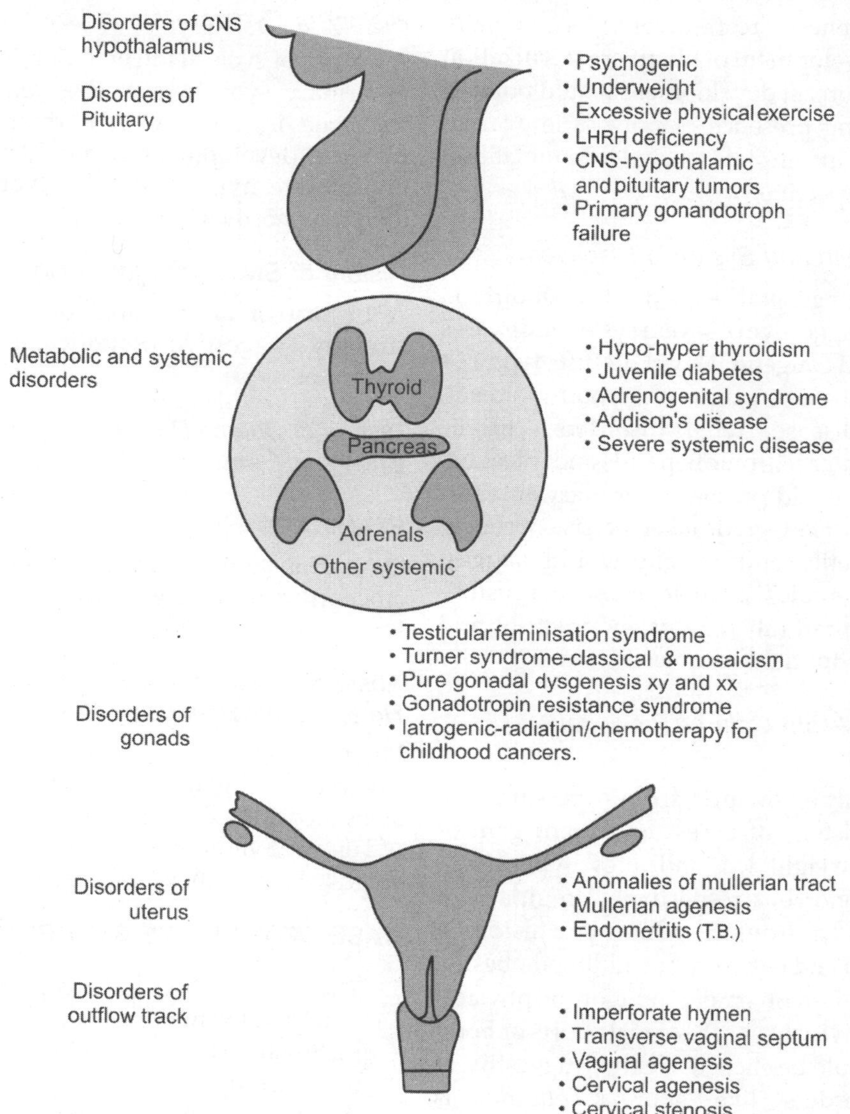

Fig. 10.1: Etiological factors of primary amenorrhea

towards underlying CNS–space-occupying lesions. Occasionally there may be a history of associated discharge from nipples (galactorrhea).

Growth and Age of Breast (thelarche) and Pubic and Axillary Hair Development (Adrenarche)

In a case of constitutional delay of growth and puberty (CDGP) there will be a history of late onset of breast development. However, her height will be appropriate for age. On the other hand in a case of arrested puberty due to CNS—space occupying lesions or severe systemic disease the tempo of otherwise normal pubertal development and growth will be affected. In such a case parents will give history of sudden cessation/retardation of progress of pubertal changes. History of absence of breast development with short or normal/tall stature for age may signify pure XX or XY dysgenesis respectively. Occasionally history of development of hirsutism/virilization with normal breast development would point to the underlying presence of polycystic ovarian syndrome or incomplete testicular feminization syndrome respectively.

General Health and Systemic Diseases

History of poor general health due to malnutrition or a history suggestive of severe systemic diseases like untreated congenital heart disease, type 1 or type 2 diabetes, primary hypothyroidism, Addison's disease, renal disorders, chronic anemias, asthma, chronic hepatitis and intestinal diseases, etc. could present as primary amenorrhea. History of low-grade fever, persistent cough, loss of appetite and weight would suggest systemic tuberculosis. However, such a history may be absent in tuberculous endometritis and may require specialized investigations.

Excessive Weight Gain or Precipitous Weight Loss

In a normally growing girl progressing into puberty a history of excessive weight gain or precipitous weight loss indicates hyperinsulinism or amenorrhea respectively. In girls with Prader-Willi syndrome there may be a history of huperphagia and early onset childhood obesity.

History of involvement in vigorous physical exercise/activity for professional sports or body building should be elicited. History suggestive of eating disorders like anorexia/bulimia is important in currently globalizing India. Morbid obesity from childhood indicates syndromic causes of primary amenorrhea (Figs. 10.2A, B, and C, Plate 1).

History of Anosmia/Hyposmia

Anosmia/hyposmia may be a symptom pointing towards the hypothalamic GnRH deficiency (Kallmann's syndrome). This history should be specifically elicited in patients with normal/tall stature and absent breast development.

History of Cyclical Pain in Lower Abdomen

A history of cyclical lower abdominal pain and/or urinary symptoms with swelling in lower abdomen in a girl with normal growth and pubertal development is highly suggestive of imperforate hymen/complete vaginal septum (cryptomenorrhea)

History of Swelling in Inguinal/Vulval Area

A history of an inguinal or vulval mass is strongly suggestive of testicular feminization syndrome.

History of Chemo/Radiotherapy for Childhood Cancers

EXAMINATION

On examination of a girl presenting with primary amenorrhea the following features must be looked for.

Absence of Normal or Presence of Heterosexual Secondary Sex Characters

Poorly developed or absent sex characters are suggestive of gonadal dysgenesis especially if associated with short stature and typical features of Turner's Syndrome (short webbed neck, cubitus valgus, short 4th metatarsa, etc.) (Fig. 10.3, Plate 1).

CASE OF TURNER'S SYNDROME

1. These girls often have cardiovascular and renal malformations. Heterosexual sex characteristics would point towards a diagnosis of incomplete testicular feminization syndrome or mixed gonadal dysgenesis. In girls with hypothamic amenorrheoea and obesity due to Prader-Willi syndrome, typical facies (dolichocephaly, narrow face, alomond shape eyes, small mouth), would be seen.
2. In presence of a history of cyclic lower abdominal pain with normal sexual characteristics, examination should include palpation for suprapubic mass and for visualization of an imperforate hymen (seen as a bluish colored bulging membrane in vagina).

3. Presence of an inguinal or vulval mass in presence of normal breast development may be a presenting feature of complete testicular feminization syndrome. These girls have a blind short vagina and absence of uterus on per rectal examination.
4. A detailed general and systemic examination should be done for evidence of any systemic or metabolic disorders. (for example, acanthosis nigricans in an obese girl with hyperinsulinemia and hyperendrogenism of Polycystic ovarian syndrome (PCOS) and depressed reflexes or bradycardia in hypothyroidism)
5. Breast examination for galactorrhea should be done in all girls with primary amenorrhea (seen in hyperprolactinemia or primary hypothyroidism).

INVESTIGATIVE APPROACH

An algorithmic approach towards investigation in girls with primary amenorrhea is depicted in Fig. 10.4.

INVESTIGATIVE APPROACH

- In. girls with heterosexual or poor/absent pubertal a karyotype would determine the type of genetic abnormality. It is important to identify the cytogenic abnormality, as 'Y' containing gonads are prone to tumor formation and malignancy.
- In case of girls with somatic abnormalities of Turner's syndrome a pelvic sonography would show absent or streak gonads and serum gonadotropins would be elevated.
- In girls with poor secondary sexual character development estimation of serum gonadotropins is advised. In presence of elevated gonadotropins suggestive of hypergonadotropic hypogonadism a pelvic sonography would reveal streak gonads suggestive of pure gonadal dysgenesis.
- However, if the ovaries are normal on USG, the clinical picture is suggestive of gonadotropin resistant ovaries. The definitive diagnosis of this rare condition can only be done at ovarian biopsy.
- Since these patients do not respond to exogenous gonadotropins, invasive procedures like laparoscopic ovarian biopsy are to be avoided.
- In girls with normal sexual character development a pelvic sonography showing uterus and presence of gonads (either abdominal, pelvic or occasionally inguinal or labial) will be seen in cases of mullerian agenesis (MA) or complete testicular feminization syndrome (TFS). Though patients of TFS will have 46XY and those with MA will have 46XX karyotypes, routine cytogenetic analysis is not mandatory. The diagnosis of TFS can be made clinically by absent axillary and pubic hair often with inguinal/labial goands.
- Girls with normal sexual characteristics, sonography would reveal any hematocolpos/ hematometra in cases of absent vagina, imperforate hymen or transverse vaginal septum in presence of typical signs and symptoms of cryptomenorrhea.
- If the pelvic sonography shows normal uterus and ovaries the patient should be further evaluated with hormonal challenge tests. A positive response to progesterone challenge is indicative of either a constitutional delay in menarche or partial hypogonadotropic hypogonadism
- Girls with PCOS and associated hyperinsulinemia and obesity have a typical USG picture of > 10 follicles at the periphery of the ovary and often an altered ratio of serum gonadotropins. These girls mostly present with secondary amenorrhea.
- In case of failure of withdrawal bleeding to progesterone challenge, an estrogen-progesterone combination is administered. A failure of withdrawal bleeding with this necessitates work-up for tuberculosis. This would include X-ray chest, Mantoux test and complete blood count with sedimentation rate. Current methods for diagnosis of tuberculosis include serum levels of anti-Koch antibodies, ELISA

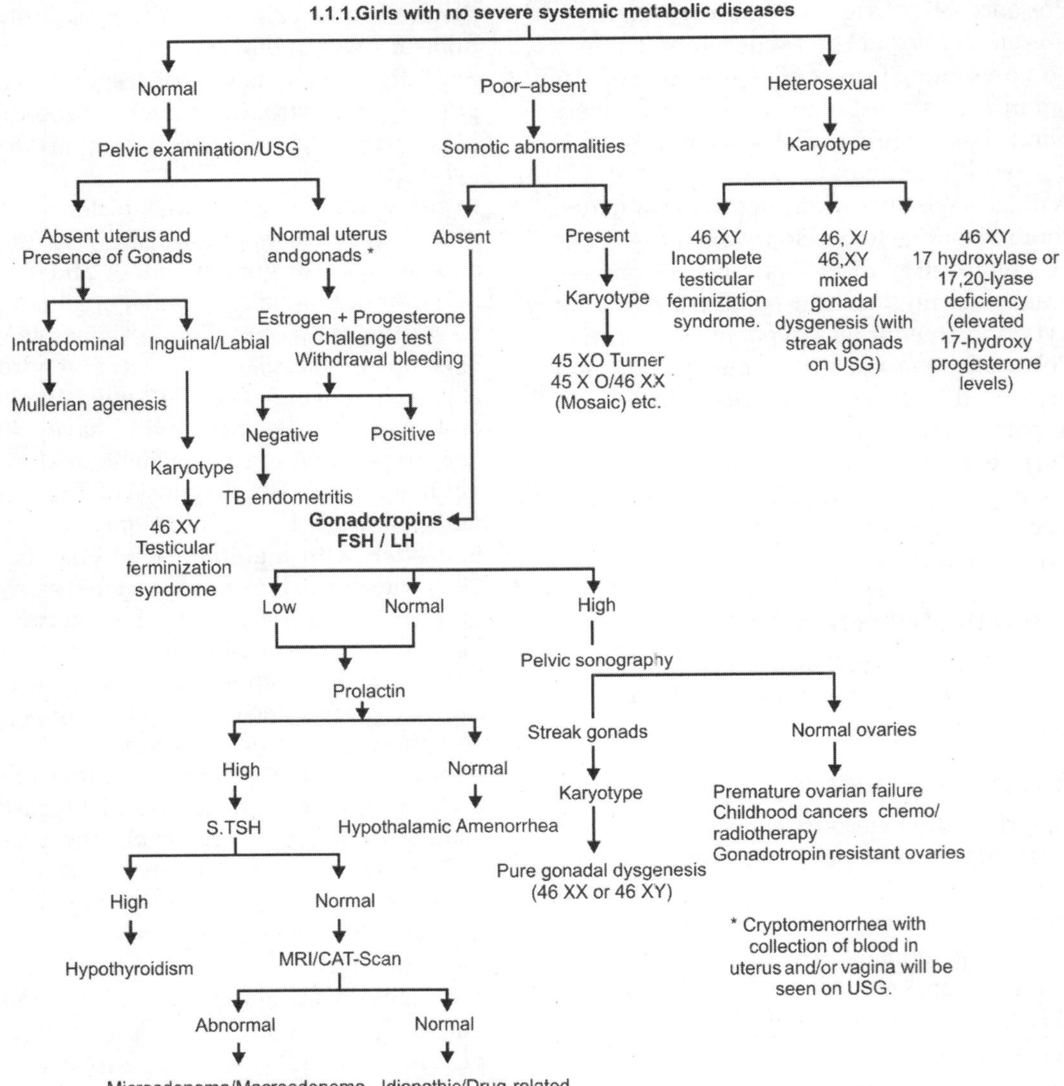

Fig. 10.4: Investigative approach for primary amenorrhea

and polymerase chain reaction (PCR) techniques for specific diagnosis of *Mycobacterium tuberculosis.*

- In girls with a positive response to estrogen-progesterone challenge, estimation of serum gonadotropins is required. If the gonadotropins are low or normal, an initial evaluation of thyroid function by serum Thyroid Stimulating Hormone (TSH) would establish a diagnosis of hypothyroidism and of lactotroph function by serum prolactin would establish whether a patient has hyperprolactinemia.
- In girls with elevated serum prolactin levels, pituitary scanning to rule out prolactinomas should be done after ruling out primary

hypothyroidism. If serum levels of both TSH and prolactin are normal other causes for hypothalmic amenorrhoea need further evaluation. A diagnosis of hypogonadotropic hypogonadism resulting from severe physical/psychological stress (in professional athletes/ballet dancers, models, etc.) and in underweight with history of anorexia/bulimia should be established by low serum gonadotropins in presence of the typical history.

- Gonadotropin Releasing Hormone (GnRH) deficiency, isolated pituitary gonadotropin deficiency, associated deficiency of human growth hormone and Prader-Willi syndrome would be other causes of hypogonadotropic hypogonadism and should be diagnosed by appropriate investigations. However, CNS space occupying lesions must be suspected in presence of atypical history of sudden cessation of growth and pubertal development with/without headaches or visual disturbances and would be diagnosed by appropriate radiological investigations (MRI/CAT scan).
- Chronic systemic or metabolic disorders in childhood which are inadequately treated can result in hypogonadism and should be diagnosed by specific tests as clinically suspected.

MANAGEMENT

Delayed puberty and/or primary amenorrhea may be the first clinical manifestation of an underlying systemic, endocrine, genetic or a CNS space-occupying lesion.

It is essential that an opportunity of early recognition is not lost.

A detailed clinical algorithm if systematically followed would avoid catalogued and lengthy list of investigations.

It also avoids premature conclusion of underlying cause.

COMMON PRINCIPLES IN THE MANAGEMENT

Identification of Underlying Diseases

Like systemic, nutritional, endocrine and cytogenetic. Serious space occupying CNS lesions should also be ruled out or diagnosed and treated. Treatment of the primary disease may reverse the process and allow progression of puberty in some of these for e.g., Bromocryptine therapy for hyperprolactinemia or adequate nutritional management in nutritionally deprived/imbalanced girls. Speciality referrals for specific underlying diseases are advocated.

Reassurance to the Child and her Parents

Regarding anticipated normal pubertal development in cases of CDGP. Short-term therapy with sex steroids (estrogens) may be needed in girls with CDGP to trigger the onset of puberty.

Induction and Maintenance of Puberty

Late initiation is beneficial in prevention of early epiphyseal closure and thus not compromising final adult height (FAH). However, to avoid psychosocial embarrassment vis-à-vis their peers, the therapy should be initiated at 13 years of age. The starting dose of ethinyl estrodiol is 1-2 mg/day, which is gradually increased every 2-3 months. The addition of progestin should be done either on full breast development or when break-through bleeding occurs. Girls with permanent hypogonadism (gonadal dysgenesis/premature ovarian failure) will need this sex steroid therapy till they reach average age of menopause in the population.

Growth Promoting, Potentiating Strategies

Abnormal physical growth like short stature in Turner's syndrome (TS) and Prader-Willi syndrome (PWS) or tall stature in Kallmann's syndrome (KS) and Swyer's syndrome (SS) can be appropriately managed. Girls with TS and PWS are known to respond to growth hormone therapy and achieve an increase in final adult height. In order to assure maximum height gain, estrogen replacement can be timely added for achieving optimum synergestic action and preventing early epiphyseal closure. In patients of KS and SS it is important to start estrogen replacement therapy (ERT) well in time to prevent eunichoid tall stature. Growth hormone therapy in girls with PWS is not only beneficial for improving stature but also for reducing obesity and increasing lean body mass and exercise capacity.

Prevention of Osteoporosis

Adolescence is critical period for bone acquisition, which is dependent upon nutrition, estrogen and lifestyle. Low bone mineral density-osteopenia/osteoporosis can result from either estrogen deprivation (nutritional, systemic cause) or permanent estrogen deficiency due to hypogonadism. Therefore, girls with permanent gonadal failure need estrogen replacement therapy not only for maintainance of puberty but also for prevention of osteoporosis.

Future Fertility

With current advances in reproductive medicine the majority of cases of pubertal disorders can be assured of future fertility. Induction of ovulation by gonadotropins in hypogonadotropic hypogonadism, advanced reproductive technology with donor eggs in hyperganodotropic hypogonadism and bromocriptine/transphenoidal surgery in cases of hyperprolactinemia, pituitary adenoma, etc. provide fertility potentiation. Even in girls with mullerian agenesis, in vitro fertilization programs employing the woman's own eggs and husband's sperm can utilize surrogate motherhood.

Surgical Therapy

Gonadectomy is indicated in cases of pure (Swyer's syndrome) or mixed gonadal dysgenesis for risk of malignancy as well as in girls with testicular feminisation syndrome (TFS). In TFS it should be done after achieving full breast development. Creation of neovagina is required in cases of TFS and mullerian agenesis.

SUGGESTED READING

1. Beck – Peccoz P, Persani L. Premature ovarian failure. Orphanet J Rare Dis 2006;1:9.
2. Birmingham, Alabama. The Practice Committee of the American Society for Reproductive Medicine. Current evaluation of amenorrhoea. Fertil Steril. 2006;86(5):S148-55.
3. Chanson P, Salenave S. Diagnosis and treatment of pituitary adenomas. Minerva Endocrinol 2004;29(4):241-75.
4. Gobel KA. Special nutritional concerns for the female athlete. Curr Sports Med Rep 2006;5(4): 187-91.
5. Jacoangeli E, Masala S, Staar Mezzasalma F, et al. Amenorrhoea after weight recover in anorexia nervosa: role of body composition and endocrine abnormalities. Eat Weight Disord 2006;11(1):e20-6.
6. Latronico AC, Arnhold IJ. Inactivating mutations of LH and FSH receptors from genotype to pheno-type. Pediatr Endocrinol Rev 2006;4(1):28-31.
7. Master-Hunter T, Heiman DL. Amenorrhoea: evaluation and treatment. Am Fam Physician 2006;73(8):1374-82.
8. Papadimitriou DT, Linglart A, Morel Y, et al. Puberty in subjects with complete androgen in-sen--sitivity syndrome. Horm Res 2006;65(3): 12631.
9. Warren MP, Hagey AR. The genetics diagnosis and treatment of amenorrhoea. Minerva Ginecol 2004;56(5):437-55.
10. Wilson GR, Haddad JE, Haddad CJ. Amenor-rhoea: common causes and evaluation. Compr Ther 2005;31(4):270-78.

11 Adolescent with Menorrhagia

Ashwini Bhalerao-Gandhi, Ashok Shukla

INTRODUCTION

Menstruation can be seen as the endpoint of an endocrine cascade that begins with thelarche and ends with menarche. All over the world, the age at menarche is decreasing. This may be attributed to many known and unknown factors. The first period occurs because there has been sufficient endometrial stimulation to result in a withdrawal bleed when there is a temporary fall in the estrogen level. Menstrual irregularities often occur in adolescent girls as cycles tend to be anovulatory. This is a stressful condition for the adolescent girl as well as her parents. As the girls cannot differentiate between normal and abnormal menstrual patterns, medical help is sought either too early or too late. Heavy periods lead to a lot of fear, anxiety and stigma.

NORMAL AND ABNORMAL MENSTRUAL PATTERN DURING PUBERTY

Till two years from menarche, most cycles are anovulatory. The length of the cycle varies from 21-40 days, the mean duration is 4-5 days, the average blood loss being 35 ml. Whenever the cycle length is less than 21 days, duration is more than 8 days and menstrual blood loss is more than 80 ml, the girl requires further evaluation and necessary treatment. Table 11.1 shows differential diagnosis in a adolescent with excessive bleeding.

Table 11.1: Adolescent with excessive bleeding per vaginum—Differential diagnosis

1. Anovulation—Immature H-P-O axis
2. PCOS
3. Stress—mental, physical
4. Eating disorders, obesity
5. Substance abuse
6. Thyroid dysfunction
7. Chronic renal disease
8. Hepatic disorders
9. Congenital adrenal hyperplasia, Cushing's syndrome
10. Hematologic abnormalities (30%)—ITP, von Willebrand's disease, Factor XI deficiency.
11. Infections—Chlamydia, Kochs
12. Genital tract injuries
13. Pregnancy related bleeding
14. Irregular intake of OCS, progesterone to post-pone/ pre-pone periods.
15. Mullerian anomalies
16. Foreign body

ETIOPATHOLOGY

Menstrual problems are common during adolescence due to slow maturation of the hypothalamic pituitary-ovarian axis and can last 2-5 years after menarche.

MENORRHAGIA

Menorrhagia (excessive bleeding PV either in duration or quantity or both) at regular intervals and metrorrhagia (cycle irregularity) are commonly seen in adolescent girls. Cervical polyp and granulosa cell tumor of the ovary may rarely cause menorrhagia. Bleeding disorders like thrombocytopenia, von Wille-brand's disease, factor II, V, VII, X and XI deficiency disorders should also be ruled out if menorrhagia starts as soon as menarche sets in. Dysfunctional uterine bleeding (DUB) causes menorrhagia in 74%; primary coagulation disorders are present in 19% and other causes account for 7%. Genital tuberculosis may cause excessive menstrual bleeding in the beginning and the disease process.

Dysfunctional Uterine Bleeding (DUB)

It is best defined as abnormal bleeding from the uterus in the absence of the organic disease of the genital tract. The bleeding may be abnormal in frequency, amount, duration or any combination of these. This is the commonest cause in adolescent girls suffering from menorrhagia. 40-50% resolve within 2 years and a better prognosis is expected when DUB starts after a period of normal menstruation than who develops it at menarche itself. In most of the girls with puberty menorrhagia, the cycles are anovulatory though in few they may be ovulatory.

Anovulatory DUB—Causes

a. Inadequate signal—Follicular development is insufficient to produce strong enough signals to induce LH surge.
b. Impaired positive feedback—may lead to proliferation and hyperplasia of the endometrium due to unopposed estrogen.

Ovulatory DUB—Causes

a. Inadequate luteal phase—The normal luteal phase is over 12-13 days with progestogen around day 20 in excess of 20 nmol/l. The inadequacy arises from inadequate follicular development, may be due to subnormal secretion of FSH.
b. Idiopathic bleeding—It is because of irregular ripening of the endometrium due to the shift in endometrial conversion of endoperoxide from vasoconstrictor PGF_2 to vasodilator PGE_2.

EVALUATION

History

- Age, Parity
- Age at menarche
- Amount, duration and pattern of menstrual bleeding
- Symptoms of endocrine/organic disease
- Use of contraceptives, if any
- Emotional stress/psychiatric disorder
- Social and personal background
- H/o drug ingestion.

Examination

- General—pallor, thyroid swelling, vital parameters
- Abdominal examination for any lump
- Local examination of external genitalia
- PS, PV, PR done rarely.

Investigations

- CBC, ESR
- Peripheral smear
- BT, CT, PT, PTT
- Platelet count
- Sr. TSH
- LFT
- USG pelvis for PCOS, fibroid, polyp, pregnancy, pelvic masses, endometrial thickness (ET).

TREATMENT OF MILD DUB

In cases with mild DUB, reassurance to the girl as well as her parents is absolutely essential. In this way the iatrogenic factors of anxiety and worry are lessened and relieved. Thus explanation and reassurance are the backbone of therapy.

Points to be Covered During Counseling

- Explain the anatomy and pathophysiology in brief and easy to understand language.

- Emphasize that puberty menorrhagia is not a very uncommon problem.
- Reassure the patient that there is nothing anatomically wrong with her.
- Sympathize with her concerns for the future including the future prospects of childbirth etc.
- High protein and iron rich diet.
- Simple hemostatic agents like gynaec CVP, RCK, etc.

TREATMENT OF MODERATE DUB

- Aims
- To stop bleeding
- To prevent recurrence
- To correct anemia, malnutrition, etc.

In these girls, PG synthetase inhibitors like mefenamic acid should be used during period to reduce the amount of bleeding. It acts on cyclo-oxygenase and blocks peripheral PG receptors leading to antiprostaglandin action, dose being 250 to 500 mg 3 times a day. Sometimes ethamsylate can be added. Iron supplementation is a must to treat anemia. Hormonal therapy in the form of OCS or progestogens is required in cases with irregular cycles. Regular evaluation of hormonal therapy is done as the H-P-O axis matures.

MANAGEMENT OF SEVERE DUB

Sometimes, hospitalization is required. Smith, et al (1998) concluded that 63% hospitalized adolescents with menorrhagia required blood transfusion. These girls should be assessed for primary coagulation disorder or any medical problem. Antifibrinolytic agents like Tranexamic acid which is a potent inhibitor of fibrinolysis should be started in the dose of 500 mg three times a day. It also can be given parenterally. Combination of mefenamic acid, tranexamic acid and/or ethamsylate may be used judiciously.

Hormonal therapy with oral contraceptive pills or plain progestogens is a must. Progestogens counter balance unopposed estrogen action. Three types of progesterones are available in the market—dydrogesterone (10 mg), medroxy progesterone acetate (5/10 mg) and norethisterone acetate (5 mg).

In moderate to severe menorrhagia, norethisterone acetate or medroxy progesterone acetate can be given in the dose of 1 BD to 1 TDS for 21 days. This therapy can be given cyclically starting from every 5th day of the period lasting for 21 days for 3 to 4 months. Once the cycles are stabilized, progestogens can be given only in the leuteal phase of the cycle, i.e. 1 BD to be started from the 14th day of the cycle for total 10 days. This leuteal phase support can be given for 3-4 months and then the girl is re-evaluated for the necessity of hormones.

In cases with mild to moderate menorrhagia, low dose contraceptive pills (OCS with ethinylestradiol 30 μgm) also can be tried in a cyclical manner for 3 to 6 months duration.

If the girl is also suffering from polycystic ovarian syndrome (PCOS), acne and hirsutism then OCS containing desogestrel or cyproterone acetate should be started. These lipid friendly progestogens help in reducing the androgenic effects as well.

What should be Avoided

- Drugs like danazol, GnRH analogues and daflon which are used in elderly women should be avoided in adolescents as danazol and GnRH analogues lead to medical menopause.
- Also, progestogen only pills (POPS) and LNG system (progestogen containing intrauterine device) are contraindicated. POPS cannot regularize the cycles and any IUD is contraindicated in nulliparous women.
- Injection depot provera is used rarely as it leads to amenorrhea or intermittent irregular bleeding.
- Unlike in women with perimenopausal menorrhagia, diagnostic or therapeutic curettage (D and C) is avoided in adolescent girls in spite of USG finding of thickened endometrium. If endometrial hyperplasia is

suspected then she is put on progesterone for a period of 6-12 months, after which she is re-assessed. Unnecessary surgical intervention may lead to infection, perforation and Ashermann's syndrome hampering future fertility.

FOLLOW-UP

Girls requiring hormonal treatment need frequent follow-up and evaluation. It may take few years before their cycles get established properly. Till then, they may require to take natural progestogens like dydrogesterone for many months. Table 11.2 shows follow-up of adolescents with menorrhagia.

Table 11.2: Adolescents with menorrhagia

1 : 5 require hospitalization
1 : 4 will have Hb of < 10 gm%
1 : 3 will require blood transfusion
1 : 2 present at menarche

DUB in Practical Gynec Endocrinology Ed Dr. Geeta Pandya and Dr. Ashwini Bhalerao-Gandhi. 1st edition Jaypee, New Delhi). ;pp 85-91,

Girls with menarche menorrhagia fall into a high risk group.

They face problems like severe anemia and blood transfusion.

In the long run, they may develop impaired reproductive potential like infertility, spontaneous abortions, etc.

They are also prone to develop endometrial hyperplasia and rarely carcinoma of the endometrium in later life if neglected.

Puberty menorrhagia sometimes can emerge as a therapeutic challenge requiring combined efforts of family physician, gynecologist, pediatrician, endocrinologist and hematologist.

SUGGESTED READING

1. Adolescent Girl—An update (2nd edition), P. Kotdawala, V. Salvi, U. Krishna; (Eds). Jaypee, New Delhi.
2. Dewhurst's practical paediatric and Adolescent Gynaecology 2nd edition by D. Keith Edmonds. Published by Butterworth and Co. Ltd. Great Britain.
3. Reproductive Endocrinology—A Clinical Approach. V. Walvekar, M. Jassawalla (Eds). et al; 2nd edition; Jaypee, New Delhi.

12 Dysmenorrhea

D Pushpalatha, L Fahmida Banu

INTRODUCTION

Dysmenorrhea is derived from a Greek word which means "difficult menstrual flow". Primary dysmenorrhea is defined as recurrent crampy pain occurring with menses in the absence of identifiable pelvic pathology.

PATHOGENESIS

Dysmenorrhea is thought to be caused by the release of prostaglandins in the menstrual fluid which causes uterine contractions and pain. Vasopressin also may play a role by increasing uterine contractility and causing ischemic pain as a result of vasoconstriction.

Risk Factors:

- Young age
- Nulliparity
- Menorrhagia
- Smoking
- Mental health problems (Depression, anxiety, disruption of social support)

DIAGNOSIS

Basically depends on detailed history taking and the process of exclusion of organic disease.

Clinical Features

The pain is characteristically colicky and located in the mid line of the abdomen and extends to other areas of lumbar region and thighs. Usually painful menstruation occurs with ovulatory cycles.

The other associated symptoms include nausea, vomiting, fatigue, light headedness, dizziness, headache, rarely syncope and fever.

Differential Diagnosis

GIT: GI tract infections

UTI: Urinary tract infections

Secondary dysmenorrhea

Endometriosis	Endometrial polyps
Ovarian cysts	Myomas
Cervical stenosis	Obstructive malformations of genital tract
PID	Adhesions

EXAMINATION

- An adolescent, who has never been sexually active and has a typical history of mild to moderate dysmenorrnea an internal (pelvic) examination is not necessary.
- All patients who have not responded to conventional therapy or have severe dysmenorrhea or when an organic pathology is suspected, a gentle pelvic examination is mandatory.

INVESTIGATIONS

- USG: Apart from routine investigations an USG of abdomen and pelvis is a useful tool for exclusion of other conditions like ovarian cysts/endometriomas/fibroids.
- MRI has limited role in primary dysmenorrhea.
- Laparoscopy should be considered when first line of therapies are ineffective or dysmenorrhea is crippling the individual's routine or tackling some pelvic pathology.

TREATMENT OPTIONS

- Non steroid anti-inflammatory (NSAIDs) drugs are the established initial therapy of treatment for dysmenorrhea. They have a direct analgesic effect through inhibition of prostaglandin synthesis and they decrease the volume of menstrual flow. NSAIDs may be the most effective when therapy is started before the onset of menstrual pain and flow although therapy need not be continued till the end of flow.
- Pills (OCP): Treatment of dysmenorrhea with OCPs is a well accepted modality.
- Treatment with monophasic formulations showed lower mean-scores than with triphasic users.

Hormonal Methods: Rarely Used

Medroxy-progesterone acetate
Danazol
Glyceryl trinitrate patches
Leuprolide acetate

Surgical Therapies

Rarely in refractory dysmenorrhea cases, laparoscopic uterine nerve ablation (LUNA) has been tried.

Future Concepts of Therapy

Vasopressin receptor antagonists
Frameless levonorgestrel IUD.

ENDOMETRIOSIS[6-8]

INTRODUCTION

Endometriosis is a disease in which endometrial glands and stroma, implant and grow in areas outside the uterus, whose growth and development depends upon ovarian steroid hormones. Thus it is most often seen in reproductive age and now a days it is a significantly contributing cause of dysmenorrhea and infertility in young adults.

PREVALENCE AND EPIDEMIOLOGY OF ENDOMETRIOSIS

- About 12-32% of women of reproductive age undergoing laparoscopy for chronic pelvic pain
- One percent of women undergoing major gynecological surgeries.
- About 9-50% of women undergoing laparoscopy for infertility.
- Fifty percent of teenagers undergoing laparoscopy for evaluation of chronic pelvic pain or dysmenorrhea.

Endometriosis appears to be less common in blacks and Asians than Caucasians. It appears to be more common in upper socioeconomic class and tall thin body habitus and women with low BMI.[1]

GENETIC FACTORS

Genetic factors probably influence an individual's susceptibility to endometriosis. If a woman has endometriosis in a first degree relative, she has a 7% likelihood of developing this disorder as compared to 1% in unrelated persons. Concordance in twins is also observed. It has been proposed that multiple genes interact with each other and with the environment to confer disease susceptibility and produce phenotype.[2,3]

PATHOGENESIS

Although endometriosis stands as one of the most investigated disorders of gynecology our current understanding of etiology and pathophysiology of the disease remains an enigma.[4]

Various theories proposed are:

Retrograde Menstruation

Sampsons theory of retrograde menstruation has gained the most supportive evidence. The reflux of menses through the fallopian tube to ectopic sites occurs especially to the peritoneal cavity. The pelvic environment may become receptive in certain women thereby allowing the endometrium to grow .Though of the 70-90% of women having retrograde menstruation only 10% develop endometriosis.[5]

- Meyer's theory of Coelomic metaplasia: Potentially undifferentiated cells of the peritoneal cavity turn into endometrial tissue. Supports the occurrence of the disease in pre menarcheal girls.
- HalBan's Lymphatic and vascular spread: This explains the occurrence of endometriosis at distant, non contagious sites, e.g. thorax, and brain.
- Immunological basis: Supports the onset of disease in particular individual though majority have retrograde menstruation.
- Impaired immune-surveillance and abnormal apoptosis: In endometriosis endometrial cells in the peritoneal fluid avoid immuno-surveillance and implant into peritoneum. Lymphocytes adhere to endometrial cells through the LFA-1 (lymphocytes function associated antigen-1), ICAM-1 (inter cellular adhesion molecule-1) and prevent recognition of the endometrial cells by the lymphocytes and prevent subsequent NK cell-mediated cytotoxicity.
- Anatomical spread: To the adjacent organs like ovary and uterus.

Inflammatory Activity in Endometriosis

Peritoneal fluid (PF) in women with endometriosis has marked increases in WBC, macrophages and their activity, increased cytokines with pleotropic biological activity.[6] Table 12.1 lists endometriotic sites.

Cytokines expressed by activated macrophages are IL-1, IL-6, IL-8 and TNF-α, while IL-8 promotes angiogenesis. These cytokines in turn modulate the stimulation of other cytokine (IL-8) and RANTES (regulated upon activation, normal T-cell expressed and secreted). RANTES is a potent attractant and activator of macrophages, T-lymphocytes and eosinophils.

Table 12.1: Endometriotic sites

Most *commonly involved*	***Less*** *commonly involved sites*	***Exceptional*** *case report*
Ovaries	Vagina	Breast
Peritoneum	Urinary bladder	Pancreas
Uterosacral ligament	Cervix	Liver

CLINICAL PRESENTATION OF ENDOMETRIOSIS IN ADOLESCENTS

- Pain: Mostly cyclical, or continuous
- Dysmenorrhea
- Dysparenunia—Painful intercourse
- Dysuria—painful urination
- Dyschezia—Painful defecation
- Vague pain in musculoskeletal regions, flanks, backache, muscle cramps.
- Infertility: primary infertility is another frequently seen condition with endometriosis: mechanism could be the disruption of pelvic anatomy, adhesions or interestingly unexplained cause.
- Various other manifestations depend upon the location of the endometriotic lesions, e.g. scar endometriosis.

PHYSICAL EXAMINATION

A complete pelvic examination may not be possible to perform in the adolescents specially in those who are sexually not active. In such individual recto-abdominal examination may be better accepted.

Adolescents rarely have uterosacral nodularity (cf. common finding in adults), adnexal pathology also felt if it exists.

LAB EVALUATION

- CBC with ESR: may suggest an acute or chronic inflammatory process.
- Urine- Routine and microscopic examination and C/S: to identify bladder infection etc.
- Pregnancy test, STD profile: wherever appropriate.
- CA 125 (5-35 IU/ml normal range)Level of >35 is often seen in endometriosis.

IMAGING STUDIES

- **USG:** Help to identify ovarian cysts, endometriomas, structural causes of chronic pelvic pain, etc. A negative sonographic report does not exclude endometriosis
- **MRI:** Helpful in some cases to better define the adnexal pathology. It is not the first line of investigation in view of its poor sensitivity for detecting peritoneal lesions
- **CT:** Also has limited role in scattered disease

DIAGNOSIS

Laparoscopy: "Gold standard" for diagnosis by direct visualization of the lesions.

Appearance: Typically appear superficial powder-burn or gunshot lesions. The endometriotic area could be black, brown, blue, pink or even yellow or clear raised areas, puckered areas, fibrosis, spots, cysts containing hemorrhage inside, etc.

Endometriomas: typically formed by thick fluid, could be densely adherent to surrounding structures like peritoneum, tubes, aterosacral ligament or bowl.

Identification of subtle endometriotic lesion which appear as clear, shiny areas on peritoneal surface. Visualization through normal saline enhances its identification.

Electrocautery, endocoagulation ultrasound (harmonic scalpel) or laser is used in ablation and resection of the lesion.

DIFFERENTIAL DIAGNOSIS

Lesions which cause confusion on visual evaluation at laparoscopy are hemosiderin deposits, hemangiomas, previous surgeries, residual suture material, fibrosis, reaction to earlier oil based radiographic studies, etc. these can be excluded by biopsy of the suspicious lesions.

Biopsy is taken whenever it is appropriate or from cul-de-sac.

The disease is staged according to site and severity of the disease. Ideally laparoscopic findings are recorded on video or DVD during surgery. Documentation on the medical record the extent of lesion, description and other features like adhesions, etc. should be included: Severity of symptoms does not correlate with the extent of the disease or location. Needing proper counseling–Pain may be severe in spite of having mild disease and vica versa.

TREATMENT OPTIONS

Empiric Treatment

Even if the definitive diagnosis is not made in adolescents, if the pain is interfering with the routine activities, the reasonable approach is to start anti-inflammatory medication .

OCP: However, analgesics cannot give relief to all patients. In such individual cyclic low dose oral contraceptive pills (OCP) are next options. The OCP suppresses ovulation and related hormonal stimulation of endometriotic areas and give relief. It will also control menorrhagia, in addition to giving contraceptive coverage in desired population. Choice of OCP depends on the severity of the patient's symptoms, the extent of disease and compliance. The adolescents need to know that pills are to be taken at scheduled time and with regularity to maintain stable hormonal level. Break through bleeding is reduced if proper time schedule is maintained. Even if break through bleeding occurs, with continuation of OCP, it is expected to resolve in six months of OCP use.

Progestin: Directly inhibit the endometriotic spots by decidualization. Inhibits pituitary gonadotropin secretion and ovarian hormone production. Potential side effects are bloating sensation, irregular bleeding, weight gain, depression. Injectable depot medroxyprogesterone acetate long-term use can cause loss of bone density in some patients.

Drug and dosage

- Norethindrone acetate: 15 mgm/day
- Medroxyprogesterone acetate: 30-50 mg/day orally
- Medroxyprogesterone acetate: 150 mg IM/ 3 monthly

When pain persists, laparoscopy for definitive diagnosis becomes essential before choosing higher modalities of treatment.

After Definitive Diagnosis Medical Treatment should be Started

The aim of post laparoscopy cauterized and ablated endometriosis is to give medication to suppress progression, thus achieving freedom for the adolescents to return to their routine work.

Gonadotropin Releasing Hormone Agonists

GnRH agonists can be used for adolescents who are at least 16 years of age.

Mode of action: By suppressing gonadotropins FSH, LH and there by estrogen, the endometriotic spots are expected to shrink but side effects like hot flashes, headache, insomnia, depression, mood swings, dryness of vagina, decrease in BMD can occur. 90% adolescents become amenorrheic or hypomenorrheic. A base line bone mineral density (BMD) assessment is documented and repeated 6 months later

Drug and dosage

- Leuprolide acetate: 11.25 mgm IM every 3 months for 6 months
- Naferelin: nasal spray or puff BD intranasally

Add Back Therapy

Add back therapy is adding estrogen/progestogens to GnRH regimes to alleviate side effects.

Drug and dosage:

- Conjugated equine estrogen (Premarin) 0.625 and norethisterone acetate 5 mg or Medroxyprogesterone acetate 5 mg daily
- Norethisterone acetate 5 mg daily

  This will improve the patient compliance.

Danazol

It is 17 α ethinynl testosterone derivative

Mechanism of action: Inhibits pituitary gonadotropin secretion

- Direct inhibition of endometriotic spots
- Direct inhibition of ovarian enzymes

Efficacy: Nearly 80% patients experience improvement of symptoms within 2 months of treatment. It is effective treatment of mild to moderate endometriosis and equivalent to GnRH agonists.

Limitations: Endometriotic cysts and adhesions do not respond well.

Side effects: dose dependent, weight gain, muscle cramps, decreased breast mass, acne, hirsutism, liver dysfunction, hot flushes, mood changes and depression.

Irreversible deepening of voice can occur. Needs proper counseling before prescription.

MANAGEMENT OF RECURRENT PAIN

In spite of medical treatment the disease may persist or progress leading to recurrent attacks of pain.

Treatment Options

- Changing to different modality of treatment
- GnRH utilization with addback therapy
- Laparoscopy-cystectomy, ablation and adhesiolysis depending upon the lesion.

SUMMARY

- Goal: To relieve pain, prevent disease progression and preserve fertility

- Detailed clinical history and gentle physical examination, keeping in mind the psychological disturbance and apprehension of the teenagers.
- Apart from routine laboratory work-up of ultrasonography and in indicated cases MRI is suggested.
- Counseling of the patient and family and explaining that there is no cure but disease can be controlled by various options explaining limitations, surgical intervention, long-term sequelae and cost.
- Treatment starts in mild to moderate disease with NSAIDs or cyclic OCP.
- Diagnostic as well as therapeutic laparoscopy may be indicated if endometriosis is suspected.
- Post-laparoscopy depending upon the seve–rity of the disease progestins, OCP, danazol or GnRH agonists selected.
- Recurrent pain is managed by change of medication, GnRH with addback therapy or surgical excision of recurrence and adhesiolysis.

CONCLUSIONS

With 15 million young and adolescent girls and more than twice the number of women of reproductive age in India, the problem of primary dysmenorrhea and endometriosis gain utmost importance. We see more often primary dysmenorrhea cases with career seeking women who postpone their married life leading to endometriosis. Hence we have to consider both short-term and long-term sequelae in management strategies.

REFERENCES

1. Harel Z, Biro FM, Kottenhahn RK, Rosenthal SL. Supplementation with omega-3 polyunsaturated fatty acids in the management of dysmenorrheal in adolescents. Am J Obstet Gynecol 1996:174:1335.
2. Dysmenorrhea Jan 15, 2005- American Family Physician.
3. Helms, JM. Acupuncture for the management of primary dysmenorrheal. Obstet Gynecol 1987; 69:51.
4. Hediger ML. Hartnett HJ louis GM association of endometriosis with body size and figure. Fertil Steril 2005;84: 1366.
5. Biscoff FZ, Simpson JL. Heritability and molecular genetic studies of endometriosis. Hum Reprod Update 2000; 6:37.
6. Kennedy S. Genetics of endometriosis Pathogenetic implications of the anatomic distribution obstetric gynecology 1986: 67:335.
7. Gnarnecia M, Olive DL. The structure and future of endometriosis research.Obstet Gynecol Clinics North America 1997, 24:455-65
8. Cramev Div Missmev SA. The epidemiology of endometriosis Ann. Acad Sci 2002;955:11-22.

13 Breast Disorders

Donald E Greydanus, Swati Y Bhave

INTRODUCTION

For adolescents breast is a very sensitive issue. When a girls develops secondary sexual characteristics the first thing they would be conscious is about the development of the breast. Some girls are very shy and will wear very loose clothes or walk with a slouch so that breasts would not look prominent. Some girls may be very proud of the newly acquired figure and wears clothes and brassieres to make them more visible.

The media has played a significant role in advertising the breast as sex symbol. Most girls are concerned and discuss about different types of brassieres and how they enhance the breasts. Girls with underdeveloped breasts want to augment them, girls with big breasts want to do reduction surgery. Every one wants a perfect size and shape.

The physiological gynecomastia can cause havoc to the psyche of a growing boy. If the gynecomastia is very pronounced the boys can undergo a lot of ridicule and humiliation

In such a background anything related to the breast may cause extreme anxiety or shyness may prevent the adolescent from seeking medical help. Nipple discharge, pain, a lump or mass, asymmetrical development all can cause distress.

Breast examination should form a routine part of examination in both boys and girls and they should be directly questioned if they have any problems or questions associated with their breasts.

Self breast examination should be taught to every adolescent and has been covered in the other chapter 10 in this section.

The impact of hormones on breast development is summarized in Table 13.1.

Congenital anomalies though rare cause a lot of distress in adolescents (Table 13.2).

Table 13.1: Impact of hormones on breast development

1. Estrogen induces:
   a. Ductal system growth
   b. Nipple maturation
   c. Areolar development (increased pigmentation and size)
   d. Induction of periductal fibrous tissue growth
2. Progesterone induces alveolar maturation
3. Prolactin allows maturation resulting in lactation

ASYMMETRIC BREAST DEVELOPMENT

Breast asymmetry development is common in many female adolescents it often improves as puberty progresses, and is noted in about 25% of adult females. It usually is a normal variant of breast growth with the smaller breast typically opposite to the dominant hand.

- A padded bra and reassurance is all that is needed in most cases.
- Once the breast development is complete on both sides, surgical correction of the asymmetry can be considered if desired and affordable.

Table 13.2: Congenital anomalies

Common anomalies

Polythelia: Extra, accessory nipples *Polymastia* is supernumerary breasts or accessory breast tissue are found along the milk lines from the axilla to the groin; however, the most common locations are below the normal breast on the chest and upper abdomen.

- A variety of nipple, areola, and glandular tissue combinations can be found, often becoming more prominent with the development of puberty, pregnancy, or lactation.
- The presence of polythelia (involving nipple and areola) is noted in 1-2% of the general population, and in some studies, is associated with cardiovascular and genitourinary defects.
- The extra nipple tissue is typically smaller than the normal nipple and may be erroneously called a mole, while the extra breast tissue can be mistaken for hidradenitis suppurative.

Inverted nipple: A nipple that does that extend beyond the breast surface.

- It is often bilateral and normally corrects itself within a few weeks after birth.
- If still noted after puberty, concerns about its appearance, frequent infection, and/or lactation problems may surface in the youth.
- Congenital nipple inversion can lead to chronic areolar abscess, characterized by nipple swelling, pain, and discharge along with periareolar erythema.
- Treatment involves local heat, antibiotics, and surgery in some cases to remove the duct system.

Rare anomalies

- *Athelia* is the absence of a nipple results from the impact of taking exogenous androgen during pregnancy.
- *Amastia is* absence of the breast), caused by mammary ridge involution involving the pectoral ridge on the affected side. It is typically unilateral and in association with defects of the chest wall. The Poland syndrome is characterized by unilateral amastia with no pectoralis muscle development, defects of the ribs, radial nerve palsy, and webbing of the fingers. *Amastia can be acquired* after birth from inadvertent breast bed biopsy, radiation damage to the breast, or other injury.
- *Symmastia* is webbing of breast tissue in the midline.
- *Depressed nipple* with lactiferous ducts opening into a depressed area in the areolar center
- *Build or split nipple*
- *Tuberous breasts:* Shape of the breasts is abnormal in which the tuberous breasts project forward without normal fullness; the areolar complex is overdeveloped, with the appearance of herniation of breast tissue into the areola. Two types are described, and surgical correction is necessary to improve the breast appearance by reconstructing the nipple-areolar complex along with breast augmentation.

Acute retraction of a nipple may suggest breast disease, as the breast cancer; fortunately, this is rare in the adolescent.

Scoliosis or defects of the rib cage can result in the appearance of breast asymmetry, or *pseudoasymmetry*.

Breast asymmetry can be the result of hypoplasia, hyperplasia, or breast anomalies.

- In aplasia or hypoplasia develops, the affected breast has no or minimal breast tissue and its shape may be abnormal; the nipple may be normal, atypical, or absent.

Unilateral breast enlargement may also be seen because of a:

- Unilateral juvenile hypertrophy
- A breast mass careful examination and follow-up is important, and biopsy done on any mass that is found.

As one breast bud develop before the other, the young adolescent may present with a unilateral mass sometimes mistaken for a tumor;

- Biopsy of this "lesion" results in damage to the yet-to-mature breast and should be avoided.

Damage to a breast bud can also result from:

- Injury to this area
- Infection,
- Anterolateral thoracotomy, and thoracostomy tube insertions in childhood.
- Burns to the chest area usually cause skin contractures with underlying breast tissue that is normal; release of these contractures in the early teen years allow normal growth of the adolescent breast.

UNDERDEVELOPED BREASTS

A common concern among adolescent females is that of small breasts (micromastia), or breasts that are much smaller than what they or society feels are normal. It is often a familial condition, and may be noted in those with a tall, thin body type with limited subcutaneous tissue in general and sometimes who have connective tissue disorders. Reassurance of the normalcy of the breasts is important, and that the "small" breasts need not interfere with her sense of femininity, sexual relations, pregnancy, or lactation. Augmentation mammoplasty can be done at some time in her life when she is emotionally, cognitively, and financially ready for such surgery.

UNILATERAL OR BILATERAL HYPOPLASIA

Unilateral or bilateral hypoplasia of the breasts may be difficult to distinguish from micromastia.

- Hypoplasia or hypomastia may be due to partial end-organ response failure, in which the breast (s) do not develop into normal breasts.
- Poor or limited breast development may also result from radiation and bilateral ovariectomy.
- Bilateral hypoplasia may result from androgen excess *in utero* or in early infant life; this may be due to congenital adrenal hyperplasia, leading to the prevention of ovarian maturation and estrogen secretion during puberty.
- The nipples are smaller, less pigmented, less estrogenized, and do not have papillae that are protuberant. The pubic hair may develop without thelarche and menarche may be delayed.
- A careful genetic and endocrinologic evaluation is necessary to exclude gonadal dysgenesis (Turner's syndrome), androgen producing tumor, preadolescent hypothyroidism, and gonadotropin deficiency (pituitary hypogonadism).

BREAST ATROPHY

Atrophy of the breasts results from significant weight loss and hypoestrogenemia, as noted in anorexia nervosa, chronic illness, postpartum depression, crash dieting, and other conditions.

- The result is loss of breast adipose tissue and often, severe acquired breast atrophy.

Scleroderma can cause local breast changes while premature ovarian failure can induce secondary amenorrhea and breast atrophy.

- The breasts become wrinkled, flattened, and old in appearance.

Treatment of breast atrophy is to correct the underlying problem.

VIRGINAL HYPERTROPHY

Thelarche in some females leads to massive diffuse enlargement of breasts to such an extent that it is termed juvenile, virginal, or idiopathic breast hypertrophy; even more massive development is called macromastia or gigantomastia.

- The cause is usually linked to individual variation, familial factors, sensitivity to estrogen and/or abnormal estrogen-progesterone ratio, and endogenous production of estrogen within breast cells.
- Obesity may play a role in some youth.

The typical history is that of thelarche at a normal time followed by very explosive breast enlargement, usually bilateral; unilateral hypertrophy can also be seen. Potential complication are summarized in Table 13.3.

Such unilateral growth can also be caused by a breast neoplasm, e.g. giant fibroadenoma.

TREATMENT

There are no medications that are acceptable to use in adolescents.

- Danazol or medroxyprogesterone can lead reduced breast size; however, there is no clear research that notes it really helps, and side effects (as masculinization and teratogenicity) prohibit their use in youth.
- Breast surgery, as breast reduction, is an option when the adolescent is mature enough

to understand this surgery and accept potential complications. It done too early, breast enlargement may continue, negating the effects of this earlier surgery. Breast reduction often involves reimplantation of the nipple-areolar complex, leading to potential lactation and nerve damage; the erotic potential of breast stimulation may be reduced.

- Potential surgical complications also include anesthesia risks, bleeding, and infection.

Complications of this breast enlargement are listed in Table 13.3. Some of these complications are worsened with a tight brassiere.

Table 13.4: Causes of breast masses in adolescent

Fibroadenoma, juvenile (giant) fibroadenoma, other fibroadenoma variants
Breast cysts, fibrocystic change, breast abscess/mastitis gynecomastia, virginal hyperplasia,
Interstitial (parenchymal) fibrosis, cystosarcoma phylloides
Intraductal papilloma (Papillomatosis) adenocarcinoma, Ductal adenocarcinoma
Nipple adenoma, nipple keratoma, mammary duct ectasia
fat necrosis lipoma, hematoma, hemangioma lymph-angioma
Intraductal granuloma, angiosarcoma dermatofibromatosis
Neurofibromatosis papilloma sarcoidosis
Sclerosing adenosis tuberous mastitis
Metastatic disease (leukemia, lymphoma, ovarian malignancy, others)

Table 13.3: Potential complications of juvenile breast hypertrophy

Embarrassment	Stretching and flattening of the areolae
Severe neck and back pain/strain,	Kyphotic posture
Skin ulceration	Dermatitis, Invertrigo
Tissue necrosis and skin rupture	Brachial plexus-induced paresthesias
Breast pain	Reduced physical and athletic function
Severe cases: Respiratory distress	or spinal curvature
Complications of surgery if breast reduction is done	

BREAST MASSES

Since malignancy is rare in the adolescent, observation of a mass over a few months is usually an appropriate clinical response. Breast cancer is noted in less than 2.5% of palpable breast masses in females under 30 and less than 0.5% in those under age 20.

70-90% of masses that are biopsied are fibroadenomas, and most of the other masses are benign cysts.

Causes of breast masses are summarized in Table 13.4.

IMPORTANT HISTORICAL POINTS IN ASSESSMENT OF A BREAST MASS

- Associated pain
- Cyclical or non-cyclical
- Galactorrhea
- Size of the lesion
- How long it has been present.

An excision biopsy is typically obtained for a mass that is hard, does not resolve, increases in size, fails to decrease over a few menstrual cycles, resumes after aspiration, and or has bloody nipple discharge.

FIBROADENOMA

A benign tumor arising from ducts and stoma of the terminal part of the breast system. most common lesion noted in post-pubertal females up to 25 years or age.

- Sensitivity to estrogen
- Effects of prolonged estrogen exposure; the tumor cells contain estrogen receptors. Biopsy reveals a histologic appearance that is similar to gynecomastia or virginal hypertrophy.
- Usually presents as a tumor that is well-demarcated, encapsulated, round, rubberty, and non-tender; it may blend into normal breast tissue or present as a oval or irregular lump that is hard or elastic on palpation.

- Are usually single and found in the upper, outer quadrant, though any quadrant may be noted.
- As many as 20% have bilateral or multiple tumors in a condition called fibroadenomatosis.
- A fibroadenoma may be 2-3 cm when first found; it remain the same size or grow rapidly to 10 to 15 cm or more.
- It may enlarge at the end of a menstrual cycle and can also increase during pregnancy; full spontaneous regression is unlikely.
- The ultrasound appearance is that of a smooth margin mass that is homogeneous.
- Does not became malignant and does not increase the adolescent's risk for malignancy later in life.
- If a lesion appearing to be a fibroadenoma does not decrease over 4 to 6 months or if it continues to enlarge, excision is usually recommended;
- Removal of a large mass may require more surgery to reduce the skin envelope for a cosmetic closure. If concern is raised about potential cancer, excision is also suggested.
- A malignancy is suggested by a tumor with tight or stretched overlying skin with superficial vein dilation and a peau d'orange appearance.

Giant (Juvenile) Fibroadenoma

A fibroadenoma is over 5 cm is often defined as a giant or juvenile type and is important because it can grow quickly to a large size, doubling itself in three to six months.

- It tends to be seen in young adolescents, has a consistency that is softer, has more dilation of superficial veins, and can cause considerable breast distortion.
- The differential diagnosis includes unilateral hyperplasia, cystosarcoma phylloides, adenocarcinoma, lipoma, and others.
- It may be confused with cancer if the histology reveals atypical epithelial hyperplasia. Though a benign tumor, it should be excised before becoming too large.

CYSTOSARCOMA PHYLLOIDES

- The most common malignant tumor of the breast reported in adolescents.
- Painless, multi-lobular tumor that is rapidly-growing, is non-fixed, and is often 8 to 10 cm when first found.
- Often presents with nipple discharge, venous dilation, and skin discoloration.
- Histology report reveals epithelial and stromal components along with multiple cysts. 10 to 15% are malignant and metastases develop, particularly to the lungs.
- A wide excision (with 2 cm margins that are tumor-free) is considered curative for benign tumors.
- Management of a malignant type includes surgery, radiation, chemotherapy, and hormonal treatment; though the prognosis is poor, it is better in adolescents than in adults.

INTRADUCTAL PAPILLOMA

- Also called papillomatosis) (Table 13.5) typically presents as a painful (but can be painless in 30%), sub-areolar mass that is unilateral in three-fourths of cases; a serosanguineous or serous nipple discharge is often described on the affected side.
- A benign tumor, though the adolescent patient should be followed carefully for the possible development of a malignant change.
- Evaluation:fine needle aspiration, breast ultrasonography, and ductography.

Table 13.5: Differential diagnosis of intraductal papilloma

Intraductal papilloma	Papillar carcinoma
Nipple adenoma	Mammary duct ectasia
Fibroadenoma	Cystosarcoma phylloides
Infiltrating ductal adenocarcinoma (rare)	

MAMMARY DUCT ECTASIA

- Also called periductal mastitis presents as a painful subareolar nodule with nipple discharge, nipple retraction, sinus tracts (or fistulae), and axillary lymphadenopathy.

- It is the most common cause of acquired nipple inversion.
- Infection with Bacteroides species is seen in adolescents, leading to inflammatory changes and periductal fibrosis and destruction of the ductal wall.
- It is usually seen in adult females at menopause who often had a history of lactation problems.
- Management includes local excision of the sinus tract or fistula along with antibiotics.

CYSTIC BREAST DISEASE

Well-known, but less common in the adolescents are single or multiple cysts of benign breast disease.

- Typically not fixed to breast tissue and aspiration reveals sterile fluid that is clear, brownish, or blood-tinged.
- Cysts can be classified in various ways, e.g. Table 13.6 including normal physiologic changes in breast size in adolescents with up to 50% size change during a menstrual cycle; these pseudolumps are normal.
- A solitary large cyst contains yellow, green, or black fluid on aspiration and may be confused with a fibroadenoma; aspiration is usually curative and the normal cytologic evaluation reassuring to patient, parents, and clinicians.
- In the postpartum period, lactiferous ducts may become distended and become galactoceles, presenting as a subareolar mass with a yellow nipple discharge; it usually disappears with lactation, but surgical excision may become necessary.
- Fat necrosis may result from trauma to the breast.

Table 13.6: Classification of breast cysts

1. Fibrocystic disease or change (with multiple small cysts)
2. Solitary large or blue-domed cysts (with bloody fluid)
3. Single cysts
4. Galactoceles
5. Normal physiologic change ("pseudolumps")

Management

- Fine-needle aspiration with cytologic evaluation to identify if it is a matter of normal physiology or overt pathology.
- The fluid is tested for the presence of red blood cells and also prepared for formal cytologic examination.
- If the lesion disappears on aspiration, it is assumed to be a cyst and the patient can be evaluated again in 2 to 3 months.
- It the lesion recurs or is solid, ultrasonography is obtained for further evaluation. Sometimes an open, exisional biopsy is necessary to identify and remove the breast lesion, if aspiration is not successful or not possible.

FIBROCYSTIC CHANGE

Previously called fibrocystic disease is noted in adolescents, but is more commonly seen in adult females over age 35 years.

- Presents as firm, movable, nodularities that are cord-like and distributed diffusely in the breasts.
- Some develop "lumpy" breasts in their young adult years that may develop into overt fibrocystic change in later adult life.
- A number of etiologies are proposed for this condition, including increased levels of prolactin, deficiency of the corpus luteum, abnormal progesterone to estrogen ratio, and others.
- Tenderness breast tenderness before menstruation and change in breast size during the menstrual cycle; sometimes, non-cyclic pain and size change may be noted.
- Cord-like, breast nodularities that enlarge and regress on a monthly basis.
- The differential diagnosis includes physiologic premenstrual mastodynia and a biopsy may be necessary to identify the actual pathology.

Management

- Good brassiere support, heat, and pain medications (analgesics).
- Oral contraceptives may offer pain relief by inhibiting progesterone secretion, as cysts

tend to be more painful in the secretory or progestational part of the menstrual cycle. Of doubtful value are vitamin E, α-tocopherol (600 IU/day) and dietary limitations of methylxanthines (and other substances).

- Danazol, bromocriptine, and tamoxifen have been tried in adult, but have no clear indication in adolescents.

BREAST ABSCESS

A breast abscess presents as a painful, cystic lesion with erythema and increased head to the skin around the abscess; there may also be a mastitis and one or multiple abscess may be noted along with fever, cellulitis, and regional lymphadenopathy. A subareolar abscess can lead to an inverted nipple causes of breast abscess are summarized in Table 13.7.

Table 13.7: Causes of breast abscess

Idiopathic	Self-manipulation
Squeezing acne lesions	Areolar hair plucking
Lactation	Foreign body
Trauma (including sexual	Epidermal cyst
Chronic illness with reduced host defenses	

Diagnosis

History, physical examination, and needle aspiration ultrasound evaluation and blood cultures may also help.

Management

- Heat with warm compresses, analgesics, incision and drainage
- If resolution does not occur, there may be an underlying, deeper abscess. Antibiotics are given seeking to cover both gram-positive and gram-negative organisms, unless a specific agent is found; for 3 to 4 weeks, sometimes given intravenously at first.
- There is a 50% recurrence rate for infections that are delayed or only partially treated. Residual scarring may develop and be mistaken for a tumor, such as a fibroadenoma. Scarring is particularly noted with underlying trauma and associated fat necrosis develops. If lactational mastitis develops, breastfeeding is usually not stopped, unless overt purulent nipple discharge develops.

MASTODYNIA

Mastodynia (mastalgia) refers to breast pain, often a hormonally-induced process that is cyclic and associated with physiologic changes characterized by nodularities and swellings.

Breast pain may occur with various breast disorders, but is more typically noted as part of normal menstrual physiology. Menstrually-induced mastodynia may be due to deficient activity of the corpus luteum producing a relative hyperestronism.

Other causes

- Breast trauma, hypertrophy, and infection
- Side effect of medications contraceptives phenothiazines, resperpine, exogenous hormones, and possible, marijuana.

The differential diagnosis of mastodynia includes costochondritis, cardiac disease, and cervical spine pathology.

TRAUMA

Trauma may lead to mastodynia, as noted with sexual activity, motor vehicle accident, sports, and various other examples of accidental trauma.

Acute Trauma

Acute trauma to the breast can lead to pain, swelling, ecchymoses, contusion, hematoma, and/or laceration.

- Basic management includes ice application for the first 24 hours followed by heat application, analgesics, firm brassiere supports, and sometimes, antibiotics.

Chronic Trauma

Chronic trauma may lead to a painful breast area or mass that is irregular of poorly defined and present for several days, even weeks.

- If the trauma was months ago, scar tissue and fat necrosis may be present in the breast.
- Sometimes the adolescent presents with a breast lesion and is concerned about having breast cancer, having forgotten the incident of trauma.
- The lesion consisting of trauma-induced fat necrosis may have physical and mammographic features suggestive of breast cancer, necessitating excision to identify the correct pathology.

MANAGEMENT OF MASTODYNIA

- Heat, good brassiere support, and analgesics (including the non-steroidal anti-inflammatory agents at ibuprofen or naproxen sodium).
- If exogenous estrogen is an underlying cause, stop this medication.
- If the pain is severe and not related to estrogen administration, cycling the menstrual periods with oral contraceptives may be helpful.
- Doubtful value are vitamin E (alpha tocopherol),and in adult female evening primrose oil not proven to help in adolescents
- avoidance of methylxanthines (found in cola, tea, or coffee), chocolate, nicotine, stress, and dairy products.
- Danazol is an androgen steroid not recommended in adolescents because it is not proven to help, and it has significant side effects, such as potential masculinization and teratogenicity.
- Also tried in adult females are bromocriptine (a prolactin antagonist) and tamoxifen (competes for estrogen receptors), there is no evidence of their benefit in adolescents.
- If breast discomfort or pain is part of swelling and weight gain associated with the menstrual cycle, diuretics may help with the breast swelling and pain.

MONDOR'S DISEASE

- Is superficial thrombophlebitis of the thoraco-epigastric vein seen with pregnancy and various types of trauma (including biopsy or breast surgery).
- It presents with painful cords of phlebitis palpated over the involved breast, typically in the upper, lateral breast area.
- It typically fully resolves in 10 to 21 days
- Management includes local heat along with oral analgesics.

Adolescent females who are runners can have nipple irritation that may lead to nipple discharge.

Causes of nipple discharge are summarized in Table 13.8.

Table 13.8: Causes of nipple discharge

Galactorrhea	Areolar (Montgomer) gland secretion
Pregnancy or abortion fibrocystic	Breast cyst (including change)
Cystic ductal hyperplasia	Intraductal papillomatosis (ectasia)
Chronic subareolar abscess	Carcinoma
Various drug effects (as marijuana, amphetamine or codeine)	
Galactocele	

Management

- Careful history regarding the the amount and color of the nipple discharge, trauma, breast manipulation, or menstrual disorders. Types of nipple discharge are summarized in Table 13.9.

Table 13.9: Types of nipple discharge

A yellow discharge	Normal physiologic effects or a galactocele
A clear, serous, or greenish discharge	Physiologic cyst
A milky discharge	Lactation, breast cancer, microadenoma, elevated TSH,, acromegaly, phenothiazine effect
A bloody discharge	cystosarcoma phylloides, papillary carcinoma, intraductal, papilloma or cystic duct Hyperplasia
A brownish discharge	Mongomery gland secretion or intraductal papilloma,
A purulent discharge	infection

- Careful examination of the breasts (including the nipples) associated breast abnormalities

- A ductogram (galactograph)
- Surgery may be necessary to remove the involved areolar duct to be sure a rare malignancy is not present, such as cystosarcoma phylloides or papillary carcinoma.

GALACTORRHEA

Galactorrhea refers to inappropriate or abnormal breast milk secretion because it occurs apart from postpartum lactation and nursing.

- The fluid may be clear, white or milky, green, or yellow; it varies in amount and a Sudan stain reveals fat globules. Most frequent causes are idiopathic (benign), self-manipulation, pharmacologic, prolactinoma, and hypothyroidism.
- It occurs most often because of pregnancy-related prolactin level increase and may occur after delivery without nursing, miscarriage or abortion.
- Idiopathic or benign galactorrhea may be seen due to end-organ hypersensitivity to prolactin levels that are normal.
- Idiopathic hyperprolactinemia can develop from various causes, including a microadenoma too small for discovery or macroprolactinemia with increased amounts of large prolactin molecules that are not biologically active.
- A variety of medications or drugs can induce hyperprolactinemia, including those that block dopamine receptors (tricyclic antidepressants, butyrophenones, and phenothiazines), deplete dopamine (as cocaine), stimulate lactotrophs (narcotics, verapamil, and high dose estrogens), and those that bind to dopamine receptors in the gastrointestinal tract (metoclopramide). Galactorrhea may be induced by oral contraceptives, reserpine, spironolactone, methyltestosterone, and others; marijuana has been implicated, but is not proven as a cause.

The adolescent who presents with galactorrhea needs a careful evaluation for the many causes that are possible (Table 13.10).

Table 13.10: Causes of galactorrhea*

Causes
Recent pregnancy terminated by spontaneous or induced abortion, with or without amenorrhea, Hysterectomy or uterine tumors, Breast (nipple) manipulation or stimulation,Chronic inflammatory disease or abscess of breast, Polycystic ovary syndrome (PCOS), ovarian tumors Contraceptive pills; including other estrogen or progesterone
Neurogenic, Herpes zoster, Spinal cord disorders and surgery, Psychogenic, including pseudocyesis and pseudonursing
Bronchiectasis and chronic bronchitis, Thoracotomy or thoracoplasty, Burns to chest wall, Chest wall disorders, Uremia, Chronic Renal Disease, Cirrhosis Nelson syndrome Acute Intermittent Porphyria Chronic crutch use, Central nervous system abnormalities, Diffuse brain disease, Coma, Pseudotumor cerebri
Encephalitis and sequelae Craniopharyngioma, Pineal tumors Other intracranial tumors, cysts and masses
Tumors, infiltrations, structural abnormalities, Neurocutaneous syndromes Histiocytosis X Sarcoidosis
Adrenal tumors and hypernephromas, testicular tumours
Pituitary Stalk section, Empty sella syndrome, Pituitary infarction and Sheehan's syndrome
Other functional pituitary tumors, Idiopathic normoprolactinemic Hyperprolactinemia with or without prolactinoma
Hypo- and hyperthyroidism, Cushing's disease, Hypogonadism
Starvation or refeeding (including anorexia nervosa) Laparotomy
Drugs: Phenothiazines, thioxanthines, other major tranquilizers, Tricyclic antidepressants
Opiates, including codeine and heroin,Monoamine oxidase inhibitors, Amphetamines, Chlordiazepoxide, Meprobamate, Metoclopramide, Bromocriptine withdrawal Cimetidine and ranitidine, Tamoxifen, Verapamil, Isoniazid, Estrogens, Opiates (including codeine and heroin), Phenothiazines, thioxanthines, other psychotropic drugs, Tricyclic antidepressants Other chemotherapy drugs (cisplatin, cytosine arabinoside, adriamycin; Others

*Reprinted, with permission from: Greydanus DE and Shearin RB: Adolescent Sexuality and Gynecology. Philadelphia: Lea and Febiger, p.145, 1990.

MANAGEMENT

- The history should be taken for drug abuse, menstrual abnormality, headaches, visual disturbances, thyroid disorder and other factors.
- If the prolactin level is elevated, evaluate for thyroid dysfunction, lesions of the pituitary

or hypothalamus, drugs or medication use, and other causes.

- Thyroid function tests are a must
- CT/MRI of the sella turcica are important tests to obtain
- Other testing is necessary, depending on the precise findings.
- depends on the underlying etiology
- Underlying thyroid dysfunction or menstrual abnormality should be treated. Management of a microadenoma is often with a dopamine agonist, as bromocriptine, and if necessary, surgery.
- Offending drugs or medications should be stopped, as should be self-manipulation if causative.
- Careful follow-up is important and consultation with experts is suggested for severe, confusing, or cases resistant to treatment.

GYNECOMASTIA

Gynecomastia refers to the development of breast tissue in males and can be seen as neonatal, prepubertal, pubertal, or postpubertal. As many as two-thirds of young males with Tanner state 2 or 3 can develop gynecomastia, probably because end-organ sensitivity triggered by a temporary imbalances in excess estrogen production with a relative testosterone deficiency.

Gynecomastia in young adolescent males usually lasts 6 to 18 months, typically fully resolved within one to two years after its onset. Usually it starts with one side and then becomes a bilateral process.

Classification

Type I Gynecomastia or Benign Adolescent Hypertrophy

This is more common and the breast development presents as a small, tender, firm, subareolar mass that is 2 to 3 cm in diameter

Type II Gynecomastia or Macromastia

This is more unusual: a larger breast development occurs, resembling Tanner stage 3 or even 4 breast development of females.It can be painful with prominent nipples that rub against clothes with resultant skin erosion and even galactorrhea. It usually does not resolve spontaneously.

Pseudogynecomastia

Pseudogynecomastia in seen in obese males who present with fat deposition resembling breasts or some may have well-developed pectoralis muscles.

Organic causes of gynecomastia should be considered especially when it develops at times other than between Tanner stage 2 and 3 in young adolescent males. These are listed in Table 13.11.

MANAGEMENT OF NORMAL PHYSIOLOGIC GYNECOMASTIA

- Reassurance and education to the male and his family about the normal benign as well as transient nature of this common condition.

Table 13.11: Organic causes of gynecomastia*

Familial gynecomastia
Klinefelter's syndrome, androgen insensitivity syndrome
Hodgkin's disease, pituitary tumor, adrenal tumor
Thyroid dysfunction (Hypo/hyperthyroidism)
Miscellaneous tumors (teratoma, seminoma, Leydig-cell tumor, hepatoma, bronchogenic carcinoma, others)
Cirrhosis of the liver, Chronic glomerulonephritis
Male pseudohermaphroditism
Leukemia, hemophilia
Traumatic paraplegia, Starvation (on refeeding)
Miscellaneous drugs
Amphetamines,Anabolic steroids, Birth control pills, estrogens
Busulfan (and other chemotherapeutic agents)
Cimetidine, Corticosteroids, Digitalis
Human chorionic gonadotropin, insulin, testosterone
Isoniazid (and other anti-tuberculosis drugs)
Marijuana, methadone, tricyclic antidepressants
Phenothiazines, reserpine spironolactone
Others

*Reprinted and modified, with permission: Greydanus DE, Shearin RB: Adolescent Sexuality and Gynecology. Philadelphia: Lea and Febiger, p.148, 1990.

- Some may need overt psychological support if they are very concerned about this condition and the teasing they may have to endure form peers.
- A careful assessment is necessary to be sure it is not organic in etiology (Table 13.11).
- If the condition does not resolve in a prompt fashion and if it is a Type II condition, referral for surgical consultation and reduction mammoplasty is often indicated. Testosterone is necessary if hypogonadism is present, as noted for Klinefelter syndrome. Antiestrogenic medications (as tamoxifen and clomiphene) have been used in some adult males with gynecomastia.

SUGGESTED READING

1. Arca MJ, Caniano DA. Breast disorders in the adolescent patient. Adolesc Med 15, 2004:473-85.
2. Behrman RE, Kliegman RM, Jenson HB (Eds): Nelson Textbook of Pediatrics—17th Ed. Philadelphia: WB Saunders Co., (Jenkins RR: "The Breast," 2004; 106: 662-3.
3. Bland KI, Copeland EM III (Eds): The Breast: Comprehensive Management of Benign and Malignant Disorders. Philadelphia, PA: WB Saunders, 2004;1694.
4. Govrin-Yehudain J, Kogan L, Cohen HI, et al: Familial juvenile hypertrophy of adolescent breast disease. J Adolesc Health 2004;35:151.
5. Greydanus DE, Matytsina L, Gains M. Breast disorders in children and adolescents. Prim Care:Clinics in Office Pract (Elsevier) 2006; 33:455-502.
6. Greydanus DE, Parks DS, Farrell EG: Breast Disorders in Children and Adolescents.Pediatric No Amer, 1989;36(3):601-38.
7. Greydanus DE, Patel DR, Baxter TL. The Breast and Sports: Issues for the Clinician. State of the Art Reviews: Adolescent Medicine 1998;9(3): 533-50.
8. Greydanus DE. "Breast and Gynecologic Disorders" In: Hofmann AD, Greydanus DE (Eds): Adolescent Medicine, 3rd Edition, Norwalk, CT: Appleton and Lange, 1997;25: 520-34.
9. Hindle WH, Pan EY. Breast disorders in female adolescents. State of the Art Reviews: Adolescent Medicine1994; 5(1): 123-29.
10. Kaul P, Beach RK. Breast disorders. In: Essential Adolescent Medicine. (Eds): DE Greydanus, DR Patel, HD Pratt. New York: McGraw-Hill Medical Publishers, 2005;27: 563-84.
11. Marchant DJ. Benign breast disease. Obstet Gynecol Clin North Am 2002;29:1.
12. McRath MH, Schooler WG. Elective plastic surgical procedures in adolescence. Adolesc Med 2004;15:487-502.
13. Sanfilippo JS: "Breast Disorders," ch. 543: 1833-1835; Rapaport R: Gynecomastia," 579: 1930-31).
14. Simmons PS, Wold LE. Surgically treated breast disease in adolescent females: A retrospective review of 185 cases. Adolesc Pediatric Gynecol 1989;2:95.
15. Smith BL. The breast. Curr Probl Obstet Gynecol Fertil 1996;19:1036.
16. Stone AM, Shenker IR, McCarthy K. Adolescent breast masses. Am J Surg 1977;134:275.
17. West KW, Resoorla FJ, Schere LR III, et al. Diagnosis and treatment of symptomatic breast masses in the pediatric population. J Pediatr Surg 1995;30:182.

14 Clinical Approach to Breast Problems in Girls

Vinay Deshmane

INTRODUCTION

- Breast diseases in adolescents are uncommon.
- Majority are aberrations of normal development and involution (ANDI)
- Breast cancer is rare in this age group
- However, breast symptoms in this group can cause major anxiety for both patient and parents
- Proper assessment and adequate counseling is essential.

Breast problems as summarized in Table 14.1.

Table 14.1: Breast problems during adolescence

Problem	*Frequency*
Related to development:	
Premenarchal development of breast bud	Common
Disorders of shape and size	Common
Virginal hypertrophy	Uncommon
Infections:	
Breast abscess	Common
Subareolar abscess (periductal mastitis)	Uncommon
Lumps:	
Fibroadenoma	Common
Giant fibroadenoma	Rare
Phylloides tumor	Rare
Cysts	Rare
Carcinoma	Rare
Others:	
Breast pain	Common
Nipple discharge	Rare

HISTORY TAKING

IMPORTANT POINTS

- Duration of problem
- Severity and nature of symptoms with their relation to menstrual cycle
- Menstrual history and LMP
- Family history of first degree relatives with breast/ovarian cancer
- Social problems related to change in shape/size
- Presence/absence of mental stress

CLINICAL EXAMINATION

- Examine patient in the lying down position as well as sitting up. With hands by her sides as well as raised above her head
- Keep a diagrammatic representation of clinical findings
- Document sites of abnormality clearly: e.g. 2 cm lump in upper outer quadrant of left breast at 3 O'clock position, 1.5 cm away from areola.
- Mention clearly presence/absence of skin changes, nipple areola changes, or lymph node enlargement.

INVESTIGATIONS

BLOOD INVESTIGATIONS

Hormonal levels, e.g. prolactin in patients with nipple discharge.

BREAST IMAGING

Breast ultrasound is the main investigation in this age group. It can help distinguish between cysts, solid masses and normal breast tissue.

Mammography is of limited use due to the dense nature of breasts, which limits visualization. However, it may be performed in the presence of symptoms or a palpable lesion to document its appearance.

MRI scan may be considered in a few select cases. It can be of benefit in evaluating dense breasts in patients with a solid palpable mass. However, but should be requested sparingly as there is paucity of data regarding its use in this population.

MANAGEMENT OF COMMON PROBLEMS

Management of comman problems are summarized in Table 14.2.

Table 14.2: Disorders of number, shape and size

Problem	*Management principles*
Prepubertal bud	Reassurance, repeated assessments, avoidance of biopsy which can permanently damage breast development.
Changes in shape and size Virginal hypertrophy	Reassurance. Referral to specialist centers. Treatment after complete development of breasts, i.e. after 18 years. Earlier, in select cases in presence of severe mental stress due to social/ peer pressure.

Table 14.3 summarized management of infections.

Table 14.3: Infections

Breast abscess	Early stage: Aspirate pus. Send for culture sensitivity. Start broad spectrum antibiotics, e.g. Amoxycillin with clavulanic acid 625 mg bd, or cloxacillin 500 mg qds with metronidazole 400 mg tds. Incise and drain only if uncontrolled or abscess starts pointing or there are systemic symptoms.
Subareolar abscess (periductal mastitis)	Inadequately treated infection can result in formation of mammary fistula. If unresponsive to usual antibiotics, this is best treated at specialist centers.

APPROACH TO AN ADOLESCENT OR YOUNG GIRL WITH A BREAST LUMP

FIBROADENOMA

- The commonest cause of a lump in this age group is a benign fibroadenoma. Types are summarized in Table 14.4.
- Malignancy, although unlikely, can be mistaken for a fibroadenoma.
- Thus accurate assessment is essential and is based on clinical breast examination, imaging (breast ultrasound) and fine needle aspiration.
- The majority of lumps may be observed provided certain guidelines are observed.
- Repeated evaluations for changes in shape or size.
- Enlarging lumps are best removed for histological evaluation.

Table 14.4: Types of fibroadenoma

Type of fibroadenoma	*Relative risk of subsequent cancer*
Fibroadenoma	1.48-1.7
Fibroadenoma with proliferative changes	3.47-3.7
Fibroadenoma with proliferative changes and atypical cells	6.9-7.29

- Lumps approaching 3 cm in size are also best excised to avoid missing phyllodes tumors and giant fibroadenomas.
- There is some associated risk of subsequent breast cancer with fibroadenomas especially fibroadenomas which are associated with proliferative changes and atypical cells. Thus accurate histological assessment of excised fibroadenomas is essential.

Approach to assessment and management of a suspected fibroadenoma

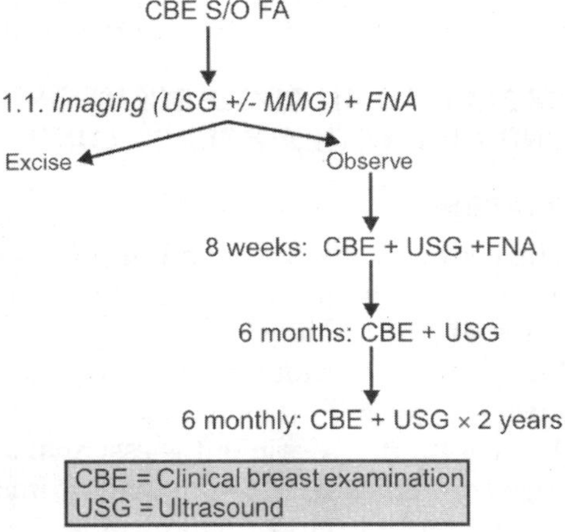

BREAST CYST

Cysts are unusual at a young age. The cause is unknown but suspected to be related to hormonal changes. Cysts can be divided into micro and macro type. Micro are those detected on ultrasound and are not palpable. These do not cause any problems and patients can be reassured. Palpable cysts can further be divided into simple and complex cysts based on their appearance on ultrasound. Complex cysts may require intervention.

An approach to management of breast cysts:

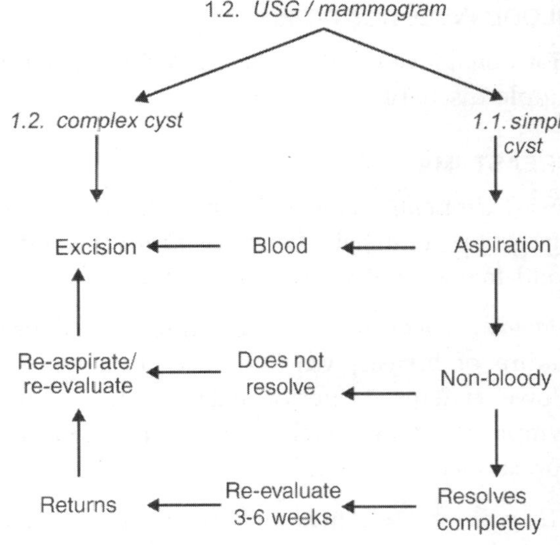

BREAST PAIN

- A common problem
- Classify into cyclical and non cyclical
- Assess severity of pain
- If pain is mild to moderate in intensity and does not disturb the patient, treatment revolves around reassurance and symptom relief with mild analgesics as required.
- Severe pain that disturbs the patient's lifestyle requires treatment.

Approach to the management of breast pain

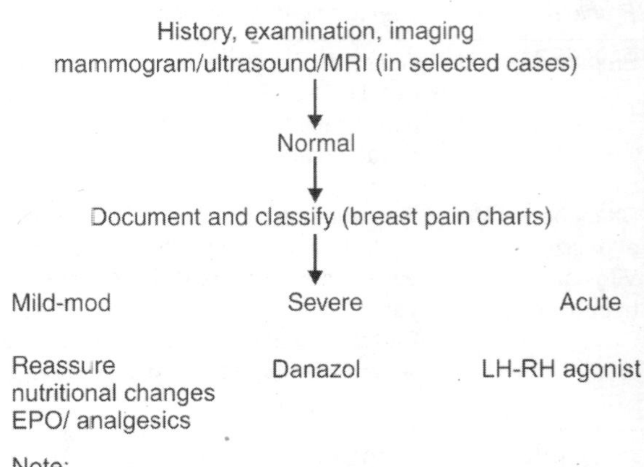

Note:
evening primrose oil: dose = 270 mg of gamma linolenic acid /day danazol 100 mg BD × 2 months
LH RH agonist 3.75 mg/month

BREAST CANCER

- Rare at an young age
- Often mistaken as fibroadenoma and treated as such
- Management involves accurate diagnosis and staging
- Management is multidisciplinary involving surgery (which can be breast preserving/mastectomy), adjuvant/neoadjuvant systemic treatment, and radiation therapy
- A detailed discussion is out of the scope of this textbook.

SUGGESTED READING

1. Devita VT, Hellman S Rosenberg SA. Cancer: Principles and Practice of Oncology. Lippincott, Williams and Williams, 2001.
2. Hughes LE, Mansel RE, Webster DJT. Benign disorders and diseases of the breast: Concepts and clinical management. WB Saunders, 2000.

15 Contraception

Mandakini Parihar, Meenakshi Bharath

INTRODUCTION

"Contraceptives should be used for every conceivable occasion"

–Spike Milligan

We currently have over 6300 million people on planet earth, and this number rises each year by around 80 million. This means, effectively, that a city for 1.5 million people has to be built every week. In addition, almost 50% of the pregnancies that occur worldwide are unplanned, and hence, the need for contraceptive awareness and newer more acceptable contraceptives is the need of the hour. The group most susceptible to unwanted pregnancies and risks of unprotected intercourse are the young adolescents.

Adolescents typically are poorly informed about how to protect their sexual health. They are less experienced and less comfortable accessing family planning and reproductive health services than adults. They are the largest target population for us to see that the unmet need of contraception is brought down dramatically. In addition, gender inequities, particularly in our country, may limit their ability to use contraceptives or seek reproductive health services.

CONTRACEPTION FOR ADOLESCENTS

Research has shown that adolescents usually do not use any contraceptive during intercourse, and those that do use, tend to use less effective methods such as withdrawal and rhythm.[3] A small proportion of adolescents who used oral contraceptive pills used them incorrectly. Adolescents tend to borrow their friend's pill, take the pill briefly or inconsistently, take the pill only during intercourse, or take the pill as if they were abortifacients.[4] Barners to use are listed in Table 15.1.

Table 15.1: Barriers to contraceptive use among adolescents

- Unexpected and unplanned sexual activity
- Lack of information and knowledge about contraceptives and where to get them
- Embarrassment and fear of lack of confidentiality
- Fear of medical procedures
- Fear of judgmental attitudes and resistance from providers
- Inability to pay for services and transport
- Fear from partner or parents
- Pressure to have children from in-laws, society
- Sexual coercion
- Poor negotiation skills
- Political, religious, cultural hurdles

Despite decline in pregnancies among adolescents in the 1990s, the pregnancy rate in this population remains high. In the year 2000, more than 840,000 adolescents became pregnant in the United States, which continues to have one of the highest pregnancy rates in the world. A substantial percentage of adolescent pregnancies in 2000 ended in induced abortion. As would be expected, both the pregnancy rate and abortion rate were highest among older adolescents, aged 18 to 19.[5] Educative programs and increasing awareness about the various methods available and the accurate information about each will help in decreasing high risk sexual behavior amongst this age group.

Adolescents need clear and accurate information about contraceptive methods, including correct use, side effects, and how to reach a health care provider with their concerns.[2] In a study in United States, it was noted that schools where there were educative programs, there was a decline in the use of methods with the highest failure rates: the use of withdrawal dropped from 20 to 13%, and the use of no method at all dropped from 17 to 13%. The use of a condom in conjunction with a hormonal method increased from 3% in 1991 to 7% in 2001.[6]

The National Family Health Survey carried out in 1995 has revealed that in India almost 78% of the conceptions that occur annually are unplanned and 25% are unwanted, contributing substantially to the 11 million abortions induced every year in India. 6-7 million are induced abortions and 4 million are spontaneous. India also has a ratio of 10-11 illegal abortions for each legal abortion performed.[1]

METHODS OF CONTRACEPTION

Adolescents can be offered various choices of contraception. Numerous current reviews and protocols for contraception are available.[7]

We should emphasize the need for contraception along with prevention of STDs for our clients. Cafeteria approach should be adopted while prescribing suitable contraceptive for the young.

In general, adolescents are healthy and they can choose from a wide range of contraceptive options, although condoms often are a clear first choice for unmarried adolescents.

Counseling for contraception should address both pregnancy prevention and STI protection.

Investigators from the Alan Guttmacher Institute assessed data from 1988 through 1995 to determine the underlying reasons for the ten point decline in the adolescent pregnancy rate during that time period (from 111 to 101 pregnancies per 1,000 women). The investigators estimated that an increase in abstinence accounted for 25% of the decline, with the remaining 75% due to an increase in contraceptive use. A further analysis of contraceptive use among adolescents showed an increase in the use of the long-acting hormonal injection and implant, which became available in the early 1990s and have the lowest failure rate of all reversible contraceptives. These methods accounted for 13% of contraceptive use among adolescents by 1995. Other trends reported included a slight increase in condom use. Given below is a brief review of the various contraceptive options that can be offered for adolescents with the important pros and cons.

ABSTINENCE

Abstinence is the most effective means of birth control. It is the only way which can provide 100% protection against pregnancy and STDs. This has to be emphasized on the minds of young girls as well as boys. The importance of this should be stressed in the educative and awareness program as the "A of ABC" of STI prevention.

Our focus should be on delaying the initiation of adolescent sexual activity until adulthood. This needs to be done without being moralistic or judgmental.

This may be implemented with adolescent sex education program like FOGSI "Growing Up" "Teen Within" and "Lets Talk" programs. These programs are helpful in preventing the young one from risky sexual behavior.

CONDOMS

The condom is the ONLY method of prevention of STI and this cannot be overstressed in all the contraceptive advice that we give the adolescents.

It needs to be reinforced repeatedly especially in the adolescents so that STI's and HIV can be prevented, along with contraceptive efficacy.

This holds true especially in adolescents with multiple sexual partners.

Adolescents must understand that the use of a condom is not optional and that a new condom must be used each time they have sexual intercourse.

They must also be instructed in the correct use of a condom. Adolescents need to understand that no other contraception method provides the same protection from STDs.[8] The male condom is a mechanical barrier method of contraception. Its effectiveness is enhanced by use of a spermicide. Latex condoms significantly reduce the transmission of STDs including HIV and should therefore be recommended for all sexually active adolescents regardless of whether an additional method of contraception is being used.

Male condoms have several other advantages.
They allow for male partner to share in the responsibility for contraception, are easily available over the counter and are inexpensive. The youngsters should be encouraged to practice dual protection to protect from unwanted pregnancy and sexually transmitted diseases.

Another method of barrier contraceptive is female condom.
The drawbacks are high cost, lack of availability and difficult insertion.[9] Table 15.2 outlines dual protection.

Table 15.2: Dual protection

Dual Protection - Condoms to prevent pregnancy and STIs. EC in event of condom slippage, breakage or failure to use.
Dual method use - Use of condom for prevention of STI by the male. A female control method for prevention of pregnancy EC as back-up.

SPERMICIDES

Spermicidal agents like nonoxinol-9 have a relatively high contraceptive failure rate when used alone and must be used with each act of intercourse without fail. The combination of spermicide and condoms is more effective means of contraception for adolescents since it provides effective contraception as well as protection from STDs. It is available without a prescription and is inexpensive.[10]

RHYTHM METHODS AND SAFE PERIOD AND WITHDRAWAL METHOD

These methods should be discouraged from being used though they are practiced widely amongst adolescents.

Their high failure rate and high risk of STI should be stressed and these methods should be avoided. However, knowledge about them should also be given with stress on its unreliability. The rhythm method provides little or no protection against STDs.

Withdrawal method is still widely used by adolescents in sexual relationships. Adolescents should be cautioned against this method due to its high failure rate. It may be emphasized that this method provides little or no protection against STDs.

ORAL CONTRACEPTIVES

Oral contraceptives are reliable and most effective for the prevention of pregnancy. They are available by prescription. Currently oral contraceptive pills are available as, the fixed-dose combination (each tablet contains the same dose of estrogen and progestin), and the mini-pill (progestin only). The newest generation of birth control pills has a low dose of estrogen (20 to 35 µgm) and new forms of progestin or anti-androgen.[11-13]

Detail medical history and examination is mandatory before commencing pills. Combi-nation oral contraceptives are beneficial for dysfunctional uterine bleeding, acne, hirsutism, etc.

Breakthrough bleeding is the most common side effect with low dose pills and usually resolves within three months. Weight gain, nausea, and headaches are infrequent.[10] Adolescents should be thoroughly counseled about side effects of pills. The pills have an edge over other methods because of its high success rate. The failure rate of oral contraceptives when used correctly is <1%.[11] However, the failure rate among adolescents may be as high as 15% because of inconsistent use.[12] This can be minimized by counseling and stressing the importance of regular intake of the tablets. Several patient populations may particularly benefit from using 20 mcg pill preparations. For example, it is quite advantageous to use 20 mcg pills for "adolescents who are very sensitive to estrogen and may have more nausea. This helps in providing effective contraception, in low doses and yet, they still receive the advantages of cycle regularity.[12]

MEDROXYPROGESTERONE ACETATE INJECTION

Medroxyprogesterone acetate is long-acting progesterone given every 12 weeks as a single 150-mg intramuscular injection. For adolescents, this contraceptive method has many benefits, such as effective pregnancy prevention, convenience and absence of estrogenic side effects. It also protects against endometrial cancer and iron deficiency anemia.

The major disadvantages of this contraceptive method for adolescents are–

Menstrual cycle irregularities
Need for IM administration
Progestational side effects like mastalgia, bloating, etc.[13]
It does not offer protection against STDs and HIV.

There was some concern about long-term use in adolescents and a decrease in bone mineral density amongst adolescents. However, the 2005 WHO meeting in Geneva has rules that if used in the correctly chosen WHO group I and II adolescents, it can be safely used, as the BMD returns back to normal after discontinuation.[14]

INTRAUTERINE DEVICES

As all copper IUCDs have a slight increase in the rate of Pelvic inflammatory disease, they are not the first choice amongst adolescents. More so, they are likely to be at higher risk because of their high risk sexual behavior. However, currently there are no contraindications for the use of IUCD amongst adolescents who are in a stable monogamous relation. Also the newer, LNG-IUS which has a decreased risk of PID may be a better option for them.

However, counseling is very important in choosing IUCD as the contraceptive option. There are some copper containing IUCD like Cu 380A, and Multiload are available in smaller size, that can be used in nulliparous girls.[15,16]

CONTRACEPTIVE ACCIDENTS

- Failed coitus interruptus
- Ejaculation on external genitalia
- Miscalculation of rhythm method
- Condom rupture, dislodgment or misuse
- Diaphragm/cap inserted incorrectly, dislodged, found to be torn or removed too early.
- Complete or partial expulsion of IUD
- Mid-cycle IUD removal due to side effects
- Missed combined pills.

EMERGENCY CONTRACEPTIVE PILLS (ECPs)

Emergency contraception is designed to prevent pregnancy after unprotected vaginal intercourse. It is also called post-coital contraception.[17-19] This method is useful for adolescents who often indulge into sexual activity without protection. It should be stressed that ECP is for emergency situations only. It should not substitute regular contraception method.

Also it can be used only twice in one menstrual cycle. It cannot be used as an abortificient and most importantly it is effective only in preventing pregnancy and will not affect if already pregnant. *The commonest method of emergency postcoital contraception.* Giving 1 dose of 750 mcg of levonorgestrel to be taken within 72 hours of unprotected intercourse followed by another dose 12 hours later.[16]

Recent evidence suggests that these can be taken within 120 hours without significantly affecting its efficacy.

The US Food and Drug Administration has indicated that the use of ECPs is safe and effective. The efficacy of ECP is 75% in the prevention of conception.[17]

Adolescents should be counseled that they should come for a follow-up after next menses and also if the period is delayed by more than 7 days.

At the Consortium on EC held in Delhi, in January 2001, this regimen has been chosen as a "dedicated product" and is now available in the market. In order to simplify LNG regimen, a single dose of 1.5 mg of LNG was tried in a WHO Multicentric Randomized Trial. It has been shown that a single dose of 1.5 mg of levonorgestrel is as effective as 2 doses given 12 hours apart upto 120 hours of exposure.[19]

In 2003, the then FOGSI President Dr. Sadhana Desai, in association with Reliance started an Emergency Help Line for promotion of EC (Phone No. 39700111). This helpline is available in more than 600 cities all over the country and the cost is that of a local phone call only. The slogan is " NUMBER LAGAO, UPAYE PAO."

COMPLIANCE AND FOLLOW-UP AFTER CHOOSING A CONTRACEPTIVE

Regular follow-up is essential to ensure correct use and counter check possible misuse of contraceptive, which is not unusual with adolescents.

At times they fail to understand the importance of contraceptive use. The clinician should be vigilant about it. The follow-up also ensure that they are using the chosen method, using it correctly and importantly if there are any unwanted side effects then the contraceptive option can be changed. If there is any risk of STI's they can be identified and diagnosed and treated promptly.

CONCLUSIONS

Despite all our collective wish that adolescents refrain from sexual activity, more than half of them will not do so. It is important to realize that a substantial number of adolescents are sexually active despite cultural norms. What is essential for all of us to ensure is that they have given the knowledge and information about and sexuality contraceptive methods so that they can protect themselves from pregnancy and disease. They lack access to information and services and the skills that allow them to effectively protect their rights and health.

Services designed for the adults may not be truly accessible to the youth due to lack of privacy, social stigma, provider attitude and various factors. Therefore, there is a need to design and implement programs that have a holistic approach and meet the requirements of the youth.

The question is "not which is an ideal adolescent contraceptive, but which contraceptive is ideal for THIS adolescent?" Giving them a basket of choices and evaluating each adolescent individually will help in increasing the contraceptive usage and acceptance and hence, decrease the unmet need of contraception in them.

REFERENCES

1. The National Family Health Survey - NFHS -2
2. Shannon, A. et al. Advocating for Adolescent Reproductive Health in sub-Saharan Africa. Washington, DC: Advocates for Youth, 1998.
3. Oodit G, U Bhowon. The use of induced abortion in Mauritius. An alternative to fertlity regulation or an emergency procedure? In A Mundigo, C Indriso (Eds). Abortion in the developing world. Sage Publishers, New Delhi, 1999.
4. Kwon TH,KH Jun SN Cho Sexuality Contraception and abortion among unmarried adolescents and and young adults: The case of Korea. In: A Mundigo, C Indriso (Eds). Abortion in the developing world: Sage Publishers, New Delhi, 1999.
5. Ventura S, et al. Estimated pregnancy rates for the United States, 1990-2000: an update. Natl Vital Stat Rep. 2004; 52 (23):1-9.
6. Santelli JS, et al. Can changes in sexual behaviors among high school students explain the decline in teen pregnancy rates in the 1990s? J Adolesc Health. 2004; 35(2):80-90

7. Grimes DA, (Ed). Contraception and adolescents: highlights from the NASPAG conference. The Contraception Report, 1995;6:4-11.
8. Hatcher RA. Contraceptive Technology. ed, 17, NY: Ardent Media, Inc; 1998.
9. Grimes DA, (Ed). ARHP meeting highlights: the female condom. The Contraception Report. 1995; 5:4-17
10. Allan Guttmacher Institute. Sex and America's Teenagers. NY: The Allan Guttmacher Institute, 1994
11. Forrest JD, Singh S. The sexual and reproductive behavior of American women, 1982-1988. Fam Plann Perspect 1990; 22:206-14
12. ACOG Committee Opinion. Safety of Oral Contraceptives for Teenagers. 1991 (No. 90)
13. Shrikhande Laxmi. Low dose pill. Contraception. Past Present and Future. 1st edition 2006, Editors – Parihar Mandakini, Bhalerao- Gandhi Ashwini. Jaypee Publications
14. D. Pushpalata. Injectable contraceptive: Progesterone only injectables. Contraception: Past Present and Future. In: Parihar Mandakini. Bhalerao- Gandhi Ashwini. (Eds). Jaypee Publications 1st edition 2006.
15. Geeta Pandya. Evolution of Intra-uterine device – the Copper IUCD. Contraception...Past Present and Future. In: Parihar Mandakini, Bhalerao-Gandhi Ashwini (Eds). Jaypee Publications. 1st edition 2006.
16. Parihar Mandakini. Levonorgestrel Intrauterine system, the generation next IUCD. Contraception...Past Present and Future. 1st edition 2006, Editors – Parihar Mandakini, Bhalerao- Gandhi Ashwini. Jaypee Publications
17. Hatcher RA, Stewart F, Kowal D, Grant F, Stewart GK, Cates W. Contraceptive Technology, 1990-1992. New York, NY: Irvington Publishers; 1990
18. Trussel J, Stewart F. The effectiveness of postcoital hormonal contraception. Fam Plann Perspect. 1992; 24:262-64
19. Ashwini Bhalerao-Gandhi. Emergency Contraception. Contraception...Past Present and Future. In: Parihar Mandakini, Bhalerao-Gandhi Ashwini (Eds). Jaypee Publications 1st edition 2006.

16 Teen Pregnancy

Ritu Joshi, Adarsh Bhargava

INTRODUCTION

Pregnancy in adolescents is one of the main problems in the world with prevalence rate varying from 2-25% in different studies. Although pregnancy is an important part of women's lives both physically and psychologically, adolescents who become pregnant present their own set of physical, psychological, and sociological considerations. Although there is consensus that adolescent pregnancy involves great cost to society and some degree of risk to young women's well being, there is disagreement regarding the most appropriate way to manage this problem.

Many attempts to prevent early pregnancy have been thwarted by vested interest groups that may be well-meaning but are often misinformed. Educators, family planning counselors, and other professionals dealing with adolescent health care must be familiar with research that will enable them to provide sound information and guidance to help adolescents make informed decisions.

This is the target population which is prone to become pregnant after marriage or before marriage. They pose a problem to the society, a hazardous event to the obstetrician. The teenage mothers bear the brunt contributing to high maternal and peri-natal mortality and morbidity in our country.

DETERMINANTS OF ADOLESCENT HEALTH IN PREGNANCY

In recent years, the prevalence of adolescent pregnancy is increasing, probably due to low puberty age, early onset of sexual activity in girls and lack of education and lack of easy availability and acceptability of contraceptives. A large number of factors determine the pregnancy outcomes in adolescence. Although these are not unique to this age but are important from therapeutic point of view.

NUTRITIONAL DETERMINANTS

An adolescent girl is a child herself with significant nutritional requirements during adolescent growth spurt. In an adolescent mother who is likely to be already malnourished the competing nutritional needs of pregnancy and growth, will affect the growth of fetus and hence the birth weight of the child. Anemia and chronic energy deficiency are important consequences of pregnancy at this age.

Anemia

Anemia is one of the primary contributors to maternal mortality (20-25%) and is significantly associated with compromised pubertal growth spurt and cognitive development among girls aged 10-19 years. Prevalence of anemia ranges from 65-75% with age specific variations.

Chronic Energy Deficiency (CED)

Young adolescent mothers have a lower body mass index (BMI) since the BMI increases markedly during adolescence as pubertal changes occur. A low BMI status, indicative of chronic energy deficiency is a particularly important aspect of the nutritional risks to women, during reproductive years. The birth weights of newborns appear to be linearly correlated with both maternal body weights. The proportion of low birth weight infants increase among mothers with low BMI. There is also some evidence to indicate that poor maternal nutritional status, as exemplified by a low BMI, is associated with poor lactation performance and poorer growth in infants.

BIOLOGICAL DETERMINANTS

Maternal mortality has been reported to be higher in adolescent pregnancies with 380-645/100,000 live births for girls between 15 and 19 years while it is 250-342/100,000 live births for women aged 20-34 years. Biological factors responsible for this include:

Physical Maturity

The development of the pelvic birth canal is slower than that of the early teenage spurt of long bones. The birth canal does not reach its mature size until several years after growth in height has ceased by the age of 18 years. As a result cephalopelvic disproportion (CP) is the commonest problem encountered during labor in teenage pregnancies, as the pelvic architecture is not yet completely formed and mature enough for delivery. Significant incidence of prolonged/obstructed labor and hypotonic uterine contractions in adolescent pregnancies have been reported by Pachauri and Jamshedji.

Age

The mother's age confounds the risk of infant death as the infant mortality rate (IMR) for adolescent mothers is 40% higher than for older mothers. Several studies have shown a direct association between maternal age and low birth weight (LBW), the incidence being 47%in adolescent age group as compared to 34% in the 20-24 years age group. It is well documented that primigravidas pose a high obstetric risk. The vast majority of teenagers are primigravidas.

SOCIAL DETERMINANTS

These factors are particularly important in India and many developing countries and include the following.

Early Marriage

In most SAARC countries nearly 60% of girls are married by the age of 18 years with one fourth marrying by the age of 15 years. In India, every third adolescent girl in the age group of 15-19 years is married. Women who marry at young age are likely to find motherhood to be the sole focus of their lives, at the expense of development in other areas such as formal education, training for employment, work experience and personal growth.

Early Child Bearing

Nearly 58% of adolescents have commenced childbearing (NFHS-1). Only 7% adolescent females use contraception. The data may not reflect the actual situation as a substantial number of pregnancies in married and particularly unmarried girls go unreported because of the high rate of deliveries at home or in places other than institutional settings.

Literacy Status

Only 7% of married women in the age group of 15-19 years have attained a higher secondary level of education as reported by second National Family Health Survey of India. Low levels of literacy adversely affect reproductive and sexual health awareness and thus quality of life. Fifty two percent of illiterate mothers gave birth to low birth weight babies suggesting that education plays a considerable role in preventing LBW.

Socioeconomic Status

The lower socioeconomic status of the mother is also associated with low-birth-weight babies. Domestic responsibilities, working for livelihood, inadequate rest along with malnutrition especially when the energy demands are increased, contribute to a large number of women delivering low birth weight infants.

Gender Inequality

Gender disparities in feeding patterns are widespread in India and take their toll on the growth of adolescent girls.

IMPACT OF ADOLESCENT PREGNANCY ON MOTHER AND CHILD

There are a large number of consequences of adolescent age on pregnancy outcomes with an increased incidence of the following:

- Anemia during antenatal and postnatal period.
- Pregnancy induced hypertension, pre-eclampsia.
- HIV: higher incidence of mother to child transmission.
- Higher severity of malaria and intercurrent infections.
- Obstructed labor.
- Preterm birth, Low-birth-weight babies and increased perinatal and neonatal mortality.
- Postpartum depression, inadequate child care and breast feeding practices.

Table 16.1: Percentage distribution of deaths due to causes related to child-birth and pregnancy recorded in the survey of causes of death

Causes	*1995**	*2001***
Abortion	17.6	19.8%
Toxemia	7.9	12-40%
Anemia	17.0	21.3%
Bleeding of pregnancy and puerperium	28.9	4-10%
Malposition of child leading to death of mother	4.0	6.0%
Puerperial sepsis	8.5	10.2%
Not classifiable	14.1	18%

Data source * UNFPA 1995, **Bhargava A. unpublished

- Children of teenage mothers are at a greater risk of behavior disorders, difficulties in school and engage in substance abuse.

COURSE OF PREGNANCY AND LABOR

There are multiple problems in the antenatal, intranatal and postnatal periods in adolescent pregnancy and include the following:

Problems in the Antenatal Period

1. *Pregnancy-induced Hypertension:* Studies report an increased incidence of the condition in young adolescents, when compared with older women.
2. *Anemia:* There is an increased risk of anemia in adolescents because of nutritional deficiencies, especially of iron and folic acid, and by malarial and intestinal parasites.
3. *Sexually transmitted infections and HIV:* Sexually active adolescents are at an increased risk of contracting STIs, including HIV infection, owing to their biological and social vulnerability. There is also the increased risk of mother to child transmission of HIV in adolescents, because the HIV infection is more likely to be recent, and therefore associated with higher viral load. The presence of other STI's (syphilis, gonorrhea and Chlamydia) with local inflammation may increase viral shedding, thereby increasing the risk of transmission during labor.
4. *Greater severity of malaria:* This is often seen in first time pregnant women (which includes many adolescents) and is a common cause of anemia in this group. This puts them at a risk and also their unborn babies at risk of intrauterine death.

Problems during Labor and Delivery

1. Preterm birth: This is common in women under twenty years of age because of immaturity of the reproductive organs, social factors such as poverty at play.

2. Obstructed labor: In young girls (below 15 years of age) this occurs due to the small size of the birth canal leading to cephalopelvic disproportion.
3. Lack of access to medical and surgical care can result in complications like vesico-vaginal and recto-vaginal fistulae and other birth injuries like cervical, vaginal and perineal tears and lacerations.
4. Above 15 years of age there is a general consensus that teenage mothers usually deliver spontaneously by the vaginal route, a few needing outlet forceps for cutting down the second stage. But incidence of cesarean sections among teenage mothers has varied from 1-6% according to Sinclair (1952) and Ghosh and Ghosh (1976).

Problems in Postpartum Period

1. Anemia is commoner and further aggrevated by blood loss during pregnancy thereby also increasing the risk of infection.
2. Pre-eclampsia– several studies report that pre-eclampsia occurs more often in young adolescents. The symptoms may worsen and at times be recognized only during the first postpartum days.
3. Postpartum depression and common mental health problems are common due to reasons described earlier. An indifferent attitude towards the neonate is common from such child mother.
4. Too early and repeat pregnancies, especially in unmarried adolescents can occur because of the difficulties in accessing reliable contraception.

Fetal and Neonatal Outcome of Teenage Pregnancy

1. Low birth weight: There is a higher incidence of low birth weight (weight < 2500 g) among infant of adolescent mothers.
2. Perinatal and neonatal mortality is increased.
3. Inadequate child care and breast feeding practices: young mothers, especially those who are single and poor, may find it hard to provide their children with adequate care. This is reflected in their poor child feeding, including breastfeeding practices.

CONSEQUENCES OF PREGNANCY IN THE UNMARRIED ADOLESCENT

There could be multiple consequences that include physical, psychological, social and economic. Some of the consequences include:

1. Higher incidence of complications of pregnancy due to lack of ANC attendance.
2. Resorts to illegal and unsafe abortions with their associated complications.
3. Ill-health or death due to complications of unsafe abortions, birth injuries and haemorrhage.
4. Guilt and depression due to social stigma.
5. Chronic illness and infertility due to complications of abortion.
6. Limited knowledge and access to contraceptive services results in early repeated pregnancy.

PREVENTION OF ADOLESCENT PREGNANCY

There are many single interventions but none alone can be effective. A multipronged strategy is required. Some of the factors that need focus in India and developing countries include:

- Educating the masses.
- Boys should be trained to respect the decision of the girl if she says 'No'.
- Provide health education
  - Information regarding problems of pregnancy in adolescents.
  - Skills to say 'NO' to sex by creative thinking, e.g. excuses like having periods, value system of family, etc.
  - Inform about contraceptive choices.
  - Inform about available services and how to access them.
  - Inform about dangers of seeking help from unskilled people.

- When pregnant, discuss about the merits involving parents/ guardians in further management.

AREAS OF CONCERN FOR THE OBSTETRICIAN

Multiple areas of concern exist for proper management of adolescent pregnancy. The concerns range from early diagnosis of pregnancy to optimal antenatal care and avoidance of obstetric complications. Optimal antenatal care include at least three antenatal check-ups. By good antenatal services complications can be diagnosed early and many can be avoided also.

Counseling during pregnancy should be mandatory for pregnant adolescents. A Sympathetic attitude towards their queries to be maintained and knowledge about postpartum care, breastfeeding and contraception should be emphasized.

KEY MESSAGES

1. An adolescent is a 'child', any pregnancy in this age is a 'child' pregnancy.
2. Adolescent pregnancy is common in India.
3. Many factors contribute to adolescent pregnancy that are mainly social and economic.
4. Adolescents with undernutrition and a high incidence of anemia are not prepared to undertake marriage and child bearing.
5. Adolescent under nutrition leads to an intergenerational effect "small mothers give birth to small babies who in turn grow into small mothers and so on".
6. An increase in maternal mortality and low birth weight, are the major adverse outcomes of adolescent pregnancies.
7. Many of the complications during pregnancy and delivery have worse outcomes in adolescents.
8. There is no long-term follow-up data on the outcome of the teenage pregnancy in Indian scenario but it is a well known fact that the overall morbidity and infant mortality among low birth weight babies are higher compared to normal babies.
9. There are important issues for health-care providers to be aware of while caring for adolescents throughout pregnancy, labour, delivery and the postpartum period.

SUGGESTED READING

1. AK Dutta, Harish K Pemde. Teenage mothers and their infants. In: Bhave's Text Book of Adolescent Medicine. Swati Y Bhave (Ed.) New Delhi: Jaypee Brothers 1st edn. 2006;178-83.
2. Fillippi V, Ronsmans C, Campbell OMR, Graham WJ, Mills A, Borghi J, Koblinsky M, Ostin D. Maternal health in poor countries: the broader context and a call for action. Lancet 2006; 368:1535-41.
3. Indian Institute of Population Studies, National Family Health Survey - 1, Mumbai 1992-93. Available from: http/www.nfhs india.org/data. Accessed November 1, 2003.
4. Mehra S, Agarwal D. Adolescent health determinants of pregnancy and child health outcomes among urban poor. Indian Pediat 2004; 41:137-45.
5. Roy TK, Arnold F, Kulkarni S, Kishor S, Gupta K, Mishra V. National Family Health Survey–2. International Institute for Population Sciences and ORG. Macro. Bombay, India., 2000; 58.
6. UNFPA. Adolescents in India: A Profile. UNFPA for UN System in India, 2004.

17 Unsafe Abortions

Ashwini Bhalerao-Gandhi, Papia Goswami-Mukherjee

INTRODUCTION

Youth around the world stand poised on the brink of a new millennium. The current generation of 10 to 19 years olds will be the largest generation in history, to make the transition from youth to adults. For young women, the years of adolescent transition are especially vital, as this is when sexual relationships, marriage and child bearing are likely to begin. Regardless of marital status, some adolescent women, who do not want to bear a child, do become pregnant. Unprotected sexual activity among adolescent girls often ends up in an unwanted pregnancy, which can be an emotionally wrenching experience. Frightened with such an unwanted pregnancy, a young adolescent girl may choose to terminate it, often through clandestine procedures by unskilled providers and under unsanitary conditions. Each year more than 75 million women worldwide experience an unintended pregnancy. An estimated 20 million of these resort to unsafe abortions, resulting in 80,000 maternal deaths and many more injuries. Approximately, 2 million adolescents risk unsafe abortions annually in the developing world, accounting for a third of hospitalizations for abortion related complications (UNFPA 1998).

INCIDENCE OF ABORTIONS IN ADOLESCENTS

Many young women become sexually active during adolescence, even if they are not married. In most of the countries of Sub-Saharan Africa, more than 70% of young women are sexually active during adolescence. Throughout the nations of North Africa, Middle East and most Asian Countries, a young woman is supposed to have sexual relationship only after she has married. The rates of sexual activity among unmarried adolescents are very low in these countries, like in India less than 10% of young girls report sexual activity, in Japan 11% of female college students report having sex before age of seventeen, although by age of eighteen about 26% have sexual relationship (The Alan Guttmacher institute 1998)[1].

INDUCED ABORTION IN ADOLESCENTS – AN ISSUE OF GLOBAL CONCERN

Unwanted pregnancy in adolescents is associated with apprehension, fear and misconception. A sizable subgroup of adolescents seek medical care late in pregnancy, often during the second trimester, due to failure to realize that they are pregnant, concealment of pregnancy and conflict with parents.[2]

To gain access to the services, this age group must surmount large obstacles like cultural attitudes, cost, travel, judgmental staff and lack of confidentiality.[3] After all these obstacles, the practitioner may not always be prompt to terminate the pregnancy due to delays for thorough investigations or hesitancy to perform the procedure for fear of medicolegal difficulties. This accounts for high incidence of second trimester terminations which have a four fold increase in complications as compared to early procedures.

Some of the induced abortions are legal whereas many are carried out illegally by unskilled providers. Women who resort to unsafe abortions put their health and lives at risk. Even where legally available, abortion remains a highly controversial procedure in much of the world, making accurate information on its prevalence difficult to obtain. Providers may be reluctant to admit that they perform abortions, and women, even those who have obtained abortions legally and safely, may be unwilling to report that they have undergone the procedure.

In recognition of the fact that most abortion–related deaths are preventable, the 1994 International Conference on Population and Development made the following recommendations (ICPD 1994).

- Access to compassionate, quality services for the management of complications arising from abortion.
- Post abortion counseling, education and family services to reduce recourse to repeat abortion.
- Where abortion is legal, access to safe induced– abortion services.

With adolescent pregnancies attracting a disproportionately higher risk of complications, these guidelines are far more relevant and demand application.

DEFINITION OF UNSAFE ABORTION

According to WHO (1993)[4], unsafe abortion is defined as "an abortion not provided through approved facilities and/or persons". What constitutes approved facilities and/ or persons will vary according to the legal and medical standards of each country. The definition does not take into consideration differences in quality, services available or the other substantial differences between health systems. Unsafe abortions are characterized by lack or inadequacy of skills of the provider, hazardous techniques and unsanitary facilities (Report of technical working group Geneva, 1992).

INDICATIONS

Unwanted pregnancy is the commonest indication for the termination of pregnancy. Lack of education, failure of contraception, financial constrain, rape and sexual relations by unmarried girls are the main factors in becoming pregnant. Social ostracism, parental disapproval, financial dependence and fear of the burden of maternity lead these young girls to opt for termination of pregnancy.

METHODS USED FOR UNSAFE ABORTIONS

Adolescent women may seek advice from traditional healers or local village "experts" on how to terminate their pregnancies. Unsafe abortions may be induced by the woman herself, by non-medical persons or by health workers in unhygienic conditions.

In attempting to self-abort, they may resort to taking a wide range of chemical agents including consuming large doses of chloroquine, drinking quinine, ergot, mercury, gasoline or toxic teas.

Abortions may be induced by insertion of a solid object (usually root, twig, or catheter) into the uterus, an improperly performed dilatation and curettage or exertion of external force. Some untrained practitioners roughly massage their abdomens or scrape out the contents of their uterus with unclean instruments.

HEALTH HAZARDS AND COMPLICATIONS OF UNSAFE ABORTIONS

Unsafe abortion is one of the most neglected problems of health care in developing countries and a serious concern to women during their reproductive lives.

Most married women seek abortion to limit family size or to space births. However in all parts of the world, particularly in urban areas, increasing proportions of those having abortions are unmarried adolescents, and in some urban centers they rèpresent majority of all abortion seekers.

The mortality and morbidity risks of induced abortions depend upon the facilities and skills of the abortion provider, method used, general condition of the woman, presence of reproductive tract infections and STDs, age and stage of pregnancy. Variety of severe complications occur following unsafe abortions. Severe complications like sepsis, hemorrhage, genital and abdominal trauma, perforated uterus or poisoning can lead to death if left untreated. Death can also result from secondary complications like gas gangrene and renal failure.

Unsafe clandestine abortions endanger the health or the very life of these young women. Terminating pregnancy in a nulliparous patient is relatively difficult and involves greater risks as compared to inducing abortions in a multipara. Also adolescent girls have higher incidence of second trimester abortions which carry greater health risks than early abortion.

PSYCHOLOGICAL ASPECTS

Adolescents are mentally immature to understand the consequences of their own acts. An unplanned pregnancy can be more frightening for a teenage girl, who may be unprepared to raise a child.

In a study on differential impact of abortion in adolescents and adults, adolescents were significantly more likely to feel dissatisfied with the choice of abortion services and, being forced by various social circumstances, they reported greater severity of psychological stress.[5]

UNSAFE ABORTIONS-INDIAN SCENARIO

The incidence of early marriage and sexual experience is quite high among adolescents in India. About 20 percent girls are already married while they are still in their teens, and many get pregnant. It is estimated that a majority of these pregnancies are unwanted and about 40 percent of all teenage pregnancies end in abortions.

However, some may be forced to continue pregnancy due to family and social pressures. A majority of adolescents do not seek contraception until they are sexually active for quite some time, in some cases up to 15-16 months after initiating sexual intercourse due to genuine ignorance, fear of parental discovery, myths of negative health consequences related to contraceptives and lack of access to newer, safer contraceptives especially in rural India.

In 1971, India became one of the countries in the world to pass legislation granting liberal, social, socioeconomical and medical grounds for the termination of an unwanted pregnancy. This legislation known as the Medical Termination of Pregnancy Act of 1971, was the government's response to the high incidence of illegal abortions taking place in India in 1960s and 1970s with grave consequences to maternal health and well-being including deaths.

Paradoxically in 1990s many more illegal abortions may be taking place than at the time of legalization. Most of these are to terminate unplanned, unwanted pregnancies. Even more distressing is the indication that illegal and backstreet abortions outnumber the legal procedures by a ratio of as much as 11-1 (Nuna and Chhabra 1995)[6], with high maternal mortality and morbidity.

According to WHO over 20,000 Indian women die of unsafe abortions every year. Global studies estimate that out of 15 million illegal abortions world wide, 4 million, the highest for any country take place in India. In 1995 the Ford Foundation study puts the figure for India at 9 million. Abortion is one of the most neglected health issues in India and women are paying a terrible price. Abortion as a cause of maternal death which was 5% in mid 1980s is at present 15% (Ford Foundation study, Chhabra 1995).[9]

Reasons for high mortality include shortage of adequately trained personnel and surgical facilities as well as recourse to highly dangerous methods of unsafe and illegal abortion. Services for MTP are mainly available at district hospitals and some community health centers. They are rarely available at primary health centers. Equipment and training are required on a large scale to make MTP services more available, complemented by efforts to inform women of their availability and making them aware that MTP is legal and safe and that such services are rendered free of charge.

LEGAL BARRIERS

Laws and policies that restrict safe induced abortion generally have the effect of creating barriers to safe abortion-related care. Even where abortion laws are less restrictive, abortion services are not always available to women, let alone adolescent women.

In India, even when the termination of adolescent pregnancies has been adequately covered by the protective umbrella of the MTP Act 1971 and abortion has been legal since 1972, limited availability and poor quality of services have kept many women from receiving safe abortion care.

Providers may be biased against adolescents, imposing moral judgments instead of providing them with the health care they need. As noted previously, adolescent women are also discouraged from seeking care for fear that providers will not respect confidentiality.

CONCLUSIONS

In India, adolescent marriages and adolescent fertility rates are disturbingly high. Premarital sexual activity has become a reality in every strata of the society. Adolescent girls have hardly any access to reproductive information as well as counseling, and are mostly excluded from free contraceptive services. It is high time we accept this reality, and understand the reproductive rights of our adolescent girls and offer them counseling as well as easily accessible quality services related to reproduction, contraception and safe-induced abortion. With changing times, economic liberalization, changing moral and social cultures, more and more adolescent girls are going to be sexually active, irrespective of their marital status. By giving them advice regarding safe sex and contraception we will help them prevent unplanned and unwanted pregnancies and also reduce the incidence of 'Unsafe Abortions', thus protecting their reproductive rights.

REFERENCES

1. The Alan Guttemacher Institute –'Into a new world'. Young womens' sexual and reproductive lives, The Alan Guttemacher Institute, 120 Wall Street, New York, 1998.
2. Chaudhari SK: Pregnancy termination. In Choudhury SK (Ed): Practice of Fertility Control-A Complete Text Book BI Churchill Livingston, 1996;207.
3. Graham A: Contraceptive clinics for adolescents. In Fox R (Ed): IPPF Medical Bulletin 1998;32(3): 4.
4. WHO/FHE/MSM/93-13, Abortion – Frequency and mortality of unsafe abortion. 2nd Edition, 1993.
5. Franz W et al: Differential impact of abortion in adolescents. Adolescence Spring 1992;27(105): 16-72.
6. Sheel C. Nuna, Rami Chhabra. Abortion in India an "Overview" R. Chhabra and S. Nuna, (Eds) Introduction, Veerendra Printers, New Delhi. page No. IV, 1995
7. Chhabra R Ford Foundation Study Abortion in India an overview". R. Chhabra, S. C. Nuna (Eds), veerendra printers, New Delhi.

18 Safe Abortions in Adolescent Girls

Jaydeep Tank, Parikshit Tank

INTRODUCTION

Teenage sexual activity is prevalent and comes with an expensive price tag – an unintended pregnancy.

An unplanned pregnancy can be emotionally wrenching for any woman, and it can be frightening for an adolescent, who may be unprepared to raise a child. In such circumstances, a young woman may choose to terminate an unwanted pregnancy.

Providing comprehensive abortion care for the adolescent goes beyond the technical aspects of an MTP. There are various issues such as the need for service provision and access, pre- and post-abortion counseling and contraceptive coverage.

INCIDENCE

In developed countries, safe abortions are available easily and the incidence reported varies from 3 procedures annually per 1000 women aged 15 to 19 years in Germany to 36 per 1000 adolescents in the United States.[1] In developing countries, safe abortions are far more difficult to come by especially for the youth.

PRE-ABORTION COUNSELING

A complete clinical evaluation is mandatory before any abortion procedure.

- Ultrasound is not required unless the gestational age is in doubt.
- Anemia is prevalent in adolescents and it is useful to check hemoglobin levels.
- Blood group should be checked and rhesus prophylaxis provided as indicated.
- Adolescents are a high-risk group in terms of sexual behaviour and drug abuse.[2] There should be counseling about sexually transmitted infections and HIV.
- The use of antibiotic prophylaxis, especially before a surgical abortion is indicated.

METHODS FOR SAFE ABORTION

The WHO, in its Technical and Policy guidance for health systems has set out the standard methods for performing medical termination of

Upto 9 weeks	*9 to 12 weeks*	*Beyond 12 weeks*
Manual vacuum aspiration	Manual vacuum aspiration	Prostaglandins or analogues
Medical abortion	Electric vacuum aspiration	Mifepristone followed by prostaglandins
Electric vacuum aspiration		Dilatation and evacuation

pregnancy.[3] This applies in equal measures to adults and adolescents. Age is not a barrier for the use of any method of abortion.

FIRST TRIMESTER

VACUUM ASPIRATION

Can be performed in the first trimester by electric or manual devices. The manual vacuum aspirator (MVA) is an excellent example of appropriate technology in the first trimester. It is a sturdy and simple equipment which can be sterilized and reused a number of times. The inherent safety of the device lies in the automatic vacuum cut off.

Where as an electric pump will continue build vacuum until it is switched off, the syringe is self-limited. This does not compromise the vacuum efficacy in any way. The MVA has a short learning curve. After loading the syringe and dilating the cervix, the cannula is inserted into the uterine cavity. On releasing the pinch valve, a rotatory motion will ensure that the pregnancy is aspirated into the syringe. There is no need for a curettage after this if signs of uterine evacuation are present.

In the younger, nulliparous women, complications of surgical abortion are related to the difficulty in negotiating the cervical canal. By priming the cervix with prostaglandins, dilatating the cervix becomes much simpler and often the canula can be inserted directly. This can be in the form of 400 micrograms of vaginal or oral misoprostol or 125 to 250 micrograms of carboprost administered intramuscularly.

Complementary use of medical and surgical methods can make abortion even safer.[4]

Medical Abortion

According to the RCOG, medical abortion is the most effective method of terminating pregnancy in the first 7 weeks.[5] Abortion with pills is allowed in our country up to 7 weeks from the date of the last menstrual period.

All the legal requirements including consent and backup facilities at a recognized center for performing MTP should be fulfilled before embarking on a medical MTP. Counseling is vital for women undergoing the procedure. Women need to be explained about the safety and efficacy of the procedure, how much bleeding to expect and when to follow-up.

They should be made aware that there may be occasional problems such as an unsuccessful procedure where one would resort to a surgical method.

Today, evidence supports the use of 200 mg of mifepristone rather than the earlier recommendations of 600 mg. This should be followed by misoprostol (800 micrograms vaginally or 400 micrograms orally) after 48 hours. The efficacy of this regimen is 94 to 97%.

Care providers should ensure suitable selection of cases especially with regards to the gestational age. There should be a mechanism to check the completeness of the procedure.

Abortions by the surgical and medical methods are comparable in efficacy. A surgical abortion is available till 12 weeks of pregnancy and requires only one visit.

Medical abortion has the advantage of avoiding anesthesia and surgical complications, demedicalizing the process and possibly being more confidential. All things being equal, the choice of method should be with the adolescent.

SECOND TRIMESTER

Till a few years ago, the method of choice for second trimester abortions was the extra-amniotic instillation of ethacridine lactate. Prostaglandins were used in conjunction to decrease the induction-abortion interval and post-abortal bleeding.[6]

Today the method of choice is vaginal misoprostol, 400 micrograms administered every three hours, to a maximum of five doses results in complete abortion in 90% of women in the second trimester.[7] The efficacy and safety of the drug is becoming well established.

Surgical methods of pregnancy termination in the second trimester have been marginalized. Hysterotomy is obsolete as a primary method today. Dilatation and suction evacuation is rarely required. It should be attempted only in the early part of the second trimester by an experienced practitioner preferably under ultrasound guidance. The standard of care for terminating a second trimester pregnancy is by medical methods.[5]

POSTABORTION COUNSELING

Prevention of teenage pregnancy is a desirable objective. Young people often know of modern methods, but may lack access or information for proper use. A "belt and suspender" approach to contraception with barrier and hormonal contraception is useful to prevent sexually transmitted infections and pregnancy.

LEGAL ASPECTS OF MTP IN ADOLESCENTS

The MTP Act is an empowering Act and allows for termination of pregnancy under specific conditions. To be protected by the Act, the practitioner should follow it in all respects. With reference to adolescents, the issues that arise are regarding age, consent and the guardian. There is no requirement for legal documentation of age. In the case of a minor(less than 18 years), consent will have to be obtained from the guardian. The concept of guardian as per the Act is amorphous at best.

CONCLUSIONS

Premarital sexual activity is a reality in every strata of society. The ideal goal of sex education for all, provision of contraception and the knowledge to use it is not always achievable. MTP in adolescents thus becomes a safety net to protect them from the hazards of unsafe abortion or early parenthood. We must bear in mind that MTP should remain a safety net and not become a method of contraception.

REFERENCES

1. Lanham MD. United Nations Educational, Scientific and Cultural Organization (UNESCO) Statistical Year Book, 1996. Bernan Press, 1996.
2. Thomas A, Forster G, Robinson A, et al. National Guideline on the Management of Suspected Sexually Transmitted Infections in Children and Young People. http://www.bashh.org/ceguidelines.html. 2002.
3. WHO: Safe Abortion. Technical and Policy Guidance for Health Systems. World Health Organisation, 2003, Geneva.
4. Singh K, Fong YF. Preparation of the cervix for surgical termination of pregnancy in the first trimester. Hum Reprod Update, 2000;6:442-8.
5. Royal College of Obstetricians and Gynaecologists. The care of women requesting induced abortion. National Evidence Based Guideline. London: RCOG; 2004.
6. Second trimester pregnancy termination using extra-amniotic ethacridine lactate. Bhathena RK, Sheriar NK, Walvekar VR, et al. BJOG 1990;97:1026-29.
7. Stubblefield PG, Carr-Ellis S, Borgatta L. Methods for induced abortion. Obstet Gynecol 2004;104:174-85.

19 Controversy Related to Consent Issues

Manisha Macha

INTRODUCTION

When we are discussing the controversies related to issues of consent and confidentiality in adolescents it will be more meaningful if we discuss some case scenarios.

Case 1: Radha, a 15-year-old girl approached a family planning clinic, unaware about the physical changes in her body that had taken place during last few weeks. She was brought by her friend on knowing that she had missed her period. On probing by the doctor, she opened the secret that she was being used by one of the family friend who used to visit her family occasionally. Radha was denied the abortion services in absence of the mother or relative to sign the consent form.

Case 2: A 13-year-old girl was brought with 6 months (24 weeks) pregnancy by her father who works as ward boy at Municipal Hospital. On repeated questioning the girl admitted that she was lured by the neighbor's driver. She worked as a domestic help full time, mother being away at native place. The girl did not realize the seriousness of the situation that she will deliver within 3 months.

Case 3: A 17-year-old unmarried girl brought by her mother (who runs *Khanawal* - a tiffin service for workers) with 20 weeks of pregnancy. Mother said she had been ignorant about her daughter's missing periods. The girl with great difficulty admitted that one of the *Khanawal* members had regular sexual relations with her in the absence of her mother. But after learning about her pregnancy he has disappeared.

Case 4: A lady brought her domestic help – 18-year-old girl for missing her periods. On examination she was found to be 8 weeks pregnant. On insisting on detailed history she finally gave the name of her "Saheb" – responsible for her pregnancy. She said please do not disclose this to "Memsaheb" or else I will lose my job.

In each of these cases, there are striking similarities in the underlying factors. They are all young girls, unmarried, with little or no knowledge on sexual reproduction, and abused by people known to them in a way. And, all of them were left pregnant at the end of it. Many more such adolescent girls face similar problems either due to lack of awareness and curiosity about sexual relationship and sometimes due to sexual abuse. They land up with unwanted pregnancies resulting in seeking abortion legally or illegally.

ISSUES SURROUNDING ABORTION

Considering that 'adolescence' is a critical period for preparation for adulthood, and that young people hold the country's future in their hands, the needs of adolescents and young adults can no longer be ignored. Lack of knowledge about reproductive health and lack of healthy attitudes towards sexuality, coupled with societal and cultural pressures make the youth more susceptible to reproductive health risks. This results in higher rate of maternal morbidity and mortality, unwanted pregnancies, increased rate of unsafe abortion. Understanding the extent to which young people know about risks of unsafe abortion, and use of contraceptives is therefore, a major concern for policy makers.

Lack of awareness about sexual and reproductive health issues among both the adolescents and parents create further taboo about the subject. Neither the adolescent nor their parents are able to discuss about the subject openly.

In one of the survey surveys carried out by Family Planning Association of India in Pune to assess the knowledge, behavior and attitudes about sexuality among youth, reveals that only 10 percent of boys' parents could discuss issues like masturbation, night emission, sexual intercourse and other related matter with their sons. About 20 percent of girls' parents were able to discuss sex related issues with their daughters. This clearly indicates that many times the young adolescent do not know several issues pertaining to their reproductive health and the consequences of their behavior resulting in unwanted pregnancies. It is interesting to study typical responses of parents to sex education (as documented in the 'SAATHI' Project report implemented by FPA India).

"Eating, sleeping and sex act ——are not to be taught…it comes naturally"

"They will learn everything after marriage why spoil them now"

"Media People are already spoiling our children you too join the wagon"

"If we talk to them about sex and sexuality we shall loose the respect we command from the youth"

"These are essential aspects of every body's life, but exposure to these issues must be at the right age"

Whether it is consensual or forced sex, the adolescent girls end up with pregnancies. However, the issue becomes even more serious when the girl in the question is unmarried. Without societal sanction, parental approval and institutional neglection, unwanted pregnancies put these adolescents in grave danger, that can be life-threatening. Women aged 15-19 account for at least 5 million of the estimated 20 million unsafe abortions that occur each year. They also make up about a quarter of the nearly 70,000 women who die every year from abortion related causes.[1] There is evidence that, in urban area unsafe abortion and abortion related death are rising among unmarried adolescent women.[2]

Almost one third of India's population is young and has significant needs related to sexual and reproductive health. This population has not been given adequate attention in the past through public delivered programs by either education or women and child development department or for that matter even health and family welfare department. The period of adolescent is increasingly recognized as a universal life phase, in which young people are especially vulnerable to health risks, particularly related to sex and reproduction. Nearly 20% of 1.5 million girls under the age of 15 years are already mothers (Census 2001). In many places, young people are becoming sexually active at younger ages or are more likely to experience sexual activity outside of marriage. As per the country paper by Ministry of Health and Family Welfare 1998, 20-30% of males and 10% of females are estimated to be sexually active before marriage. This sexual activity is increasingly occurring in the midst of an HIV pandemic that disproportionately affects youth under 24 years of ages.

NON-CONSENSUAL SEXUAL ACTIVITY AMONG ADOLESCENTS

As many studies acknowledge that as a taboo subject, sexual violence is rarely reported or studied. Hence, it is difficult to estimate how many young people suffer from sexual abuse, violence, coercion, incest, rape or sexual trafficking, yet there is no denying the fact. One of the key issues among adolescents is the non-consensual or forced sex, and their consequences. Studies report that adolescents may be more likely to experience sexual violence than older women. A street children study in Bangalore by Ramakrishna et'al' found that some 74 of 121 street boys aged 9–21 were sexually experienced and 40 had their first sexual experience by age 12. A large proportion of boys reported coercive experiences, both as victims and perpetrators, often involving exchange of money, gifts or other favours, as well as physical force. Sexual coercion is so pervasive on the streets that street boys rated rape and forced sex as among the most pleasurable ways of seeking sexual gratification.

Another study by Sodhi and Verma among low-income adolescents in Delhi stated that 32 out of 71 youth interviewed described widespread verbal harassment of women, sexual coercion, including forced sex. A study of 811 higher secondary school children with an average age of 16 revealed that nearly one-third of students—both male and female—reported a coercive experience in the past year, and 6% reported forced sexual intercourse.

Disturbing findings of these studies strongly underline a need for cohesive national level framework for providing SRH services, education, timely assistance in abortions, and an institutional support system for the affected.

NO HELP ON HAND

Adolescent tends to delay obtaining an abortion and often seek help from a non-medical provider, leading to higher rates of complications. Self-induced abortion is also common in many countries.[3] It is important to influence the health seeking behavior of adolescent in order for next decade to witness the rapid improvement in the health indicators. An analysis of the sexual and reproductive health needs of adolescents reveals several issues that pertain to both unmarried and married girls and boys.

i. There is a lack of representative data on the SRH needs of adolescents as evidence comes largely from the micro studies.
ii. Prevalent sociocultural norms constrain adolescent in many ways through restricted mobility of girls, early marriage and limited access to information and services, lack of parental support and gender discrimination.
iii. Issue of lack of underutilization of services resulting from myths and misconceptions, insufficient economic resources, absence of support from family and service providers
iv. Lack of privacy and judgmental attitudes of service providers contribute to limited access of adolescents to services.

THE UNMET NEED

The unmarried adolescents remain out of the ambit of family welfare programs in terms of contraceptive access and services, particularly the abortion services. Prevalent sociocultural norms constrain adolescents from seeking help. For instance, unmarried pregnant girl faces shame, social isolation, interruption of school or employment, increased economic hardship and diminished opportunity to marry. For these reasons abortion is the most common solution to an unwanted pregnancy for an unmarried adolescent girl in most part of the world.[4]

Reproductive health needs especially adolescent reproductive health needs, are poorly understood and addressed in India. Studies addressing issues of sexual behavior in general and adolescent sexual behavior in particular are few and mainly exploratory. Further, there is no precise estimate of the total number of induced abortions in India because government data only account for abortions performed in government-approved facilities, which are a fraction of the total number of abortions that occur every year.[5] Very few studies represent the rural populations or low income adolescence. At the same time, studies have varying methodologies, and there are questions about the potential biases and how representative the findings are and the reliability of responses in a population as conservative as in India (Jejeebhoy 2000).

ADOLESCENT ABORTION—A NEGLECTED ISSUE

Although enough has been debated about the abortion among the adolescent, not much has been done to increase access of SRH services to adolescent. While government and NGOs increasingly addressing prevention of adolescent pregnancies, a gap exists in policy making and programming to address the consequences of unwanted pregnancies, including abortion related care.

Even when abortion is legal, the procedure may be expensive or too difficult for an adolescent to obtain without the involvement of family or neighbors. As a result regardless of abortion's legal status, non-married adolescent girls most often seek unsafe abortion services from non-medical providers.[6]

One also needs to understand that young women from low socioeconomic status are at an increased risk of injury and death due to unsafe abortion in comparison to others. Teenage abortion patients are almost twice as likely to experience cervical lacerations during abortion compared to older women. This increased risk is thought to be due to the fact that teens have a smaller cervix which is more difficult to dilate or grasp with instruments. They are also at higher risk for postabortion infections such as pelvic inflammatory diseases (PID). Researchers believe that teens may be more susceptible to infections because their bodies are not fully developed.[7]

LEGAL QUAGMIRE

That safe abortion services must be promoted particularly for adolescent girl and services must be accessible, cannot be emphasized enough. However, for such a policy framework to exist, the laws must be progressive, humane and contextual. Increasing number of adolescents experiencing sex before marriage and gradually diminishing average age of first sexual experience, both demand recognition. Combined with prevalence of STIs and HIV/AIDS, lackadaisical policy approach can create a huge public health issue in India.

Though Indian MTP Act has made abortion legal in India, there are several clauses in the Act that makes it restrictive. For instance, Act requires the consent of the parent or guardian for abortion if an adolescent girl is below 18 years of age. This can be a challenge. For example, at the Kutumb Sudhar Kendra (Family Planning clinic) of FPA India, adolescent girls who visited the clinic to seek the abortion services always faced difficulties as they never wanted their mother to be aware of the pregnancy.

There also used to be the fear of loosing job, since they were working as domestic workers and pregnancy occurred as the male in the family abused the adolescent girl. Even if in the best interest of the child one wants to help the teenage girl, the law creates barriers. On the other hand, the confidentiality is at stake if the issue is disclosed to the parents, which also is against the ethics of the organization. In such circumstances the service providers cannot do much other than referring the girl.

Studies have also shown that the major factors that affect seeking abortion services are the stigma attached to it, the fear of abuse by the parents.

The rights of young people to reproductive health education and services are recognized in international treaties and agreements, for example the Convention on the Rights of Child. In many countries young people's rights are still a controversial issue and parents are considered to be responsible for informing their children about sex and personal relationship.

However, many parents around the world are unable or unwilling to provide this information to their children. Those opposed to sexuality education and services for adolescents often state that it increases the sexual activity of young people. However, the WHO and UNAIDS surveys clearly indicate that there is no evidence for this.[8]

ROLE OF GOVERNMENT AND NGOs

The Program of Action adopted at the International Conference on Population and Development (ICPD) in Cairo in 1994 stipulates a number of objectives and action related to sexual and reproductive health and rights.

The ICPD Program of Action was the first international document to explicitly affirm the concept of reproductive rights, which provided a 20-year plan of action agreed by 179 countries. As part of this POA, abortion and adolescent are considered as the major segment that demands an immediate attention.

India being the signatory to these international treaties, many steps have been taken in the above direction by the Ministry of Health and Family Welfare, yet much needs to be done.

- The government should recognize that adolescent have more unwanted pregnancies. In order to eliminate unsafe abortion and early childbirth, there is need to ensure access to legal and safe abortion services for adolescents.[9]
- Rather than mandating parental involvement, government should ensure that health care providers are trained to assess the capability of adolescents to make reasonable, independent, and confidential decisions regarding their reproductive health.
- Government should also ensure that adolescent have access to appropriate high quality abortion services. Women's health care services should be equipped to meet the health needs of adolescents. In addition, health professionals should be trained to provide information to adolescents about preventing and terminating pregnancy.
- The NGOs must ensure to have sexuality education as part of their programs for young people. They must also establish linkages with other GO/NGOs for the services for adolescents and to create advocacy for the rights of adolescents.
- The health professionals may create a dialogue with parents of adolescents particularly those who are regular visitors to the clinics. Also IEC material on SRH displayed in the clinics will not only guide the parents but also the adolescents themselves. This way the private practitioners can create awareness among the people as well as contribute to the government's programe too.

REFERENCES

1. UNFPA,State of the World Population 2004 Supra note 2 at 76.
2. World Health Organisation(WHO). Unsafe abortion 17 (2004), available at www.who.int/reproductive-health/publications/unsafe_abortion_estimates_04/estimates.pdf
3. IPAS, Adolescents. Unwanted Pregnancy and Abortion 10, available at www.ipas.org/publications/en/ADOLPOL_E04_en.pdf, 2004.
4. Centre for Reproductive rights. Adolescents Need Safe and Legal Abortion available at www.reproductiverights.org.
5. Women of the World: Laws and Policies Affecting Their Reproductive Lives, edited by the Centre for Reproductive Rights, 'Chapter 2 India'.
6. Centre for Reproductive rights, Adolescents Need Safe and Legal Abortion available at www.reproductiverights.org.
7. Amy R Sobie, David C Reardon. Detrimental Effects of Adolescent Abortion. Available at http://www.afterabortion.info/PAR/V9/n1/teens_vs_older.html, cited on Nov 19, 2006.
8. Passion for Rights. Ten years of fighting for sexual and reproductive health, published by RFSU.
9. Centre for Reproductive rights. Adolescents Need Safe and Legal Abortion available at www.reproductiverights.org.

20 Controversy about Consent at 16-18 Years–Clinician's Perspective

Parag Biniwale

INTRODUCTION

Consent is a common medical procedure for an adolescent in the context of sexual and reproductive health. Consent enables a person to allow or disallow any act; may it be sexual relationship or any surgical procedure like termination of pregnancy. Informed consent implies that the person giving consent understands the benefits and risks of treatment—or of refusing treatment. Thus the issue of controversy arises.

In two recent Delhi High Court cases, judges recorded that, girls below the age of 18 may willingly enter into marriage. This judgment in 2005 raises two questions. First, do minor girls, particularly those below the age of 16 years, have the competency to make such decisions? And, second, to what extent do minor girls in the Indian sociocultural context have the opportunity to make "free, voluntary and informed decisions"? Currently, according to Indian law, only those who have attained majority (above 18 years), can give consent for medical procedures like medical termination of pregnancy and HIV testing. It is presumed that adolescents are not competent to make such decisions and that their parents or legal guardians will act in the best interest of their children.

LET'S CONSIDER SOME CASE SCENARIOS

1. A sixteen-year-old girl visits teen clinic. She gives history that she is sexually active and desires to know more about contraception. The doctor explains her various options and also makes her aware about STIs and HIV. She decides that her partner will use condoms and demands a prescription for the same.

   The clinician is in dilemma whether contraceptive supply should be given or not especially in rural area where there are a lot of community pressures if a medical officer decides to help the adolescent.
2. A seventeen-year-old unmarried girl comes to the clinic with missed periods. On examination, she is found to be 8 weeks pregnant. She tells the doctor that she wants termination of pregnancy. Doctor explains her the procedure and asks her to get adult guardian. She is hesitant and says that she cannot get any relatives.

   What should the girl do? She has two options; she discloses this to her relatives and invites criticism for herself or she seeks abortion from a quack and faces grave consequences of an unsafe abortion.
3. A-sixteen-year-old married Muslim girl comes to out patient clinic. She is 6 weeks pregnant and insists on termination of pregnancy. She is explained the possible risk of termination and she desires to undergo abortion.

If a married adolescent seeks abortion, is it mandatory for her to obtain consent of an adult? Is it not her right to decide whether she wants to continue pregnancy or not?

These are not uncommon scenes in the out patient clinic. In all the above case scenarios, the client is an adolescent girl in the age group of 16 to 18 years. They want to decide about themselves but there are barriers in policy, which prevent them from doing so.

WHY CONTROVERSY?

Before considering the issues related to consent, let's note some very interesting but important facts.

1. Any kind of sexual activity, voluntary or coerced, with a girl below the age of 16 amounts to rape.
2. Any sexual relation between a man and his wife, who is 15 years or less, amounts to rape.
3. It is right of adolescent to decide whether she wants to continue pregnancy or not.
4. A girl below 18 years of age who wants termination of pregnancy must be accompanied by an adult guardian or parent.

In short, by law, an unmarried adolescent girl can give consent to sex before the age of 18 years but if she becomes pregnant, cannot give consent for an abortion.

LET'S LOOK AT THIS CONTROVERSY AND TRY TO ANALYZE IT. WHAT ARE THE SCENARIOS WHERE ISSUE OF CONSENT ARISES?

PARENTAL CONSENT FOR THE TREATMENT OF MINORS

Till few years ago, minors were considered incapable of entering into binding legal contracts, including contracts with physicians, or to give informed consent to medical care. Thus, parental consent for health-related issues is required.

It is thus mandatory for the physician to obtain the informed consent of a parent or guardian before the physician can treat a minor. There are various reasons for the same. First, minors are generally thought to be incapable of making their own medical decisions and must be protected from their own mistakes. Thus the law authorizes parents to give consent because parents are considered to have the intelligence, maturity and experience needed to make these important decisions, and are believed to have the same interest as the minor in the adolescent's health.

A second reason for obtaining parental consent is that it promotes both the state's and the family's interest in encouraging parental participation in minors' lives. Promoting family autonomy and parental control strengthen the family as an institution.

Finally, the parents are also responsible for paying for necessary service of the health care provider since most of the minors lack the financial resources to pay for medical care. Thus the parents do have a role in decision making for the adolescent's health as to how and which treatment should be given.

The past few years have seen change in the role of parents. The parental consent requirement, however, has been modified considerably. The law now recognizes that minors are often competent to understand the implications of medical decisions and are frequently reluctant to seek treatment for "sensitive" issues if they are required to involve their parents. The evolution of the law has resulted in determining alternatives and exceptions to the requirement of parental consent for medical treatment.

WHEN PARENTAL CONSENT IS NOT REQUIRED: EMERGENCIES

A health emergency is "a condition which may require urgent treatment to protect the patient's life or health." In a health emergency, a physician or other health care provider may treat a minor without parental consent. The rationale behind this is that in an emergency, time management is of utmost importance and any wastage of time may endanger life or health if prompt medical attention is not given thus jeopardizing the minor's life or health. In the United States, a number of state legislatures have accepted the medical emergency exception.

ALTERNATIVES TO PARENTAL CONSENT

There are many situations where the consent of someone other than a parent is either required or is considered legally sufficient for the treatment of a minor patient. Law has a special provision for group of adolescents, who are under the jurisdiction of the juvenile courts or is in the care of a child welfare agency. In these situations state law usually authorizes the juvenile court or the child welfare agency to authorize medical care. The reason behind this is that absence of parent should not jeopardize health and life of adolescent. Thus, the state acts as a substitute for the parent in caring for the minor.

WHEN MINORS MAY GIVE CONSENT

A health care provider must obtain a patient's informed consent before providing medical care. In general, a physician must obtain that consent from a parent or guardian for the care of a minor. When an adolescent reaches the age of majority, usually age 18 years, she may give her own consent. Other exceptions as given in the US law are

Emancipated Minors

There are cases in which a minor is sufficiently independent to be legally free of parents' control and to make many decisions, including medical decisions, on the same basis as adults.

Mature Minors

Adolescents who have the intellectual capacity, experience, and knowledge necessary to make a choice and the consequences of the choices that can be made.

MARRIED MINORS

Religion has an important role in married adolescents. Once girls reach puberty, which is presumed to occur at 15 years of age, they are considered marriageable. This makes girls more prone for becoming pregnant at an early age however they are not empowered to take any decisions and cannot give consent for any surgical intervention. There is a need for such adolescents to give consent for themselves.

PREGNANT MINORS

It is still doubtful whether a married adolescent can decide about her own pregnancy.

MINORS WHO ARE NOT LIVING WITH THEIR PARENTS

In India, such separate groups are not identified. Our adolescents still require consent of an adult for most of the procedures. The MTP act demands such consent. However, efforts are being made to enable married adolescents to give consent for procedures like termination of pregnancy.

EXCEPTIONS FOR SPECIFIC HEALTH SERVICES

In the US, some or all states have laws, which permit minors to consent for one or more of the following services. However, in India these laws are not clear.

- Pregnancy related care
- Contraceptive services
- Abortion
- Diagnosis and treatment of sexually transmitted disease
- HIV testing or treatment
- Diagnosis and treatment of reportable infectious, contagious, or communicable disease
- Treatment of drug or alcohol problems
- Diagnosis or treatment for sexual assault
- Outpatient or inpatient mental health counseling

Pregnancy, contraception and abortion are the common areas of concern in adolescent health. Hence, they need to be addressed individually.

PREGNANCY-RELATED SERVICES

Adolescents have a right of privacy. They have a right to access contraceptive services if they indulge in sexual activity and they can maintain their privacy. In the case of minors' access to both contraception and abortion, the Supreme Court includes the parents' interests in its analysis of the exercise of a fundamental right. Parents do have a guiding role in upbringing the children thus having its impact on freedom of minors.

CONTRACEPTIVE SERVICES

Adolescents do not need parental consent to access contraceptive services. However, health care provider should see to it that the adolescent understands various choices. Parents may be informed if the adolescent wishes so. In our country, it is still socially unacceptable in most of the communities that an adolescent, especially unmarried, accesses contraceptive services.

SAFE ABORTION SERVICES

A number of cases address the issue of parental consent or notification and minors' access to abortion. It is legally mandatory in our country that parents/ adult guardian accompany a girl between 16 and 18 years of age.

Validity of consent of an adolescent still remains unsolved issue. It may take few more years for our system to change and accept the rights of adolescents. Only then, this controversy will come to an end.

SUGGESTED READING

1. A Guide for School-Based and School-Linked Health Centers http://www.advocatesforyouth.org/publications.
2. The Journal of Legal Medicine by American College of Legal Medicine.
3. Indian Journal of Medical Ethics.

21 Special Issues in Boys

Swati Y Bhave

INTRODUCTION

When we talk about ARSH issues it is mainly the girls we think about. The reasons for working especially for boys is important from a gender perspective

1. *Gender specificity:* Adolescent boys respond differently than adolescent girls in certain situations and have specific needs that require attention. These include specific sexual and reproductive health concerns, violence, substance abuse, educational difficulties, etc. Most public health programs work with boys in gender specific health issues.
2. *Gender equity:* If we want boys and men to understand and empathize with the ASRH issues in women, we need to involve adolescent boys. This will have a positive impact on adolescent girls and on women in future. There are a very few programs that promote greater gender equity.

Working from a gender perspective will help to assist boys to develop into healthy and responsible citizens, partners and fathers. No doubt both genders are equal and "Nurture versus nature" will soon obliterate these thin lines between genders in the coming years, but even today there are still certain gender differences that would need different handling of an adolescent boy versus a girl. As clinicians we need to be aware of these issues.

Most programs deal with adolescent boys from a "deficit "perspective and focus solely only on their problems, We need to understand their potential and positively use their strengths. The needs of adolescent boys and young adult men are similar, and that there exists a need to provide continuity in work to built up healthy men. For example, instilling a feeling of respect for women in adolescent boys should bring down the incidence of crime and violence against women including rape and domestic violence.

We need to remember that though boys and girls should have equal rights there are still some significant differences in their brain development, maturity at various ages, how they relate and emote differently in the same set of circumstances. By adopting the method of raising the boys and girls in a similar way and handling them in a similar fashion we are encountering increasing problems in society.

Reaction to stress and problems is different. Girls internalize by becoming depressed or anorexic or get pregnant early. In contrast boys externalize by becoming delinquent: bully other boys, join gangs or destroy property.

DEVELOPMENT CHARACTERISTICS OF BOYS

The influence of testosterone needs quick physical release of tension and is associated with higher levels of aggression. Sports are a good outlet for testosterone as they involve physical aggression. The male brain is better at spatial orientation hence sports', involving moving an object-a "ball-through space" which the male brain is good at is best liked by adolescent boys.

When community programs harness this aggression of boys there is less incidence of violence. Boys, who are not trained in self-discipline, can cause harm to self and society, as they are physical risk-takers. The energy of boys has to channelized so that it can develop and expended in healthy, appropriate ways from a very young age. The ancient games and competitions held in the roman and Greek arena allowed expression of aggression and used up energy in a constructive fashion. In India young boys underwent a thread ceremony and were sent to stay in a "Gurukul" away from the family with boys of same age. In African tribes boys undergo initiation rites when they undergo puberty and are then trained as a group in various skills needed for an adult male. Today the adolescent boys are not trained on what to do with their sexuality nor are they trained in self-discipline or care of the soul. Boys need positive male role models in home and outside a "strong father figure" which is necessary to keep boys from straying is sadly lacking to day. This is needed to counter the media images and distinguish fantasy from reality; TV shows and pornography versus real life.

The media has a tremendous impact on how adolescent boys will think and act. It is very important to monitor the TV and internet use. Drinking and driving and substance abuse is far more with boys .There is need to have family discussions with the boys to clarify and interpret these issues. Girls are more likely to have open discussion with parents on various issues.

A Boy need to know the role he has to play as a partner and father. Premarital counseling is very important for a successful marriage.

Most girls get a lot of sexuality knowledge from their mothers at least about menstruation and pregnancy. Most fathers are embarrassed to discuss sexual issues like masturbation, night emissions with their sons. Many adolescent boys do not understand the fertility cycles in females, nor are they having ready to use or confident of using a condom, leading to a increasing number of unwanted teenage pregnancies. Today between puberty and marriage there is a very long gap. Increasing premarital sex there are a large number of adolescent fathers in the western society who may or may not be married to the mother of their child, which has a negative impact on the upbringing children and ultimately on society. Let us hope this situation does not take place in India in near future.

If we want marriages to be stable and happy we need to make adolescent boys understand that love is not just having sex but there is an art of love making and forming a physical and emotional bond with the partner. All the sex education given in schools does not teach the skills necessary for this to, his lack of knowledge can cause poor self confidence of getting consent from a female. This can explain the increasing number of rapes by adolescent boys today. In the ancient cultures, formal and informal sexual education was given to boys. There are no socially endorsed means of teaching an adolescent boy how manage the first sexual encounter in today's situation. As adolescent specialists we need to derive a consensus on how to impart this knowledge by proper premarital counseling to both boys and girls.

Though we should always emphasis on abstinence as the best method of safe sex, we will have to keep in mind the need to empower sexually active boys with the means of controlling unwanted pregnancies and safety from sexually transmitted disease. We need to empower them to understand the ill effects of pornography and internet sex.

In 2000, WHO reviewed programs for adolescent boys in six regions.

- It was seen that majority of programs are related to sexual and reproductive health, either through the provision of information or clinical services.

- Non-governmental organizations (NGOs) are largely responsible for introducing and experimenting with innovative programming from a gender perspective.
- University-based (including both public and private sector) research and the work of health centers play an important role in introducing new services. Their main focus is on (1) health education or health promotion, (2) counseling, (3) clinical services, (4) training of health professionals to work with adolescent boys.
- Other services look after specific needs like shelters for homeless or transient populations, vocational training and employment, educational support for school drop out, school difficulties, life skills, men sex with men (MSM), commercial sex work, juvenile justice system, and homeless or transient young men, etc.

The analysis of these six regions showed that:

A. The *overall* needs of adolescent boys are:
   1. Vocational training and employment
   2. Counseling or spaces to talk
   3. Reproductive/sexual health concerns
   4. General health care, including self-care/hygiene
   5. Educational support, i.e. activities supporting boys in completing their formal education
   6. MISC: intimate relationships gender roles, vocational training and employment, educational support, violence/injury prevention.

B. Important *health* needs of adolescent boys are:
   1. Reproductive/sexual health care needs
   2. Self-care and hygiene
   3. Substance use
   4. Counseling
   5. Violence prevention
   6. MISC: special services for general health, environmental and occupational health, sports-related medicine, physical therapy for disabilities, and substance use prevention.

It has been documented that girls are more receptive to preventive counseling and information and follow-up. Most girls are aware of self-care, hygiene and preventive health issues; boys need to be given such information. Most adolescent boys go to clinics only when they have a problem. They are very poor in coming for follow-up and do not take responsibility for their own or their sexual partners' health. Follow-up is specially poor in mental health problems

Well trained gynecologists are avaible to deliver services to adolescent girls but finding doctors who have had special training for working with adolescent boys is difficult. It is costlier to set up a clinic for boys. The cost per clinic visit for adolescent boys is also higher because of fewer numbers attending.

Boys get bored of lecture formats and need multiple themes, more role plays and high-energy activities. A cafeteria approach has to be tried to recruit boys into attending services. While discussing topics related to sexual reproductive health it is seen that boys prefer to focus on HIV/AIDS while girls prefer to discuss reproductive health. Boys are more comfortable asking questions in same sex group specially about homosexuality. However to promote gender equity, it is very important for adolescent boys to listen to what adolescent girls think. Most cultural norms require sexual segregation, so one should begin with same-sex groups and once the group is functioning well, to begin work with both sexes groups very cautiously.

It is essential to have staff of both genders while delivering services to adolescents. It is better to begin with the same sex but ultimately ability and personal characteristics are more important than the gender of the staff. Male staff can work in the evenings, which is a prime time to reach adolescent boys, while women staff usually do not or cannot work evenings.

DIFFICULTIES IN WORKING WITH ADOLESCENT BOYS

1. Boys do not have a positive attitude for health promotion programs.

2. Lack of awareness and misconceptions about the needs of adolescent boys by various programmers.
3. Lack of resources, trained staff, and program ideas for working with adolescent boys.
4. Difficulty in sustaining behavioral changes and providing accessible and suitable services for adolescent boys.
5. Awareness about the needs of adolescent boys is fairly low in public sector and generally highest among NGOs.

Girls can be easily reached for programs which are community or home bases. It is far more difficult to reaching adolescent boys. They have to reached through workplaces, shelters for homeless or transient populations, centers for vocational training, employment, army training, juvenile justice centers bars, discos, taxi stands, commercial sex work areas, drug houses via peer promoters. Health promotion information has to target them with drama, telephone hotlines, sports clubs, youth clubs, summer camps and religious groups.

Majority of research that has been done with boys in the field of sexual and reproductive health, with street and working youth, examining violence, maltreatment and substance use. Changing nature of masculinity is a very important issue to address; several studies have highlighted the lack of fathers and positive adult male role models and the general lack of positive identities for low income boys. Adolescent boys need more leisure-time activities. Many adolescent boys lack parental supervision as they are away due to higher education, migration for employment, family break-up, or emotional distanced due to poor communication psychological impacts of sexual dysfunctions, the impact of the media on sexual behavior of adolescent boys, (MSM)/ sexual orientation, are special issues be considered .

SUMMARY

In conclusion clinicians have to understand the adolescent boys need to be involved in issues of ARSH for gender equity and need special handling.

SUGGESTED READING

1. Barker G. WHO survey on programmes working with adolescent boys and young men: Summary report. Latin America, Caribbean and USA. Geneva, WHO, 1999.
2. Bhave Swati Y, Bansal CP. Adolescent Boys In: Bhave's Textbook of Adolescent Medicine 1st edn. In: Swati Y Bhave (Ed). New Delhi: Jaypee Brothers Medical Publishers, 2006;7.4:261-64.
3. Fraternity Gang Rape New York: New York University Press, 1990.
4. Resnick MD, Bearman PS, Blum RW, Bauman KE, Harris KM, Jones J, Tabor J, Beuhring T, Sieving RE, Shew M, Ireland M, Bearinger JH, Udry R. Teen Childbearing Trends: Which Tide Turned When and Why? Pediatrics 1998; 102:1205-06.
5. Working with adolescent boys: Programme Experiences, Ross Hempstead (Eds): Consolidated findings from regional surveys in Africa, the Americas, Eastern Mediterranean, South-East Asia, and Western Pacific Department of Child and Adolescent health and Development World Health Organization WHO/FCH/CAH/00.10'.

22 Genital and Sexual Problems in Boys

Vijay Kulkarni

INTRODUCTION

The adolescent boy to young adult age group is in a phase of transition- physically, psychologically and sexually. Sex related problems are abundant in this group. Sexually transmitted infections and endocrinological problems are important aspects related to genital problems in this age group which have been covered in other chapters. Hence the repetition is avoided here. However the treating physician should be conversant with some common queries and conditions which come across in urological, andrological and sexual-medicine practice, and the same are covered here.

If one talks to the parents and doctors, it is realized that the adolescent age-group is a difficult group to deal with. Besides the physical growth, psychological and emotional upheavals, endocrinological changes in the body, there are sexual urges and curiosities which are compounded by social taboos, cultural and religious upbringing, peer influences. The outcome often is a confused adolescent boy or a young adult who has no clear knowledge of sexual anatomy, physiology and hygiene. Worse still, are the misguided ideas and unrealistic expectations brought about by peers as well as by easily available pornographic material.

Worst of all, they have nobody to turn to in order to ask, explain and clarify their ideas or problems.

In our practice, we see scores of youngsters who hesitantly come to us and awkwardly ask questions about their perceived sexual problems. These frequently asked questions (FAQs) give us the insights into their lack of knowledge, misconceptions, anxieties and fears. Hence the health provider, i.e. Pediatrician, General practitioner, Family Physician, Guides or Psychologists at Adolescent guidance centers or clinics should be familiar with these queries, understand psychological background which brings about such queries and should have a firm scientific knowledge to answer them confidently and convincingly. Also, he or she should be familiar with some of the surgical conditions which occur in this age group.

Hence this topic of genital problem is dealt with in the practical sequence of question, scientific background for the health provider who has to answer the question and then the self-explanatory answer itself; rather than simply providing textbook-like data.

DOCTOR, I THINK I HAVE A SMALL PENIS. CAN YOU GIVE A MEDICINE TO MAKE IT BIGGER ?

Very often the boy is referring to the penile size when it is flaccid.

The penis has two functions- passing urine and depositing sperms into the female tract for procreation.

For the former, length is immaterial. In fact in females, the urine is passed without penis at all. So the penile length during flaccidity is inconsequential.

For the latter function, one requires the length of penis only for penetration into the female tract during sexual intercourse. Eight centimeters and above of erect penis is adequate for this purpose. Length of an erect penis corresponds to the stretched length of flaccid penis, measured from pubic symphysis to mid-glans.

Demonstrate this length to the patient and reassure him.

THERE IS NO MEDICINE TO MAKE PENIS BIGGER.

I GOT INTO A BAD HABIT OF MASTURBATION- I) CAN I HAVE NORMAL SEXUAL LIFE AFTER MARRIAGE? II) IT HAS SPOILT MY HEALTH, I FEEL WEAK

Masturbation is a form of sexual behavior. In sexual intercourse, penis is enveloped by vagina. In masturbation, it is enveloped by a cup of hand.

It has no bearing on sexual life after marriage.

It has no bearing on health either, as the nature has designed specific tasks for specific set of glands, e.g. lacrimal glands for tears, salivary glands for saliva, testes with accessory glands (seminal vesicles and prostate) for semen.

One does not become blind by crying or suffer from malnutrition by spitting. Similarly masturbation does not have any effect on sexual life.

As for the loss of secretion, just like tears and saliva, seminal secretions would be made up by the body. There is nothing holy or precious about seminal secretions. Notions like **HUNDRED DROPS OF BLOOD ARE EQUIVALENT TO ONE DROP OF SEMEN, ARE A MYTH.**

I DON'T KNOW HOW TO STOP MY 'WET DREAMS.' EVEN IN DAYTIME, I SOIL MY CLOTHES BY PASSING SEMEN. I PASS DHAT WHILE PASSING STOOLS. IT HAS RUINED MY HEALTH

Secretions from testes, seminal vesicles, prostate are in a continuous process of formation. When the storing capacity of the dilated end-portion of vas, i.e. ampulla, is full, it 'overflows'.

This is nocturnal emission or a 'wet dream'. It is totally physiological.

Besides the passage of urine and semen, another antegrade discharge from the external urethral meatus is that of urethral secretions.

It is often misunderstood as semen and the patients are quite upset about this frequent passage of 'Dhat' (semen) which is looked upon as 'precious' fluid, thus ruining their health by wasting it. Its value to the body is same as that of a spittle.

Urethral glands keep the mucosa moist, just like saliva keeps the mouth moist. When one sees or smells good food, there is watering of mouth.

When one is sexually excited by sight or a fantasy, there is 'watering' of urethral passage, misconstrued as semen. During defecation, well-formed stools press past the urethra, squeezing the secretions antegrade. These are transparent, watery secretions; far different from whitish, thick semen.

Explaining these facts along with anatomical pictures goes a long way in allaying the fears and misconceptions of the distressed youngster.

WHAT IS CIRCUMCISION? WHEN IS IT NECESSARY? IS IT TRUE THAT CIRCUMCISED MAN HAS MORE SEXUAL POTENCY?

Surgically excising the prepuce (a free skin-fold overlying the glans penis) and exposing the glans permanently, is called as circumcision.

The indications are two—Religious reasons and Medical reasons.

For religious purpose, it is done as a part of religious ritual.

For medical reasons, it is done when prepuce cannot be pulled back over the glans penis, especially during erection. Prepuce should be retractable over the glans for cleaning the glans penis which other wise would collect inspissated secretions called 'smegma'. It is foul smelling, whitish encrustations over the glans and behind coronal sulcus.

Retracting the prepuce and cleaning underneath, is a part of genital hygiene which must be done daily.

Also during sexual intercourse, if it cannot be pulled over the glans, it can cause pain to the male. In addition, there are other medical conditions like diabetes which cause repeated infections and render the prepuce tight that would need circumcision.

There is no difference between the sexual potency of a circumcised male and that of an uncircumcised male.

DOCTOR, MY ONE TESTIS IS BIGGER THAN THE OTHER. IS IT A PROBLEM?

Following conditions cause swelling of one or both sides of scrotum.

Hydrocele—Unilateral or Bilateral

It is a fluid collection within two layers of testicular covering called tunica vaginalis. It may be congenital (usually so in children) or acquired in young adults. It is harmless. It requires surgical excision of the fluid-containing sac and NOT of testis. In specified case, a clinician may need to determine the cause of the fluid, e.g. tuberculosis.

Hernia—Unilateral or Bilateral

It is protrusion of abdominal contents like intestines into the scrotum. It may be congenital or acquired. It is NOT harmless at this age and can lead to serious complications. Hence once diagnosed, should get early (not urgent) elective surgery done. There is no treatment other than surgery for hernia in this age group.

Varicocele

These are varicosities of pampiniform plexus of veins of the spermatic cord. There may be dragging pain, not acute. The testis may undergo atrophy compromising fertility in later life. Hence microsurgical excision of the dilated veins sparing testicular artery is recommended in adolescent varicocele.

Malignancy

A very uncommon cause can be a malignancy of the testis like Non-Seminomatous Germ Cell Tumor. But remember, it is far less common than hernia and hydrocele.

WHAT ARE THE CAUSES OF SEVERE PAIN IN SCROTUM?

Any young man or an adolescent boy or his parents reporting of his getting severe pain in scrotum, has to be seen as an emergency case. Following conditions can cause such pain needing urgent treatment and have significant consequences in the adult life.

Torsion of the Testis

The onset is sudden with pain and swelling. Here the testis undergoes rotation in its vertical axis. The twist in the cord starts compromising the blood supply of the testis, leading to ischemia and if unrelieved, even to gangrene. Hence it is necessary to suspect this condition, refer him to a specialist for early diagnosis and the necessary surgical treatment .Note- the unaffected testis is also fixed to prevent undergoing similar torsion.

Acute Infection

The onset of pain is not as dramatic as in torsion and is invariably accompanied by fever. There is pain and swelling. Needs to be differentiated from torsion, hence a specialist must see the case as early as possible. The treatment is antibiotics with analgesics.

Strangulation of Hitherto Unknown Hernia

A small hernia might have gone unnoticed or ignored, till it strangulates and draws attention. It is a surgical emergency.

MY PENIS IS NOT STRAIGHT WHEN ERECT. WILL I BE ABLE TO HAVE INTERCOURSE?

A flaccid penis becomes erect when two corpora cavernosa become fully engorged with blood. Depending upon its crural (proximal end of cavernosa) attachment to the under-surface of pubic rami and length of fibrous ligament of penis, the angle of erection would change, i.e. at 90 degrees, tilting upwards or downwards. Similarly, two corpora, like two fingers of both hands, are not identical. Hence when erect, may cause a small tilt to either side. The resultant 'bending' as the patient tends to call it, is totally inconsequential to his ability to have intercourse.

However, the clinician must examine the patient to make sure that he has no congenital anomaly like abnormally placed opening of the external urinary meatus (e.g. hypospadias). If present, it can give rise to true bending (chordee) of an erect penis. This condition requires surgical correction.

DOCTOR, I AM SUFFERING FROM IMPOTENCE

Today, a lot of adolescent boys and girls are sexually active. One of the common problems following initial failure to have penetrative intercourse is to have serious doubts about his potency.

Lack of knowledge of genital anatomy, lack of privacy, restrictive social circumstances, fear of pregnancy and of pain on female's part are commonest reasons to have failed penetration at intercourse.

Initial failure has a strong psychological impact on the young male, giving rise to severe performance anxiety; which further induces erectile dysfunction.

The young adult must have a detailed psychosexual counseling as first line of treatment.

In this age group, the erectile dysfunction is almost always psychogenic in origin.

However, the treating physician must be aware that in exceptional cases, ED can be organic, e.g. congenital vascular dysplasia, trauma.

The specialized tests available for differentiating organic ED from psychogenic ED are:

1. Pharmacologically Induced Erection (PIE) test
2. Nocturnal Penile Tumescence and Rigidity (NPTR) monitoring by a dedicated device called Rigiscan.
3. Colour Duplex Doppler with injection of vaso-active drug like Papaverine.

CAN A MALE ALSO BLEED DURING THE FIRST INTERCOURSE ?

There is a small fold of skin on the under-surface of glans penis, attaching the glans to the skin, called Frenum. Lack of lubrication, vaginismus, vigorous thrusting movements can tear the frenum and can cause bleeding.

SUMMARY

Growing boys have a lot of anxiety and questions related to sexual and reproductive health. Unlike mothers who freely discuss issues of menstruation and pregnancy with their daughters, most fathers are not comfortable discussing masturbation and wet dreams with their sons. These issues can bother a adolescent boy greatly even to the extent of causing anxiety and depression. A adolescent boy may come directly with the above questions but more often they are very shy and embarrassed to do so. The presenting complaints may be acne, headache, body ache, poor performance in studies, etc. while the main problem is usually a sexual one. The clinician must establish a rapport and gently probe into the history. A non-threatening atmosphere and simple questions like "is any other issue is bothering you? Do you want information on some issues?" May open the flood gate.

SUGGESTED READING

1. Education in Human Sexual by Dhun Panthaki, Published by FPAI (Family Planning Association of India) and IPPF (International Planned Parenthood Federation).
2. Human Sexual Response, by Masters and Johnson, Published by Little Brown And Co., USA.
3. Sex and You, by Dr. Prakash Kothari MBBS, PhD. Latest edition being published by Penguines Publishers (for release in Jan 2007).

23 Intersex

Kanchan S Kewalramani, PH Chauhan

INTRODUCTION

To establish a cause for intersex and thereby formulate a management plan is probably one of the most challenging situations for the practicing pediatric and gynecological endocrinologist and appropriate surgical colleague.

Genetic issues dominate the pathophysiology of intersex, and genetic counseling should be available to families needing advice about recurrence risks, carrier detection and options for prenatal diagnosis and perhaps prenatal treatment.

Management in the long-term needs the skills of counselors trained and experienced in psychosexual issues affecting children and adolescents.

DEFINITION

Intersex is a condition of incomplete or disordered genital or gonadal development leading to a discordance between genetic sex, gonadal sex and phenotypic sex.

The approach to investigate and manage intersex requires an understanding of normal prenatal sexual development.

SEXUAL DIFFERENTIATION

Mammalian sexual differentiation is a sequential process that begins with the establishment of chromosomal or genetic sex at fertilization. The Y chromosome or the genetic sex then directs gonadal differentiation (so-called gonadal sex), which in turn determines the secretion of hormones that masculinize nongonadal tissues, resulting in phenotypic sex. In those infants bearing a 'Y' chromosome, the expression of SRY in sexually undifferentiated genital ridge cells initiates testicular development at approximately 5 weeks of gestation.[1]

The testes secrete Anti Mullerian Hormone (AMH) at 6 weeks which causes regression of mullerian structures and testosterone at 7 weeks which stabilizes and further differentiates the Wolffian ducts along with masculinization of the external genitalia and other body tissues. In the absence of SRY, ovaries develop, the Wolffian ducts regress and the mullerian ducts mature (Fig. 23.1).

INTERSEX SIMPLE CLASSIFICATION

According to this method of classification, there are four major categories of intersex patients (Table 23.1)..

MASCULINIZED FEMALE

Congenital Adrenal Hyperplasia (CAH)

More than 90% of cases of CAH are caused by 21–hydroxylase deficiency.[2,3] The degree of virilization of the external genitalia can be so

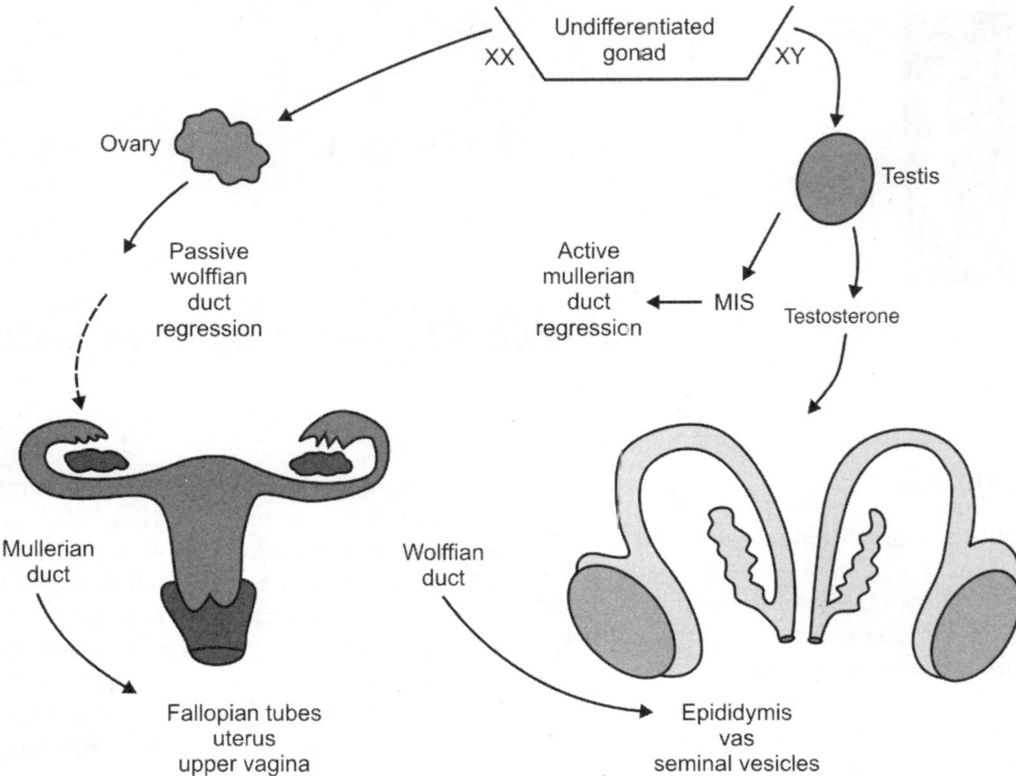

Fig. 23.1: The differential of the wolffian and mullerian ducts

Table 23.1: Intersex a pragmatic classification

Type/cause	*Result*
Masculinized female	
Fetal androgens	CAH, placental aromatase deficiency
Maternal androgens	adrenal tumors, ovarian tumors
Under-masculinized male	
Defects in androgen biosynthesis and	17 β-OH—dehydrogenase Metabolism deficiency 5 α-reductase deficiency
Resistance to androgens	Androgen insensitivity syndromes (AIS) complete AIS partial AIS
True hermaphroditism	
Presence of both testicular and ovarian (with follicles) tissue	XX, XY, XX/XY
Mixed gonadal dysgenesis	
Presence of testis and streak gonad	45XO/46XX XO/XY mosaicism

marked that infants born with such findings are investigated early. Generally in CAH, there is clitoromegaly, rugosed and pigmented labio-scrotal folds and a single perineal opening representing a urogenital sinus.[2]

Prenatal treatment needs to start as soon as an at-risk pregnancy is confirmed and prenatal tests are undertaken on a sample of chorionic villi.[4,5] These include the karyotype and mutuational analysis of the 21 hydroxylase gene, CYP21. Only mothers carrying an affected female need continuation of dexamethasone treatment. Virilization of the external genitalia is completely prevented in many instances and the remainder require no surgery or minimal intervention.

The question whether surgery should be early (2-6 months) or later (1-2 years) is still a matter of debate. There appears to be even more debate about whether girls needing clitoroplasty and vaginoplasty should have this performed as a one-stage procedure in infancy, or as a two-stage procedure with the vaginoplasty delayed until late childhood or early adolescence.[6-8]

The medical management of CAH in infancy is relatively simple. This includes glucocorticoid and mineralocorticoid replacement together with salt supplements to the oral feeds initially.

Transplacental Exposure to Androgens

Rarely, a female fetus may be virilized as a result of either a maternal androgen-secreting tumor involving the adrenals or ovaries or due to transplacental transport of excess androgens from mother to the fetus (aromatase deficiency)[9] (Fig. 23.2, Plate 2).

UNDER-MASCULINIZED MALE

This is a 46XY patient with inadequate virilization of the external genitalia of a varying degree due to deficient biosynthesis of testosterone (TST), inadequate conversion of TST to dihydrotestosterone (DHT) (lack of 5α-reductase) or inadequate androgen action (Fig. 23.3, Plate 2).

TRUE HERMAPHRODITISM

In this disorder the patients possess both ovarian and testicular tissue in various combinations. Their karyotype also varies, i.e. 46XX, 46XY or mosaic 46XX/46XY. True hermaphrodites make up approximately 10% of the intersex cases (Fig. 23.4, Plate 2).

MIXED GONADAL DYSGENESIS

Ambiguous genitalia of the newborn may occur as a result of chromosome abnormalities or from a partial form of XY gonadal dysgenesis. The commonest chromosome abnormality is 45XO/46XY mosaicism associated with mixed gonadal dysgenesis. The phenotype may include signs consistent with features of Turner's syndrome (particularly short stature) as well as the abnormal genital development. The concomitant streak gonad should be removed because of the risk of malignancy.

CLINICAL EVALUATION

There is no substitute for an initial adequate history and physical examination. The medical history should include questions about the genetic and ethnic background of the parents and the potential for consanguinity. The parents should be questioned to determine whether any others in the family have had genital ambiguity, virilization, sudden infant death syndrome, pubertal problems, or infertility. Medications used during pregnancy should be documented, and the presence of any maternal virilization during pregnancy should be ascertained.

PHYSICAL EXAMINATION

The initial physical examination should define and document the degree of genital development. All intersex infants should undergo a routine physical examination and description of the genitalia which includes:

1. Vitals: Temperature, pulse, blood pressure
2. Anthropometric—length, weight, and head circumference
3. State of hydration and perfusion
4. Dermatological findings—generalized or genital hyperpigmentation
5. Dysmorphic features

The appearance of the genitalia should be documented which includes the phallic configuration, the presence of chordee, the position of urethral meatus, the presence and position of the gonads (to be palpated for in the labio-scrotal and inguinal regions), the width and length of the stretched phallus, and the symmetry of the external genitalia. The Prader scale classification can be useful in documenting the overall extent of ambiguity.[10] Fig. 23.5.

LABORATORY INVESTIGATIONS

The initial investigations which should be undertaken are:

- Buccal smear (if available with accuracy)
- Plasma17-OH-progesterone assay, plasma renin activity, plasma androstenedione
- Plasma electrolytes

These three investigations will provide definitive evidence of CAH, which is the most frequent intersex disorder, in which case no further investigation is needed.

In rest of the cases the laboratory work-up will proceed as follows:

- Karyotype
- Plasma LH, FSH and testosterone assay pre and post-hCG administration. The hCG stimulation test is particularly helpful in differentiating the main syndromes of male pseudohermaphrodites and in evaluating the Leydig cell potential and the potential for phallic growth which is essential if the baby is to be assigned male sex.
  Abdominal ultrasound (U/S) to visualise possible internal genital organs.
- A contrast medium genitogram to visualize urethral or urogenital sinus morphology.
- Urethral or urogenital sinus endoscopy under general anesthesia, provided the examiner is experienced in interpreting the findings.
- Biopsy of gonadal material.

The decision for appropriate sex assignment is then made taking into account the precise etiological diagnosis and the functional potential of the genitalia. Schematically the following practical outline can be applied.

- Female pseudohermaphrodites (i.e. CAH) should be reared as females since genitoplasty can correct virilization, and spontaneous puberty.

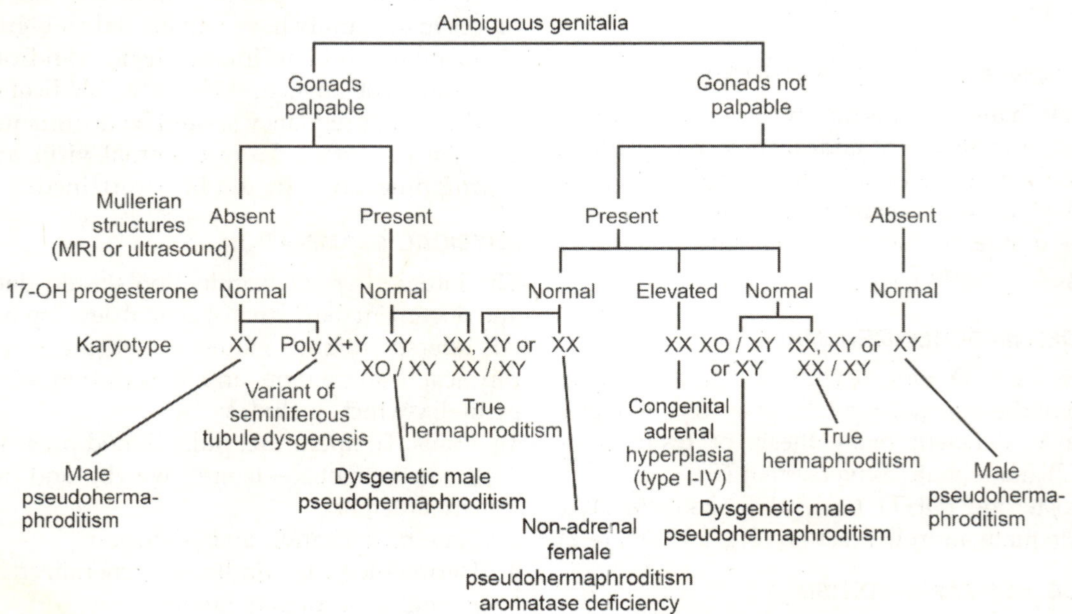

Fig. 23.5: Steps in the diagnosis of intersexuality in infancy and childhood

- Male pseudohermaphrodites with an inadequate phallus should be given androgen therapy, i.e. systemic testosterone therapy and those with a poor clinical response should be reared as girls. The only exception is that of 5α-reductase deficiency, 17α-hydroxysteroid deficiency and some cases of partial androgen insensitivity syndrome in whom masculinization is expected at puberty, and they may be reared as male.
- True hermaphrodites are preferably reared as girls as they have adequate mullerian structures, i.e. vagina and potential for pregnancy.
- Patients with mixed gonadal dysgenesis with an inadequate phallus and intraabdominal testes are usually reared as girls. Male sex may, however, be chosen when the phallus is of adequate size with corpus cavernosum, and the testis is palpable, inguinal or scrotal.

CONCLUSIONS

Intersex or ambiguous genitalia of the newborn is a rare disorder which needs prompt investigation, locally based on a sound knowledge of normal sex determination and differentiation. The complexity of the problem requires a multidisciplinary team working in specialist centers.

REFERENCES

1. Koopman P. The molecular biology of SRY and its role in sex determination in mammals. Reprod Fertil Dev 1995; 7 (4): 713-22.
2. Acerini CL, Hughes I. 21-Hydroxylase deficiency defects and their phenotype. In: Huges IA, Clark AJL (Eds). Adrenal Disease in childhood: Clinical and Molecular Aspects. Basel: Karger, 2000: 93-111.
3. White P C, Speiser P Congenital Adrenal Hyperplasia due to 21-hydroxylase deficiency. Endocr Rev 2000; 21: 245-91.
4. Forest M. Prenatal diagnosis, treatment, and outcome in infants with congenital adrenal hyperplasia. Curr Opin in Endocrinol Diabet 1998: 4: 209-17.
5. New MI, Carlson A, Obeid J, et al. Prenatal diagnosis for congenital adrenal hyperplasia in 532 pregnancies. J. Clin Endocrinol Metab 2001; 86: 5651-57.
6. Farkas A, Chertin B, Hadas-Helpren I. 1- stage feminizing genitoplasty. 8 years of experience with 49 cases. J Urol 2001; 165: 2341-46.
7. Melton L. New perspectives on the management of intersex. Lancet 200; 357: 2110
8. Hrabovsky Z, Hutson J.M. Surgical treatment of intersex abnormalities: a review. Surgery 2002; 131: 92-104.
9. Grumbach MM, Auchus R J. Estrogen: Consequences and implications of human mutations in synthesis and action. J Clin Endocrinol Metab 1999; 84: 4677-94.
10. Christopher P. Houk, Intersexed states: Diagnosis and management Endocrinology And Metabolism Clinics of North America, Sep 2005; 34: 800-801.

SUGGESTED READING

1. Charles Brook—Paediatric Text book of Endocrinology 5th Edition.
2. Melwin M. Grumbach, Disorders of sex differentiation; William's Textbook of Endocrinology 10th edition.

24 PCOS in Adolescent and Young Girls

Duru Shah, Reena Wani

INTRODUCTION

Polycystic ovarian syndrome is one of the commonest endocrine disorders, diagnosed in 5-10% of women between adolescence and menopause. It has an impact not only on the physical but also on the mental health of the young girl. Female adolescence is normally accompanied by the increased adrenal and ovarian production of androgens. It is not uncommon in early to mid puberty to see typical features of PCOS.

There is a spectrum of symptoms which may be associated with polycystic ovarian disease. At present no single test can differentiate girls in whom this process will be self limiting from girls who will progress to adult PCOS with its consequences.

PCOS is associated with increased androgen secretion, hirsutism, menstrual irregularities and infertility. Many women have the onset of symptoms during adolescence, therefore it is essential that health care providers for adolescents be familiar with the evaluation and treatment of this disorder.

HISTORY TAKING AND EXAMINATION

It has often been said that there is no substitute for a detailed history while evaluating a patient. This is more so in young girls, who are often also a little reticent and need to be encouraged to come out with what is bothering them. Just going into the history can often guide the further management of the case. It is important to clarify, in a sensitive manner, whether she is sexually active or not, particularly in cases of menstrual irregularity or amenorrhea. Pelvic examination is often not possible and may not be necessary. General examination for obesity, acne, hirsutism and anemia should be done. Per abdominal examination, evaluation of Tanner's staging, and looking for galactorrhea and thyroid enlargement is important.

DEFINITION AND DIAGNOSIS

CLINICAL DEFINITION

PCOS is characterized typically by a history of chronic anovulatory bleeding in combination with some evidence of androgen excess, such as hirsutism, acne, elevated serum androgen concentrations or a combination of these. This is based on the Consensus Conference of the National Institute of Health and National Institute of Child Health and Development held in 1990.[1]

The consensus was that there are "definite or probable" criteria for the diagnosis of polycystic ovary syndrome. *Definite criteria* included menstrual dysfunction and androgen excess and excludes congenital adrenal hyperplasia and other causes. *"Probable criteria"* include factors like insulin resistance, elevated ratio of luteinizing hormone (LH) to follicle stimulating hormone (FSH) and ovaries appearing polycystic on ultrasonography.

PHYSICAL EXAMINATION

Includes measurement of weight and the waist-to-hip ratio, and an assessment for clinical signs of hyperandrogenism (including hirsutism, acne, or signs of virilization) and insulin resistance (acanthosis nigricans) can be helpful in establishing the diagnosis of PCOS. One should evaluate for clinical signs of other causative disorders to exclude their diagnoses.

CLINICAL MANIFESTATIONS IN ADOLESCENTS

Studies of the clinical manifestations of PCOS in the adolescent are sparse.

SIGNS OF HYPERANDROGENISM

Hirsutism and acne are the most common manifestations and can be a cause of embarrassment among female adolescents.

Hirsutism is defined as the growth of pigmented coarse hair in androgen-dependent areas such as the face, chest, back, and lower abdomen. The distribution and severity of the hirsutism can be quantified using the Ferriman and Gallwey score, with a score of 8 or greater signifying significant hair growth.[2] Ethnic and racial differences exist in body hair type and distribution and should be taken into consideration when assessing hirsutism. The leading cause of hirsutism in adolescence is PCOS.[3] Premature adrenarche and hirsutism that occur before puberty also have been associated with PCOS in adolescents.[4,5]

Acne is common in adolescents with PCOS. More than one third of women presenting to a dermatology clinic with acne are diagnosed with PCOS.[6]

INSULIN RESISTANCE

Acanthosis nigricans is a marker of insulin resistance. It is presence of raised, velvety, hyperpigmentation of the skin seen in the axilla, neck, and intertrigenous areas. Prepubertal girls with acanthosis nigricans and premature adrenarche have significantly decreased insulin sensitivity when compared with prepubertal girls without acanthosis nigricans.[4]

MENSTRUAL IRREGULARITY

Menstrual irregularity is a significant component of PCOS. Secondary amenorrhea, oligomenorrhea, and dysfunctional uterine bleeding are some of the menstrual irregularities seen with anovulation. Menarche typically begins at a normal age but can be delayed in girls with PCOS. Irregular menses, most commonly oligomenorrhea, persisting from the time of menarche well into adolescence is a common feature of adolescent PCOS.[7,8] Because menstrual irregularities are commonly seen in adolescents, it may be difficult to make the diagnosis of PCOS unless there are concomitant signs of hyperandrogenism.

OBESITY

Obesity is often associated with PCOS. Nearly 50% of hyperandrogenic anovulatory women are obese. The weight distribution is centripetal, with increased waist-to-hip ratios of greater than 0.85. A study of adolescents with PCOS in Singapore revealed a 27% incidence of obesity (defined as weight >120% of ideal body weight), with 9% of the population being thin (weight<85% of ideal body weight).[9]

INVESTIGATIONS

ULTRASOUND OF THE PELVIS

Polycystic-appearing ovaries on ultrasound, defined as more than 10 follicles 2 to 8 mm in diameter located peripherally on the ovary, are commonly seen in patients with PCOS (Fig. 24.1). Van Hooff and colleagues found the incidence of polycystic-appearing ovaries to be 45% in oligomenorrheic girls compared with a 9% incidence in normally menstruating adolescents.[10] Nevertheless, polycystic ovaries also can be seen in 33% of normally menstruating adolescents[7] and prepubertal girls, and in other conditions, such as congenital adrenal hyperplasia, hypothalamic amenorrhea, and hyperprolactinemia. Because polycystic ovarian morphology can be seen in a variety of pathologic conditions as well as in normal individuals, ultrasound is not useful in the diagnosis of PCOS. In our personal experience[12] of adolescent girls over 1996-2003, the prevalence of polycystic ovaries on ultrasound was approximately 36.5%. Amongst the girls having polycystic ovaries on ultrasound, 78% had evidence of hyperandrogenism [hirsutism and/or acne], 52% were obese, and 87% had menstrual irregularity [regular or delayed periods and secondary amenorrhea].

LABORATORY DIAGNOSIS

The laboratory evaluation of an adolescent with suspected PCOS varies with the symptoms and clinical findings. To establish the diagnosis of PCOS, the goals are to *confirm ovarian hyperandrogenism* and *exclude other causes of hyperandrogenism and menstrual dysfunction,* such as adrenal or ovarian tumors, nonclassical adrenal hyperplasia, Cushing's syndrome, hyperprolactinemia, and thyroid disease.

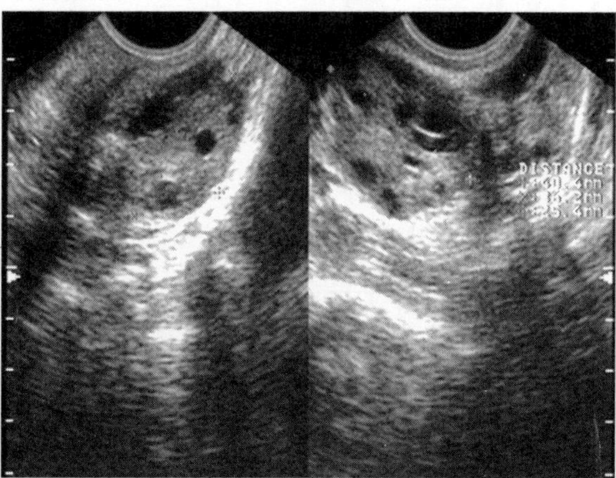

Fig. 24.1: Ultrasound appearance of PCOS

HORMONE ASSAYS

- Free and total testosterone and dehydroepiandrosterone (DHEA) are commonly performed to confirm the diagnosis of PCOS and to exclude other causes of hyperandrogenism.
- Assays for prolactin and thyroid-stimulating hormone are recommended to exclude the diagnoses of hyperprolactinemia and hypothyroidism, both of which can present with menstrual irregularities and anovulation.
- Determination of FSH levels may be required to exclude the diagnosis of premature ovarian failure in adolescents with primary or secondary amenorrhea without signs of hyperandrogenism. LH-to-FSH ratios are not useful in the diagnosis of PCOS given that as many as 40% of women with PCOS have normal ratios.

DIABETES MELLITUS SCREENING

Diabetes mellitus screening should be performed in all patients with PCOS owing to the risk for glucose intolerance and diabetes in this population. A fasting glucose level should be obtained in all adolescents with PCOS. A 2-hour, 75-g oral glucose tolerance test (OGTT) is more sensitive for diagnosing impaired glucose tolerance . The OGTT may be prudent in high-risk adolescents, because the results from the recent diabetes prevention trial have shown that treatment of impaired glucose tolerance decreases the risk for diabetes.

EVALUATING FOR INSULIN RESISTANCE

Evaluating for insulin resistance is not mandatory but may be helpful in directing therapy. Adolescents with obesity and acanthosis nigricans should be screened for insulin resistance. A fasting glucose-to-insulin ratio of less than 4.5 has been shown to indicate insulin resistance in women with PCOS. This ratio may also help identify adolescents at risk for type 2 diabetes mellitus.

As discussed earlier, ultrasound findings alone are not useful in the diagnosis of PCOS. If one is unable to perform an adequate pelvic examination to rule out ovarian pathology, or if an ovarian tumor is suspected, an ultrasound evaluation is warranted.

TREATMENT

Therapeutic approach depends on patient symptoms, etiologic considerations, motivation and whether the patient is seeking immediate fertility. If fertility is not an immediate goal, as in adolescent girls, then treatment goals fall into two broad categories.

1. **Short-term goals** include the regulation of menses, the control of hirsutism and acne, and the stabilization or reduction of weight.
2. **Long-term goals** are less pressing to the adolescent and include the prevention of diabetes, endometrial hyperplasia, obesity, heart disease, and infertility. Weight loss is the most natural method for increasing insulin sensitivity.

Traditional treatment of PCOS has focused on the suppression of symptoms of androgen excess and anovulation. Newer therapies with insulin-sensitizing agents are intended to correct the underlying metabolic disorder. Currently, no studies have compared the effectiveness of these two approaches. Randomized controlled trials are needed to determine whether insulin-sensitizing drugs are better than traditional therapies and, if so, to determine which patients would benefit from these medications.

ILLUSTRATIVE CASE SCENARIOS

Case 1: Presentation with Menstrual Irregularity

An 18-year-old girl presents with a history of heavy, irregular, delayed periods. She achieved menarche at age 15 years and has usually no more than four or five periods each year.

Approach:

- Detailed history about menstrual pattern, weight change, any treatment taken and family history
- Examination to determine BMI, body hair distribution, exclusion of associated endocrine disease (thyroid, adrenal).
- Induction of withdrawal bleeding by progesterone (after urine pregnancy test, if relevant) may be required before further testing.
- Endocrine profile on day 5 of menstrual cycle, and ultrasound scan to confirm the diagnosis of PCOD.

Treatment

Regulation of menses is important, because the anovulation seen in PCOS is associated with the development of endometrial hyperplasia and carcinoma.

In addition, irregular menses and abnormal bleeding can be troublesome for the adolescent.

Cyclic progestin and oral contraceptives (either combined or progestin-only formulations) can be used to resume menstrual regularity.

Newer OCS containing lipid friendly progestogen like desogestrel can be used to reduce acne and hirsutism.

In contrast to oral contraceptives, cyclic progestins do not suppress ovarian androgen production.

Depomedroxyprogesterone acetate (Depo-Provera) is an injectable alternative to oral contraceptives that can effectively decrease ovarian activity. Ovarian suppression with Depo-Provera is much greater than that achieved with oral contraceptives.

Case 2: Hirsutism

A 16-year-old girl presents with complaints of excessive hair growth, weight gain and irregular menstruation. She is most worried about her appearance as she is starting college soon.

When assessing this patient, first we need to answer the question, is it truly hirsutism or is it hypertrichosis? Detailed examination, and Ferriman-Galloway scoring is done.

- *Hirsutism* indicates the presence of excess terminal hair growth in areas of the body that are androgen-sensitive such as the face, chest, areola, lower back, buttock, inner thigh and external genitalia.

- *Hypertrichosis* indicates excess terminal hair growth in areas of the body that are not androgen-sensitive such as forehead, forearms, tops of the hands.

Laboratory Investigations specific to this case
- Total testosterone levels greater than 200 ng/dL in the setting of rapid progression of hirsutism and the presence of virilization are consistent with an androgen-producing ovarian tumor.
- DHEA levels greater than 7000 ng/dL are indicative of an adrenal tumor. The diagnosis of most tumors can be based on history and physical findings as opposed to biochemical levels.
- Nonclassical adrenal hyperplasia can be excluded by obtaining a basal 17-hydroxyprogesterone level during the follicular phase of the cycle (or at any time in an anovulatory patient). An adrenocorticotropic hormone stimulation test should be performed if an elevated 17-hydroxyprogesterone level is found (>2 ng/mL).

Treatment for hirsutism: Goals of therapy are to control current hair growth and to prevent growth of new hair. Mechanical hair removal techniques and counseling are an essential part of management.Hirsutism and acne are difficult problems for an adolescent, because they have a significant effect on image and self-esteem. One should address these concerns even if symptoms are mild. Once hair is present, it is hard to remove; therefore, therapy should be initiated early when the adolescent is beginning to have symptoms rather than waiting until hair growth is significant. The risks and benefits of starting therapy in a young adolescent must be weighed carefully with this goal in mind.

Drug therapy for hirsutism is directed towards decreasing the production of androgens, blocking the action of androgens at the receptor, and slowing hair growth. Various options are:
- Combination oral contraceptives
- Anti-androgen therapy
- Gonadotropin-releasing hormone agonists

Combining mechanical hair removal techniques with drug therapy achieves the best results. Because the growth cycle of hair is relatively long, especially for hair on the face, the results of treatment may not be observed for as long as 6 months. The adolescent should be counseled about realistic expectations of therapy to encourage compliance and avoid disappointment.

Case 3: Acne

A 15-year-old girl comes with the main complaint of nodulo-cystic lesions on her face and neck, which heal with scars.

Acne is a common problem among adolescents with PCOS. As is true for hirsutism, treatment should include drug therapy to reduce circulating androgens and to decrease their effect on the pilosebaceous unit.

Treatment goals are:
- To heal existing lesions
- Stop new lesions from forming
- Prevent scarring
- Minimize the psychological stress and embarrassment caused by this disease.

Options for acne include:
- Over-the-counter (OTC) medicines
- Prescription topical medicines applied to the skin
- Prescription systemic medicines taken by mouth

Consultation with a dermatologist is advised for nonhormonal treatments such as antibiotics, benzoyl peroxide, and 13-cis-retinoic acid.

COMBINATION ORAL CONTRACEPTIVES

The combined oral contraceptive pill effectively controls symptoms of PCOS. Oral contraceptives regulate menstruation and prevent endometrial hyperplasia. They are also effective in the treatment of hirsutism and acne by suppressing FSH and LH, which decreases ovarian androgen production, and by increasing the hepatic production of sex hormone–binding globulin, which decreases circulating free androgens.

There is no significant difference in clinical efficacy among oral contraceptives despite inherent differences in progestin androgenicity. *Low-dose oral contraceptives* containing 20 μg of ethinyl estradiol have been shown to be effective in the management of acne.

ANTIANDROGENS

Antiandrogens are frequently used in combination with oral contraceptives, because their mechanism of action is different, and their combined effect is additive.[18] In addition, oral contraceptives have the added benefit of preventing side effects of irregular bleeding seen with antiandrogens.

The most commonly used antiandrogen is *spironolactone*, an aldosterone antagonist that was originally developed to treat hypertension but found to be more effective as an antiandrogen. It is a weak diuretic with antiandrogenic properties, and effective doses used to treat hirsutism are 25 to 100 mg twice daily. This effect is dose dependent,[19] with a 30 to 40% decrease in hirsutism score achieved with 50 mg twice daily .Therapy with spironolactone should be initiated with a dose of 25 mg daily and increased in a progressive fashion over several weeks to avoid side effects. Side effects are mild and can include menstrual irregularity, hypotension, lethargy, urinary frequency, and hyperkalemia. One-time monitoring of potassium is suggested following the initiation of therapy.

Cyproterone acetate is a potent progestin that exhibits antiandrogen activity and suppresses ovarian androgens. Cyproterone acetate is available in combination with ethinyl estradiol as the oral contraceptive Diane (cyproterone acetate, 2 mg; ethinyl estradiol, 35 μg). Treatment with Diane results in a significant decrease in hirsutism scores over 6 months.[21]

Drosperinone is a derivative of spironolactone and is contained in the new combined O C pill, Yasmin, which appears to be well-tolerated in women with PCOS.[22]

OBESITY

In addition to improving appearance, weight loss can significantly benefit patients with PCOS by improving peripheral estrogen and ovarian androgen production.

Weight loss has been shown to be effective in decreasing androgen levels and resuming menstruation. A 7% decrease in body weight has been shown to decrease testosterone levels and lead to resumption of menses.

Lifestyle modifications, including restriction of calories and performance of exercise, can decrease waist circumference and improve insulin sensitivity and fasting insulin levels in anovulatory women with PCOS.

First-line therapy for PCOS in the obese adolescent should include counseling regarding the importance of diet and exercise in the management of this disorder. Emphasis should be placed on healthy eating habits and exercise rather than rapid weight loss. A nutritionist can be helpful. In this manner, the symptoms of PCOS will improve, and the consequences of obesity may be avoided.

INSULIN-SENSITIZING AGENTS

With emerging evidence suggesting that insulin resistance has a significant role in the pathophysiology of PCOS, insulin-sensitizing agents have been proposed as treatment for this disorder. Although most current regimens treat the symptoms of PCOS, insulin-sensitizing agents are intended to correct the underlying metabolic defect of this syndrome, potentially conferring a treatment advantage. The classes of agents that have been investigated include the *biguanides, thiazolidinediones, and d-chiro-inositol.* These drugs are not approved by the FDA for this indication. Although insulin-sensitizing drugs show great promise in the treatment of PCOS, long-term randomized controlled studies are needed before they can be recommended as first-line therapy in adolescents.

Metformin

The biguanide metformin inhibits hepatic glucose production and increases peripheral tissue sensitivity to insulin. In doses of 1500 to 2000 mg per day, metformin has been shown to decrease androgens, decrease insulin, improve ovulatory rates, and lead to resumed menstrual cyclicity.[21] Most studies have involved a small number of select patients, are observational in design, and are of short duration (12–26 weeks). The effect of metformin on hirsutism has not been studied adequately. One long-term study showed no improvement in hirsutism scores with metformin therapy,[21] whereas another showed a significant improvement in a small number of adolescents.[20]

Few studies have evaluated the use of metformin in adolescents; however, its use seems safe in small observational pilot studies. Glueck et al evaluated metformin therapy administered in combination with a high-protein, low-carbohydrate diet for 6 months in 11 adolescent girls with PCOS.[23] Menstrual cyclicity resumed in 91% of girls, and 9 of 11 girls lost weight. Ibanez et al studied 10 nonobese adolescent girls using metformin for 6 months and found resumption of regular menses in all subjects, as well as a decrease in hirsutism, testosterone levels, and the free androgen index.[23] Furthermore, metformin therapy in 18 nonobese adolescents with PCOS resulted in ovulation in 78% of subjects.[24]

Treatment with metformin has been compared with the oral contraceptive containing cyproterone acetate in obese women with PCOS.[25] Both therapies decreased serum testosterone levels following 6 months of treatment. In addition, metformin resulted in improved menstrual cyclicity and a significant decrease in the waist-to-hip ratio and insulin concentrations, whereas the oral contraceptive resulted in significant improvement in hirsutism.

SUMMARY

PCOS is much more than just oligomenorrhea, amenorrhea, or infertility. PCOS encompasses many long-term health problems such as the development of cardiovascular disease, type 2 diabetes mellitus, and prolonged exposure to unopposed estrogen, which can lead to endometrial hyperplasia and endometrial carcinoma.

The recent line of approach for the management of the adolescent with PCOS is a multidisciplinary one.[26] Treatment must be provided in a supportive environment. Because adolescent females are concerned about their appearance and body image, short-term treatment goals are usually directed toward the amelioration of hirsutism, acne, and irregular menstruation. Although not immediately concerning to the adolescent, the prevention of long-term sequelae from anovulation and hyperinsulinemia is also important. Multiple concomitant therapies are often necessary to address the variety of symptoms and achieve better results.

KEY POINTS FOR CLINICAL PRACTICE

Treatment strategies include:

- Weight loss and exercise
- Healthy approach to eating
- CO C or progestin to reduce testosterone levels and regulate the menstrual cycle
- Insulin-sensitizing agents
- Anti-androgens
- Topical treatment for acne and excess facial hair
- Collaboration between health professionals and sensitivity during treatment are important in management
- Awareness of future health hazards will make Gynecologists, Pediatricians and Family Physicians (Primary Care Physicians) manage them correctly and effectively, so that teenagers enjoy a healthy future.

REFERENCES

1. Zawedzki JK, Dunaif A. Polycystic ovary syndrome.377 Boston: Blackwell Scientific, 1992.
2. Ferriman D, Gallwey JD. Clinical assessment of body hair growth in women. J clin Endocrinol Metab 1961;21:1440-47.
3. Plouffe Jr. L. Disorders of excessive hair growth in the adolescent. Obstet Gynecol Clin North Am 2000;27:79-97.
4. Oppenheimer E, Linder B, Dimartino-Nardi J. Decreased insulin sensitivity in prepubertal girls with premature adrenarche and acanthosis nigricans. J Clin Enodocrinol Metab 1995;80(2):614-18.
5. Ibanez L, Potau N, Zampolli M, Prat N, Virdis R, Vicens-calvet E, et al. Hyperinsulinemia in postpubertal girls with a history of premature pubarche and functional ovarian hyperandrogenism. J Clin Endocrinol Metab 1996;81:1237-43
6. Timpatanapong P, Rojanasakul A. Hormonal profiles and prevalence of polycystic ovary syndrome in women with acne. J Dermatol 1997;24(4):223-29.
7. Michelmore KF, Balen AH, Dunger DB, Vessey MP. Polycystic ovaries and associated clinical and biochemical features in young women. Clin Endocrinol 1999;51:779-86.
8. van Hooff MAH, Voorhorst FJ, Kaptein MBH, Hirasing RA, Koppenaal C, Schoemaker J. Relationship of the menstrual cycle pattern in 14–17 year old adolescents with gynaecological age, body mass index and historical parameters. Hum Reprod 1998;13:2252-60.
9. Dramusic V, Goh VHH, Rajan U, Wong YC, Ratnam SS. Clinical, endocrinologic, and ultrasound features of polycystic ovary syndrome in Singaporean adolescents. J Pediatr Adolesc Gynecol 1997;10:125.
10. van Hooff MHA, Voorhorst FJ, Kaptein MBH, Hirasing RA, Koppenaal C, Schoemaker J. Polycystic ovaries in adolescents and the relationship with menstrual cycle patterns, luteinizing hormone, androgens, and insulin. Fertil Steril 2000;74(1):49-58.
11. Franks S. Polycystic ovary syndrome. Arch Dis Child 1997;77:89-90.
12. Shah Duru. PCOS and adolescents. Personal series. Unpublished data 1998- 2003.
13. Azziz R. The time has come to simplify the evaluation of the hirsute patient. Fertil Steril 2000;74:870-72.
14. DiMartino-Nardi J. Pre- and postpubertal findings in premature adrenarche. J Pediatr Endocrinol Metab 2000;13(5):1265-69.
15. Lewy VD, Danadian K, Witychel SF, Arslanian S. Early metabolic abnormalities in adolescent girls with polycystic ovarian syndrome. J Pediatr 2001;138(1):38-44.
16. Macut D, Micic D, Cvijovic G, et al.Cardiovascular Risk in Adolescent and Young Adult Obese Females With Polycystic Ovary Syndrome (PCOS). J Pediatr Endocrinol Metab. 2001;14(suppl 5):1353-1359.
17. Balfour JA, McClellan K. Topical eflornithine. Am J Clin Dermatol 2001;2:197-201.
18. Tartagni M, Schonauer LM, De Salvia MA, Cicinelli E, De Pergola G, D'Addario V. Comparison of Diane 35 and Diane 35 plus finasteride in the treatment of hirsutism. Fertil Steril 2000;73:718-23.
19. Moghetti P, Tosi F, Tosti A, Negri C, Misciali C, Perrone F, et al. Comparison of spironolactone, flutamide, and finasteride efficacy in the treatment of hirsutism: a randomized double-blind, placebo-controlled trial. J Clin Endocrinol Metab 2000;85:89-94.
20. Ibanez L, Potau N, Marcos MV, de Degher F. Treatment of hirsutism, hyperandrogenism, oligomenorrhea, dyslipidemia, and hyperinsulinism in nonobese, adolescent girls: effect of flutamide. J Clin Endocrinol Metab 2000;85(9):3251-55.
21. Moghetti P, Castello R, Negri C, Tosi F, Perrone F, Caputo M, et al. Metformin effects on clinical features, endocrine and metabolic profiles, and insulin sensitivity in polycystic ovary syndrome: A randomized, double-blind, placebo-controlled 6-month trial, followed by open, long-term clinical evaluation. J Clin Endocrinol Metab 2000;85:139-46.
22. Palep-Singh M, Mook K, Barth JH, balen AH. An observational study of Yasmin in the management of polycystic ovary syndrome. J Fam Plan Reprod Health Care 2004; 30; 163-65.
23. Glueck CJ, Wang P, Fontaine R, Tracy T, Sieve-Smith L. Metformin to restore normal menses in oligo-amenorrheic teenage girls with polycystic ovary syndrome (PCOS). J Adolesc Health 2001;29:160-69.

24. Ibanez L, Valls C, Potau N, Marcos MV, de Zegher F. Sensitization to insulin in adolescent girls to normalize hirsutism, hyperandrogenism, oligomenorrhea, dyslipidemia, and hyperinsulinism after precocious pubarche. J Clin Endocrinol Metab 2000;85:3526-30.
25. Morin-Papunen LC, Vauhkonen I, Koivunen RM, Roukonen A, Martikainen HK, Tapanainen JS. Endocrine and metabolic effects of metformin versus ethinyl estradiol-cyproterone acetate in obese women with polycystic ovary syndrome: a randomized study. J Clin Endocrinol Metab 2000;85:3161-8.
26. Pfeifer SM, Dayal M. Treatment of the adolescent patient with polycystic ovary syndrome. Obstetrics and Gynecology Clinics 2003;30(2).

25 HIV/AIDS

Swati Y Bhave

INTRODUCTION

Nearly 25% of new HIV cases occur below 22 years of age. India has 5.1 million people living with HIV, and 34% of the reported cases are in the age group of 15-29 years. (NACO). Considering India's large population, a mere 0.1 percent increase in the prevalence rate would increase the number by over half a million people.

Adolescents migrate to cities either for education or for employment. They live without parental supervision and have money to spend. Many lead a life style with high risk sexual behavior. Older men choose increasingly younger sexual partners. Adolescent girls are more vulnerable biologically and socially for HIV/AIDS. There is increasing incidence of HIV/AIDS in women in India 21.3% AIDS of cases (1997).

Teenagers have the highest rates of sexually transmitted diseases (STDs) of any age group, with one in four young people contracting an STD by the age of 21 (DHHS, 1998). STDs, including HIV, can damage teenagers' health and reproductive ability. Adolescence are more likely to have sex with multiple and high risk partners and rearely use condom To protect them from infection efforts should be made to delay the age at which young people first have sex.

CLINICAL APPROACH AND DIAGNOSIS

In addition to the usual presenting symptoms which makes a clinician ask for HIV testing any adolescent who is sexually active needs to be evaluated for possible risk of HIV infection

The detailed history of risk taking behaviors is necessary as their management is as important as HIV management.

History of blood transfusion and unsafe injection practices like tattooing, body piercing and sharing of needles for IV drug injection and sexual orientation has to be elicited Some adolescents may present with an acute seroconversion illness.

Rarely perinataly acquired infection may sometimes have a slow progression and be detected during adolescence.

The adolescents should be staged evaluating their CD4+ counts, which are felt to be close to the adult normal values. Treatment includes a comprehensive package of care including opportunistic infection prevention, and treatment, nutritional programs, and psychosocial support. Treatment program should also combine full range of HIV prevention efforts to continue to decrease new infections.

Table 25.1 shows WHO staging system for HIV infection and disease in adolescents and adults.[9]

Table 25.1: WHO staging system for HIV infection and disease in adolescents and adults[9]

Clinical Stage I • Asymptomatic • Generalized lymphadenopathy Performance scale 1: asymptomatic, normal activity
Clinical Stage II • Weight loss <10% of body weight • Minor mucocutaneous manifestation(Seborrhic dermatitis prurigo, fungal nail infection, recurrent oral ulcerations, angular cheillitis) • Herpes zoster with in last five years • Recurrent upper respiratory tract infections (bacterial sinusitis) And /or performance scale 2: symptomatic, normal activity
Clinical Stage III: • Weight loss > 10% of body weight • Unexplained prolonged fever (intermittent or constant), >1 month • Unexplained chronic diarrhea, >1 month • Oral candidiasis (thrush) • Oral hairy leucoplakia • Pulmonary tuberculosis • Sever bacterial infections (pneumonia, pyomyositis) And /or performance scale 3:bed ridden <50 %of the day during last month
Clinical Stage IV • HIV Wasting syndrome* • *Pneumocystis carinii* pneumonia • Toxoplasmosis of the brain • Cryptosporidiosis with diarrhea > 1 month • Cryptosporidiosis extrapulmonary • Cytomegalovirus disease of an organ other than liver, spleen or lymph node, e.g. retinitis • Herpes simplex infection, mucocutaneous (>1 month) or visceral • Progressive multifocal leucoencephalopathy • Any disseminated endemic mycosis • Candidasis of esophagus, trachea, bronchi • A typical mycobacteriosis, disseminated or lungs • Non typhoid *Salmonella* septicemia • Extra pulmonary tuberculosis • Lymphoma • Kaposi's sarcomas • HIV encephalopathy** And /or performance scale 4: bed ridden >50 % of the day during last month.

* HIV wasting syndrome: weight loss > 10 % body weight, plus unexplained chronic diarrhea (>1 Month) or chronic weakness and unexplained prolonged fever (>1 month)

** HIV encephalopathy: clinical findings of disabling cognitive and/or motor dysfunction interfering with activities of daily living, progressing over weeks to months, in the absence of a concurrent illness or condition other than HIV infection which could explain the findings

ARV THERAPY IN ADOLESCENT AGE GROUP

WHO staging should be used to decide ARV therapy. Stages I and II HIV disease, the presence of CD4 cell count < 200 mm^3 is an indication for treatment (Table 25.2).

Stage III conditions a threshold of 350/mm^3 has been chosen as the level below which immune defiency is clearly present such that patients are eligible for the treatment when their clinical condition portends rapid progression.

Table 25.2: Starting ARV therapy WHO

Clinically advanced HIV disease:
WHO Stage IV disease, irrespective of the CD4 cell count
WHO Stage III disease with consideration of using CD4 cell count < 350/ mm^3 to assist decision making.
WHO Stage I or II
HIV disease with CD4 cell count <200 /mm^3

Stage IV disease, a CD 4 cell count is not be an essential criteria, however where available, this test can be helpful in categorizing patients with stage III conditions with respect to their need for immediate therapy, e.g. pulmonary TB can occur at any CD4 cell count and if CD4 count is well maintained above > 350 mm^3, it is reasonable to defer ARV therapy and continue to monitor patient.

Because of the cost and complexity of viral load testing, WHO does not currently recommend its routine use in order to assist with decisions on when to start therapy.

First line ARV Regime for Adolescents

For adolescents who are Tanner stage 1 or 2, pediatric dosaging should be followed.

Adolescents who are Tanner 3 and 4 should be carefully monitored on adult dosing guidelines.

Globally, NNRTI –based regimen are now the most widely prescribed combinations for initial therapy. They are potent and relatively simple. EFV and NVP are both potent NNRTIs with demonstrated clinical efficacy when administered in appropriate combination regimens.

ARVs in fixed dosage combinations and blister packs have potential advantages and are helpful tool to simplify treatment and promote adherence.

This is summarized in Tables 25.3 and 25.4. The second line therapy is summarized in Table 25.5.

Table 25.3: ARV regimes in various situations NACO [1]

ARV regimen	*Major potential toxicities*	*Usages in women of child bearing age or pregnant*	*Use in TB co-infection*	*Available as FDC*	*Lab monitoring required*
d4T/3TC /NVP	d4T neuropathy, pancreatitis and liportrophy NVP –hepatotoxicity and severe rash	Yes	Yes in rifampicin free continuation phase	Yes	No
ZDV/3TC /NVP	ZDV—anemia, neutropenia, GI intolerance NVP-hepatotoxicity and severe rash	Yes	Yes in rifampicin free continuation Phase	Yes	Yes
d4T/3TC /EFV	d4T neuropathy, pancreatitis and lipotrophy. EFV—CNS toxicity, potential teratogenicity	No	Yes, but not to women in child bearing age	No EFV + d4T/3TC	No
ZDV /3TC EFV	ZDV –anemia, neutropenia, GI intolerance. EFV—CNS toxicity, potential teratogenicity	No	Yes, but not to women in child bearing age	Yes, but not to women in child bearing age	Yes

Table 25.4: Dosages of ARV medications for adolescents NACO[1]

Drug class/drug	*Dose*
Nucleoside RTI	
Abacavir (ABC)	300 mg twice daily
Didanoside (ddl)	400 mg once daily ; 250 mg once daily if< 60 kg
Lamivudine (3TC)	150 mg twice daily or 300 mg once daily
Stavudine (d4T)	40 mg twice daily: if < 60 kg 30 mg twice daily
Zidovudine (ZDV)	300 mg twice daily
Nucleotide RTI	
Tenofovir (TDF)	300 mg once daily
Non NucleosideRTI	
Efavirenz (EFV)	600 mg once daily
Nevirapine (NVP)	200 mg once daily for 14 days ; then 200 mg twice daily
Protease Inhibitors	
Indinavir /ritonavir(IDV/r)	800 mg /100 mg twice daily
Lopanavir /ritonavir (LPV/r)	400 mg/100 mg twice daily 533 mg/133 mg twice daily when combined with EFV or NVP
Nelfinavir (NFV)	1250 mg twice daily
Saquinavir/ritonavir(SQV/r)	1000 mg /100 mg twice daily or 1600 mg /200 mg once daily

Table 25.5: Recommended second-line regimens in adolescents NACO

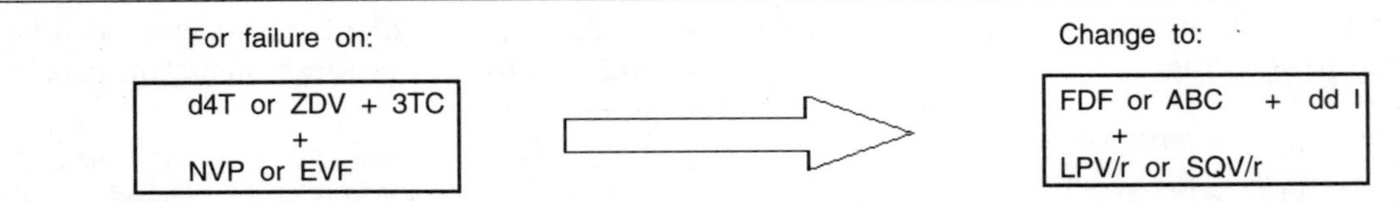

MONITORING CLINICALLY

In resource-limited settings WHO recommends that the basic clinical assessment before the initiation of ART should include documentation of past medical history, identification of current and past HIV related illnesses, identification of co-existing medical condition that may influence the timing of initiation and choice of ART (such as TB and pregnancy), and current symptoms and physical signs.

Active TB should be managed in accordance with National TB Control Programs.

MONITORING BY LABORATORY INVESTIGATION

This is to ensure the efficacy and safety of the drug regimen but should not place undue limitations on the scale-up efforts.

Clinical and laboratory assessments are considerations at base line (pre-ART) and on treatment.

CD4 cell testing is the backbone of ART therapy, but even if CD4 cell count testing is unavailable, simple tools such as hemoglobin measurements and TLC can be used as laboratory markers.

SPECIAL ISSUES IN ADOLESCENTS

A clinician should remember that while treating HIV/AIDS in adolescents certain special issues have to be kept in mind.

THE ADVERSE EFFECTS OF ART ON DEVELOPMENT OF ADOLESCENTS AND PREGNANCY STATUS

When prescribing to ART to a sexually active adolescent girl, it important to remember that EFV and NVP may *interact with estrogen based contraceptive pills.*

Adolescents on who are on ART should avoid pregnancy by effective and appropriate contraceptive methods.

If a adolescent with HIV/AIDS is pregmant the following should be kept in mind.

- If a PI based option is preferred to then SQV/r or NVF should be chosen as they are safer in pregnancy.
- EFV should be avoided in early pregnancy due to potential danger of *teratogenicity.*
- Dual NRTI combination of d4T/ddI should be avoided in pregnancy, because of the increased potential of *lactic acidosis.*

ADOLESCENTS WHO ARE INJECTING DRUG USERS

If such adolescents are to be started on treatment they require to have the HAART (Highly aggressive anti-retroviral Therapy).

Methadone with EFV, NVP or RTV results in decreased plasma levels of methadone and signs of opiate withdrawal.

INCREASING ADHERENCE IN ADOLESCENCE

Drug compliance is poor in adolescents in any chronic disease. The same applies in treatment of HIV/AIDS. All efforts must be made to ensure that they take the treatment properly and regularly.

The concrete thought processes of adolescents make it difficult for them to take medications when they are asymptomatic, particularly if the medications have side effects. It is very challenging as they do not want to be different from their peers. Hiding the disease from parents makes it difficult to get or take medications on a regular basis Homeless adolescents have no place to store medicine. HIV infected adolescents often have unstructured and chaotic lifestyles, and may cope poorly with their illness due to a low self-esteem, and lack of familial and social support.

The most common reason for non-adherence in this cohort was "too many pills", hence the regimes should be simple with minimal pills.

DISCLOSURE OF THE DIAGNOSIS

Adolescents are afraid of disclosure to parents for fear of rejection and abandonment. In our country the laws are such that we cannot do HIV testing in adolescents below 18 years of age unless parental permission is obtained. If adolescents as a older sexual partner they are afraid to lose him/her as often the sexual partner is the only supportive and loving person in the adolescent's life.

COUNSELING

In our country HIV testing has to be done with informed consent and hence pre and post HIV test counseling is vital. This counseling is done at the VCTC (Voluntary counseling and testing centers) set up all over the country.

Counseling helps individual to cope with stress, emotional and social issues related with HIV infection. Where medical therapy is not available counseling is the only tool available to the management of HIV/AIDS.

Counseling can be *primary preventive counseling* to prevent HIV infection or *secondary preventive counseling to prevent* transmission. It can be *Primary supportive counseling* to support the HIV affected person or *secondary supportive counseling* to support of those affected directly and indirectly by HIV. This helps to alter high risk behaviour. Counseling, testing, and referral can lead some people to change their behavior to avoid transmitting HIV to others.

Protective lactors for reduction in transmission are summarised in Table 25.6.

Table 25.6: Protective factors for reduction in transmission

- Positive and connected family atmosphere
- Closely knit and supportive social and community environment
- Awareness programs for sex education
- Positive peer pressure by peer educators
- Positive media campaign impact:
- Behavior modification

SUMMARY

If we want to prevent and reduce the HIV/AIDS in our country it is important to concnetrate on the adolescent age group as more than 50 % new cases of HIV occur in this populatione. Girls are specially vulnerable both in and out of wedlock.

All programs designed to increase awareness and prevention of HIV/AIDS should have a good focus on adolescents. Lack of awareness, risk taking behavior and negative peer pressure are major factors in transmission Peer education and family support are protective factors.

WHO guidelines are available for diagnosis and treatment which help standardization of policies all over the world in India all persons dealing with adolescent HIV/AIDS should be well aware of NACO (National AIDS Control organization) policies and guidelines.

Research has shown that School based interventions for life skill education and awareness knowledge about HIV/AIDS does not cause promiscuity or early sexual experimentation but empowers adolescents to delay sexual activity and/or practice safe sex.

SUMMARY

Adolescent HIV/AIDS is a ever increasing problem. A clinician should be update with the special issues while treating an addescent and also have acess to various treatment protocols.

ACKNOWLEDGEMENTS

Tables 25.1 to 25.6 reproduced with permission from Jaypee Brothers, New Delhi, Chapter 6.5 Bhave SY, Pensi T. HIV/AIDS in adolescents in "Bhave's Textbook of adolescent Medicine. Bhave Swati Y (Ed): 2006 p184-99.

SUGGESTED READING

1. Bhave SY ,Pensi T " HIV /AIDs in adolescents in "Bhave's Textbook of Adolescent medicine. Bhave Swati Y, Publisher Jaypee Brothers Medical Publishers New Delhi 2006 184-99.
2. Bhave Swati Y, Gurnanai P. Counseling in HIV in children and adolescents in IAP ITPAH 2002 course manual part II chief editor Bhave Swati Y. Cambridge Press New Delhi 2002; 36 p221-24.
3. DHHS Guidelines for the use of antiretroviral agents in HIV-1 infected adults and adolescents. Available from URL; http; // AIDS info.nih.gov /guideline.
4. Joint United Nations Programme on HIV/AIDS (UNAIDS) and World Health organization (WHO) AIDS epidemic update; Geneva UNAIDS. Available from URL;http;// www.who.int/hiv/pub/epidemiology 2004.
5. NACO. Combating HIV/AIDS in India. and Antiretroviral Therapy Guidelines Ministry of Health and Family Welfare, New Delhi: 1999-2000.
6. UNPAN. National AIDS Prevention and Control Policy (India) 1997.
7. Satpathy SK, Shaukat M. HIV/AIDS in India-The present scenario. In: Aggarwal OP, Sharma AK, Indrayan A, (Eds.), HIV/AIDS Research in India ,New Delhi 1997; 4-7.

26 Reproductive Tract Infections and Sexually Transmitted Diseases

Swati Y Bhave

INTRODUCTION

Research data from world over is showing increasing incidence of STD in young. The causes of high incidence of STIs in Adolescents are multifactorial. Major reason is the adolescent high-risk behavior which include high rates of sexual activity with multiple and "high risk" sexual partners, commercial sexual episodes and homosexual experimentation, drug abuse, tattooing, body piercing. Inability to deal with peer pressure due to lack of life skill training is a major component. There is a high incidence of sexual exploitation, sexual abuse, coercive or forced sex.

Care free attitude of adolescent age results in thinking they are invincible and diseases happen to others. Most adolescents start sexual activity before acquiring adequate knowledge and skills. Sexual intercourse is generally unplanned, impulsive; on the spot decision which generally results in indulging in unprotected sex. They have lack of awareness and limited knowledge about transmission and prevention of STIs.

Biological factors like increased vulnerability in female adolescents due to immature cervix and vagina also are additive factors

They have fear of confiding in parent's about these issues and lack easy accessibility to medical care due to issues of confidentiality and consent for testing. This results in going to quacks. Hence, clinicians dealing with adolescents have a great role to play in dissemination of knowledge regarding prevention and early treatment of STDs.

Girls are more susceptible to STI as compared to boys adult vaginal epithelium has good mucous secretion and low vaginal pH increasing the resistance to infection. Until ovulation begins the cervical mucus production and humoral immunity are absent. The columnar epithelium of the immature cervix is more vulnerable for infections like *Neisseria gonorrheae* and for oncogenic effects of. Human papilloma virus (HPV).

Fortunately, many STDs are curable and majority are preventable, provided early and adequate antibiotic therapy is used. Standardized management protocols are available for STD management. Due to lack of knowledge and embarrassment and various psychosocial factors, adolescents show considerable delay in seeking treatment for STDs. This leads to transmission to others and more chances of sequele in the infected adolescent.

All infections of reproductive tract, whether transmitted sexually or not, are defined as "***Reproductive tract infections (RTI's.***)"Vaginal infection due to bacteria and fungus are RTI they can be a result of change in vaginal flora or iatrogenically introduced by IUD insertion, unsafe abortions, and improperly managed reproductive tract problems.

"Sexually transmitted infections" (STIs) include infections transmitted primarily by sexual routes from person-to-person. They may also be transmitted by blood transfusion and vertical transmission from mother to child.

STDs that are not curable need more emphasis on prevention, e.g. viral STDs. These include herpes simplex virus(HSV) human immunodeficiency virus(HIV), hepatitis B virus, (HBV) and human papilloma virus, (HPV)

Curable STDs include trichomoniasis, gonorrhea, chlamydial infection, chancroid, syphilis, lymphogranuloma venereum and donovanosis..

APPROACH TO A CASE OF STD IN ADOLESCENTS

It is very important to establish rapport and assure confidentiality if a clinician wants to achieve success.

Adolescents will be hesitant to give details of their sexual history. By being non-judgmental in attitude and asking open ended questions one can elicit a detailed history regarding their sexual behavior. The clinician should not lose the opportunity to educate about safe sex, contraception and prevention of transmission of STI. It is important to emphasize that sex partners should be identified and treated as well.

Immunization should be given for hepatitis B, hepatitis A (specially for males having sex with men and intravenous drugs users). In near future one will have to advise HPV vaccine.

Symptoms with which the adolescents with STD can present are: vaginal discharge, urethral discharge, pruritis vulva, dysuria, pain in the lower abdomen, swelling in the groin and genital ulcers (sores).

The four most common STIs in India are chlamydial infection, gonorrhea, syphilis and trichomoniasis.

Ideally a good lab set-up is necessary for proper diagnosis of STI's. Where lab facilities exist it is always better to confirm the diagnosis with appropriate testing. However, in many places in India laboratory facilities are not available. It is important to give treatment at the patient's first contact with health services, hence the syndromic management of STIs by WHO and NACO is a good protocol to follow (Table 26.1).

WHO SYNDROMIC MANAGEMENT FOR STI

STI diagnosis is based on the identification of a consistent group of symptoms and easily recognizable signs (syndromes) and the provision of effective treatment that will deal with the majority of the organisms responsible for producing each syndrome.

The seven syndromes of STI

Syndrome 1	Urethral discharge
Syndrome 2	Genital ulcer
Syndrome 3.1	Vaginal discharge (without speculum examination)
Syndrome 3.2	Vaginal discharge (with speculum examination)
Syndrome 4	Scrotal swelling
Syndrome 5	Lower abdominal pain in the female
Syndrome 6	Inguinal bubo
Syndrome 7	Ophthalmia neonatorum

SYNDROME 1 URETHRAL DISCHARGE

The common causes of uretheral discharge are *N. gonorrheae* and/or *C. trachomatis.*

If no discharge is seen, massage along the ventral aspect of penis towards the meatus to look for discharge.

Treatment

For both Gonoccocal and Chlamydial infections
Azithromycin 2 gm orally single dose.

Only Gonococcal infection
Cefixime 400 mg orally, single dose or Inj. Ceftriaxone 250 mg IM single dose

Only Chlamydial infection
Doxycycline 100 mg orally, 2 times daily for 7 days

Table 26.1

Organism	*Symptoms*	*Disease*	*Routine and special tests*	*Treatment*
N. GONORRHOEAE	purulent or mucopurulent Urethral or cervical discharge, dysuria, frequency, and hesitancy. dyspareunia	Pharynx urethra, cervix, rectum, Pelvic organs epididymis disseminated disease	Smear Culture Antibody detection	Azithromycin, cefixime, ceftriaxone doxyclyine
C. TRACHOMATIS	Mildly purulent Urethral or cervical mucoid-discharge	Conjunctivitis urethra cervix, salpingitis	Culture Nucleic acid amplification test	Azithromycin, cefixime, ceftriaxone doxyclyine Erythromycin
TRICHOMONAS VAGINALIS	Severe itiching or asymptomatic discharge can be frothy and /or discolored,dysuria and dyspareunia	Cervicitis and vulvovaginitis	smear Antigen testing	Metronidazole Tinidazole
BACTERIAL VAGINOSIS	Discharge	Cervicitis Volvovaginitis	Smear culture	Metronidazole Azithromycin Ceftriaxone Doxycycline
HERPES SIMPLEX VIRUS HSV 2 is much more common than HSV1	Mucopurulent discharge Genital lesions start as an area of pruritus leading to small vesicles with red bases. painful ulcers with inguinal lymphadenopathy.	Genitals can disseminate Encephalitis Conjunctivitis	Scrapings of lesion, Antigen detection Need to Rule out HIV/AIDS syphilis	Acyclovir varacyclovir famciclovir
HUMAN PAPILLOMAVIRUS	Asymptomatic infection, condylomas;	Causes over 90% of cervical cancer noted in females < 30	Pap smear Colposcopy	Cyrotherapy Surgery Intrlesional Interferon
SYPHILIS	Chancre Painless ulcer Lymphadenitis	Genitals systemic	Smear VDRL Trepanomal antibody tests	Benzathine Penicillin Doxycycline Erythromycin
CHANCROID	Painful, multiple Genital ulcer and Lymphadenopathy	Ulcer non healing	Smear culture IF Antibody	Azithromycin Ceftriaxone Ciprofloxacin
LYMPHOGRA-NULOMA VENREUM	Inguinal painful buboes painless transient papule genitals	Genitals swelling in groin genitoanorectal syndrome	Smear serological testing of aspirate	Doxycycline Tetracycline Erythromycin

For patients with drug allergy to above drugs use' Erythromycin base/stearate 500 mg orally, 4 times daily for 7 days.

Treat for Trichomoniasis.
If discharge persists even after full treatment for gonococcal and chlamydial infections.

SYNDROME 2 GENITAL ULCER

The most common STIs presenting with genital ulcer(s) are syphilis, chancroid, and genital herpes. Treat adequately to cover both syphilis and chancroid or genital herpes depending on history and examination.

Treatment

Ask all patients to wash genital area with soap and water.

If vesicles are seen or/and history of recurrences given.

First episode
Acyclovir 200 mg orally 5 times daily for 7 days.

Recurrent episodes
Acyclovir, 400 mg orally, 3 times daily for 5 days.

There is no known cure of herpes but the course of the symptoms can be modified by acyclovir.

If vesicles are not seen and no history of recurrences given. Treat for both syphilis and chancroid.

Recommended regimen Inj. benzathine penicillin, * 2.4 million units IM, in 2 equally divided doses. Give injection in each buttock, after testing for sensitivity for penicillin (to treat syphilis) + Azithromycin 1 G, single dose, orally under supervision (to treat chancroid).

Alternate regimens

- Option 1—Inj. benzathine penicillin, * 2.4 million units I.M, in 2 equally divided doses; give one injection in each buttock, after testing for sensitivity for penicillin (to treat syphilis) + Inj. ceftriaxone, 250 mg, single dose I.M (to treat chancroid)
- Option 2 . (Do not use in pregnant women) Inj. benzathine penicillin, * 2.4 million units, IM in 2 equally divided doses. Give, one injection in each buttock, after testing for sensitivity for penicillin (to treat syphilis) + Ciprofloxacin 500 mg two times a day orally for 3 days (to treat chancroid)

**In individuals allergic/intolerant to penicillin*
Doxycycline 100 mg, 2 times daily, for 15 days, but in pregnant women allergic/intolerant to penicillin.

Erythromycin base/stearate 500 mg, 4 times daily for 15 days.

Ask these women to bring the newborn baby for treatment within 7 days of birth.

SYNDROME 3.1 VAGINAL DISCHARGE (WITHOUT SPECULUM)

Vaginal discharge is commonly due to vaginitis and/or cervicitis. Cervicitis is caused by N. gonorrhoeae and *C.trachomatis* while vaginitis is caused by *Candida albicans, Trichomonas vaginalis,* and bacterial vaginosis, However, clinical differentiation between the two conditions is difficult.

An assessment of the female's risk status may help in making a diagnosis of cervicitis. If risk assessment is negative treat for vaginitis. Where it is not possible to differentiate and/or the risk assessment is positive, treat patients for both cervicitis and vaginitis.

Treatment
Cervicitis
Recommended regimen
Azithromycin, 2 gm orally, single dose, under supervision (to treat both gonococcal and chlamydial infections).

Alternate regimens

- Option 1—Cefixime 400 mg, orally, single dose, under supervision (to treat gonococcal infection) + Doxycycline* 100 mg orally, 2 times daily for 7 days (to treat chlamydial infection).

- Option 2—Inj. Ceftriaxone 250 mg IM, single dose (to treat gonococcal infection) + Doxycycline* 100 mg orally, 2 times daily for 7 days (to treat chlamydial infection).

Vaginitis
Recommended regimen
Metronidazole** 2 gm orally, single dose, under supervision (to treat trichomoniasis and bacterial vaginosis).+ Fluconazole 150 mg orally, single dose (to treat candidiasis).

Alternate regimen
Metronidazole** 400 mg orally 2 times a day, for 7 days. (to treat trichomoniasis and bacterial vaginosis).+ Clotrimazole 500 mg vaginal pessary once only (to treat candidiasis).
**In individuals allergic /intolerant to doxycycline and in all pregnant woman give erythromycin base/ stearate, 500 mg orally, 4 times daily, for 7 days instead of doxycycline.*
***Do not give Metronidazole during the first trimester of pregnancy.*

SYNDROME 3.2 VAGINAL DISCHARGE (WITH SPECULUM EXAMINATION)

Treatment remains same as in 3.1 but one is sure that cervicitis is present or absent.

SYNDROME 4 SCROTAL SWELLING

A serious complication of gonococcal and chlamydial urethritis is epididymo-orchitis.

The patient often gives a history of urethral discharge. The scrotum becomes swollen, warm, and painful. If quick and effective therapy is not given, destruction and scarring of the testicular tissues may occur, causing sub-fertility.

Other causes of sub-fertility are mumps virus infection and filariasis.

Treatment

Treat for both gonococcal and chlamydial infections.

Recommended regimen
Azithromycin 2 gm orally, single dose under supervision (to treat both gonococcal and chlamydial infections).

Alternative regimen
- Option 1—Cefixime 400 mg orally, single dose under supervision (to treat gonococcal infection) + Doxycycline* 100 mg orally 2 times daily for 14 days (to treat chlamydial infection).
- Option 2—Inj. Ceftriaxone 250 mg IM, single dose (to treat gonococcal infection) + Doxycycline* 100 mg orally, 2 times daily, for 14 days (to treat chlamydial infection)

** In individuals allergic/intolerant to doxycycline, Erythromycin, 500 mg, 4 times daily orally, for 14 days.*

Supportive therapy
To reduce pain advice bed rest, scrotal elevation with a scrotal support (T-bandage) and analgesics

SYNDROME 5 LOWER ABDOMINAL PAIN IN FEMALES

Lower abdominal pain is often the presenting feature of women with pelvic inflammatory disease (PID). PID is defined as an infection of the female genital tract above the cervix and may include endometritis, salpingitis, tubo-ovarian abscess and peritonitis. It occurs as a result of ascending infection from the cervix and is caused by anaerobic bacteria. *N. gonorrhoeae, C. trachomatis* and occasionally, it may be caused by *Mycoplasma hominis*. Infertility due to tubal occlusion and ectopic pregnancy are serious complications..

Treatment
Treat patient for gonococcal and chlamydial infection as well as for anaerobic bacteria.

Recommended regimen
Azithromycin 2 gm orally, single dose under supervision (to treat both gonococcal and chlamydial infections).+ Metronidazole** 400 mg orally, 2 times daily, for 14 days (to treat anaerobic bacteria).

Alternate regimen
- Option 1—Cefixime 400 mg orally single dose under supervision (to treat gonococcal

infection) + Doxycycline* 100 mg orally, 2 times daily, for 14 days (to treat chlamydial infection) + Metronidazole** 400 mg orally, 2 times daily, for 14 days (to treat anaerobic bacteria).

- Option 2—Inj. ceftriaxone 250 mg I.M, single dose (to treat gonococcal infection) Plus Doxycycline* 100 mg orally, 2 times daily, for 14 days (to treat chlamydial infections), + Metronidazole** 400 mg orally, 2 times daily, for 14 days (to treat anaerobic bacteria)

**In individuals allergic /intolerant to doxycycline and in all pregnant/lactating women use erythromycin base/stearate, 500 mg orally, 4 times daily, for 14 days instead of doxycycline.*

***Generally, metronidazole is not recommanded during the first trimester of pregnancy.*

However, it should not be withheld from a highly acute case of PID, which always represents an emergency.

SYNDROME 6 INGUINAL BUBO

This is a painful swelling of the lymph nodes in the inguinal region. A bubo may occur in chancroid or lymphogranuloma venereum (LGV). It can also result from any kind of acute infection in the pubic area, genitals, buttocks, anus, thighs, legs feet and toes.

Treatment

Recommended regimen

Doxycycline 100 mg orally, 2 times a day for 21 days.

Alternative regimen

- Option 1—Tetracycline 500 mg orally, 4 times a day for 21 days.
- Option 2—(for pregnant and lactating women) Erythromycin base / stearate 500 mg orally, 4 times a day for 21 days.

If bubo becomes fluctuant, aspirate pus with a wide bore needle and syringe. Make entry into the bubo through adjacent normal healthy skin over a non-dependent area. Never incise and drain.

SYNDROME 7 OPHTHALMIA NEONATORUM

Ophthalmia neonatorum is the condition, where the baby develops purulent conjunctivitis in one or both eyes within four weeks of birth. Though is much rarer than in the past when seen it is a medical emergency and unless treatment is initiated within 24 hours there could be permanent damage to the eyes resulting in blindness.The discharge from the eyes may be caused by *N.gonorrhoea* or *C.trachomatis* and less frequently by other bacteria.

Treatment

Clean the eyes with distilled water or saline.

Recommended regimen

Inj. ceftriaxone 50 mg / kg body weight, IM single dose, up to maximum of 125 mg (to treat gonococcal infection), + Erythromycin syrup 50 mg / kg body weight orally, daily in 4 divided doses for 14 days (to treat chlamydial infection)

Alternate regimen

Inj. Kanamycin 25 mg / kg body weight IM single dose, up to a maximum of 75 mg (to treat gonococcal infection), + Erythromycin syrup 50 mg / kg body weight orally, daily in 4 divided doses for 14 days (to treat chlamydial infection)

Since adolescents are not able to pay for themselves and would not like to tell parents it is important that a single-dose regime is selected and administered immediately parental consent is a ethical and legal issue that will have be dealt with case by case.

HIV INFECTION AND STD

There is 10 fold increased risk of HIV transmission in the presence of genital ulcer or disease with discharge. Early diagnosis and effective treatment of STIs can contribute reduction of HIV transmission. Some STI pathogens are more virulent in the presence of HIV infection. It is recommended that HIV testing may be considered in patients with severe or therapy-resistant forms of STIs and should be done only after obtaining the consent and with proper pre-and post-test counseling. There should be guarantee for confidentiality.

SEQUELE AND COMPLICATIONS OF RTI AND STD

Pelvic disease: Chronic pelvic inflammatory disease results in an increased risk of recurrent pelvic infections and a higher risk of hysterectomy. It also causes chronic pelvic pain

Pregnancy: It has considerable maternal and child morbidity if associated with STI. They can result in ectopic pregnancy. *Neisseria gonorrhoeae* and *Chlamydia trachomatis* cause morbidity both in mother and neonate.

Treponema pallidum, can cause congential syphilis.

Infertility: can result from gonococcal or chlamydial infection that may be asymptomatic or ignored by the female. This may not be of much significance in a older woman who is already a mother but can mean a destroyed life for a young girl who has never borne children.

Urethral strictures: One out of seven males with gonorrhea in developing countries, has recently been reported to develop urethral stricture.

Cervical cancer, is caused by human papilloma virus.

In the developing world, infertility and bad obstetric history results in social stigma.

Personal damage can result in divorce and strained relationships.

Marital instability caused by infertility leads to sexual mobility and further spread of venereal disease punishment with violent and abusive behavior on knowing about an STD in the married partner specially female is common

SUGGESTED READING

1. Bhave Swati Y, Bansal CP. Sexually transmitted diseases in adolescents in Recent advances in Pediatrics Special issue on adolescents chapter Gupte, Swati Y Bhave, Jaypee publications New Delhi 2006 pp
2. Clottey C, Dallabetta G. Sexually transmitted diseases and human immunodeficiency virus, epidemiologic synergy? Infect Dis Clin North Am 1993;7:753-70.
3. Greydanus DE, Bhave Swati Y, Patel D: STD and RTI in adolescents in Bhaves Text book of adolescent medicine 1st ed 2006 Chief ed swati YBhave Jaypee Brothers Ltd New Delhi India chapter 6.7–199-221
4. Syndromic management of STI by NACO www.nacoonline.org
5. WHO/64. Sexually transmitted diseases three hundred and thirty-three million new, curable cases in 1995. Geneva: World Health Organization, 1995.
6. www.who.int/reproductive-health/publications/ trainingmodules_syndromic_mngt_stis/ m2.pdf3
7. www.who.int/reproductive-health/rtis/ training.htm.

27 Immunization Relevant to Reproductive Health

Harish K Pemde, Swati Y Bhave

INTRODUCTION

Although several vaccines are recommended during adolescence only few vaccines are important in relation to reproductive health. General immunization is summarized in Table 27.1.

CLASSIFICATION

The vaccines related to ARSH can be divided into two categories:

A. Vaccines that prevent sexually transmitted diseases or related adverse effects:
   1. Hepatitis B
   2. Human Papilloma virus vaccine

B. Vaccines that are related to preventing morbidity and mortality in the fetus /neonate and or mother:
   1. Rubella.
   2. Tetanus.

HEPATITIS B VACCINE

Hepatitis B can be transmitted by either percutaneous or mucous membrane contact with infected blood or other body fluids. The virus is found in highest concentrations in blood and

Table 27.1: General immunization in adolescents

Vaccines	*Previously immunized adolescent*	*Previously NOT immunized adolescent*
Hepatitis B	No need	Three doses at 0, 1, 6 months
MMR	No need. Some countries recommend second dose at 12-13 years of age.	Single dose at 12-13 years of age
Rubella	No need	Single dose to girls at 12-13 years of age
TT or Td	Booster doses at 10 and 16 years and thereafter every 5 years	At 0, 1, 6 months and thereafter every 5 years
Typhoid	Vi polysaccharide vaccine every 3 years	Vi polysaccharide vaccine every 3 years
Varicella	No need	1 dose up to 12 years of age and 2 doses at the interval of 4-8 weeks after 12 years of age
Hepatitis-A	No need	2 doses at 0 and 6 months
Human papilloma virus vaccine	No need	6 months prior to initiation of sexual activities or at 11-12 years of age in girls. May be given between 9-25 years of age.

serous exudates (as high as 108 to 109 virions/ ml); 1 to 2 log lower concentrations are found in various body secretions, including saliva, semen, and vaginal fluid.

Perinatal transmission occurs at the time of birth; in uterotransmission is relatively rare, accounting for less than 2% of infections transmitted from mother to infant in most studies. There are 70 to 90% chances of developing chronic HBV infection in children born to HBeAg positive mothers and less than 10% from those who are born to HBeAg-negative mothers. Most perinatal HBV infections occur among infants of pregnant women with chronic HBV infection.

Unprotected sexual contact is a very efficient way of transmission of HBV. This accounts for a high proportion of new cases in adolescents and adults in areas with low endemicity. Multiple sexual partners (> 1 partner in a 6-month period), history of a sexually transmitted disease (STD), or sex with a known infected person are the risk factors for transmission in heterosexual persons. Very high risk of transmission is seen in men having sex with men(MSM)or in anal intercourse.

Schedule and Dose

For adolescents who have not received this vaccine earlier, the preferred schedule is three doses of 1 ml (20 mg) at 0, 1, 6 months This should be given intramuscularly in the deltoid. The Gluteal area should be avoided as lit has been shown that excess of fat hampers proper absorption.

Postexposure Prophylaxis in ARSH for Hepatitis B Vaccine

This is needed after unprotected penetrative sex, when the partner is suspected or known to be infected with Hepatitis-B virus.

Hepatitis Immunoglobulins (HBIg) should be given intramuscularly, with first dose of Hepatitis B vaccine at a different site. HBIg should be given as early as possible after the exposure to Hepatitis-B virus, preferably within 48 hours. No benefits are likely if administered after 7 days of exposure. Adults 1000-2000 IU. This is the maximum dose that can be used in adolescents.

Thereafter 2 doses of Hepatitis B should be given after one month and six months to complete the schedule

When HBIg is not available, rapid immunization with Hepatitis B vaccine at 0, 10 and 21 days or 0, 2, and 6 weeks followed by a fourth dose at 1 year can also be used. The dose should be increased to 40 mg per dose in immunocompromised individuals, i.e. double the routine dose (2 ml).

HUMAN PAPILLOMA VIRUS VACCINE

The HPV causes various diseases in humans, the important being genital warts and various cancers. The HPV is associated in 90% cases of genital warts. Other cancers linked to HPV are non-melanoma skin cancer, and cancer of conjunctiva.

Cancers of the Reproductive Tract

The causal role of HPV in all cancers of uterine cervix has been confirmed biologically and epidemiologically. Most cancers of vagina and anus are also caused by HPV. Some of the cancers of vulva, penis, and or pharynx are also caused by HPV infection.

The HPV 16 and 18 accounts for about 70% of cancers of cervix, vagina and anus and for 30-40% of cancers of vulva, penis and oropharynx.

The HPV type most prevalent globally is HPV-16, which is found in 50-60%, of cervical cancer, followed by HPV-18 found in 10-12% of cervical cancer.

The HPV is a necessary cause but not the self-sufficient cause meaning thereby that other risk factors are required for progression form HPV infection to cancer.

These factors are long-term use of contraceptives, high parity, tobacco smoking, nutritional deficiencies, *Chlamydia trachomatis,* co-infection with HIV and herpes simplex virus type -2, and immunosuppression.

Indian Scenario

Various studies from India have confirmed the association of HPV with cervical cancers. HPV was found in 50-87% of specimens having cervical cancers. One study found HPV-DNA in 77% of patients with oral cancers. In community studies HPV was found in 10-14% of cervical specimens from asymptomatic women.

HPV Vaccine

Currently, in India, one phase III trial of bivalent vaccine (HPV 16, 18) is on and a trial of quadrivalent vaccine is planned.

The HPV vaccine is likely to get license in India based on these trials.

The quadrivalent vaccine contains strains HPV types 16 and 18, (which cause cancers) and less virulent HPV 6 and 11 (which are responsible for common genital warts).

Thus, both male and female would benefit from vaccination. The efficacy varies between 95-100% against HPV types 6, 11, 16, 18.

Indications for HPV Vaccination

HPV is the commonest sexually transmitted infection in USA. Nearly half the sexually active men and women become infected at the same time. Prepubertal females will be benefited the most with this vaccine. Young men should be vaccinated as they are the carriers and can infect their partner.

Schedule for Administration

The vaccine has been approved by FDA (USA) for use in the age group of 9-26 years in girls and woman. The schedule is three doses at 0, 2, and 6 months. This vaccine should be given about 6 months prior to beginning of sexual activity. It is generally given at 11-12 years.

However, females are not protected if they have been infected with that HPV type(s) prior to vaccination, indicating the importance of immunization before potential exposure to the virus and hence it can be started at 9 years of age.

Since the vaccine is new, more studies need to be done to decide about the need of booster doses. The FDA has not yet come out with a recommendation.

RUBELLA VACCINE

Rubella is a mild exanthematous viral infection in children and young adults. However, it assumes greater importance in pregnant women, from whom the causative virus is often transmitted to their fetuses. All organs of the fetus are affected, resulting in a number of abnormalities in fetus. These abnormalities continue to develop in later life also and diabetes mellitus and thyroiditis have also been linked to congenital rubella infection. The time of infection during pregnancy is important in relation to the fetal outcome. Early infection results in serious ocular or cardiac disease, whereas infection late in the first half of pregnancy is likely to result in deafness.

The rate of transmission to the fetus during the first trimester of pregnancy is about 80%. Preconceptional rubella rarely results in fetal infection, but rashes that occur within 12 days of the last menstrual period carry proven risk.

In one study from India, 26% of 90 infants investigated for congenital malformations had serologic evidence of congenital rubella syndrome. Two other Indian studies 117, 118 showed that 10-25% of children with nontraumatic cataracts and 15% of infants suspected of having congenital infection were rubella positive.

Indications

To control the congenital rubella syndrome a two dose policy should be adopted. One dose should be given at 15-18 months of age as MMR vaccine. The second dose (as Rubella Vaccine or as MMR) can be given to post pubertal girls at 12-14 years of age.

Older women who have not received any of these vaccines can also be given rubella vaccine. Although a better policy would be to a serological test to check rubella titres which may be protective and achieved by a exposure to a natural rubella infection. Natural infection provides life long immunity Women testing negative can be given the rubella vaccine.

Dose: Single dose of 0.5 ml given subcutaneously.

Contraindications

Pregnancy is an absolute contraindication for rubella vaccination.

Immunodefficiency is the contraindication for all live vaccines including rubella vaccine.

Common Side Effects

Mildrubella, including rash, lymphadenopathy, fever, sore throat, and headache. The incidence of each of these side effects varies directly with age, being almost absent in infants but present in up to 50% of women. Rarely, serious side effects like arthritis, neuropathies and thrombocytopenia can occur.

TETANUS VACCINE

Tetanus neonatorum has been reasonably controlled by vaccination strategies of providing primary vaccination to all children in the form of diphtheria, pertusi, tetanus (DPT) and diphtheria and tetanus (DT) and to pregnant women in the form of tetanus toxoid (TT) vaccine in the antenatal period.

Increasing incidence of diphtheria has been reported in adolescents and in adults too. To control this diphtheria, it has been proposed to use Td vaccine in place of TT vaccine in all vaccinations wherever TT is indicated, i.e. as vaccination of adolescents, vaccination after trauma, and vaccination during pregnancy.

TD VACCINE

Schedule and Dose

Td vaccine contains the same amount of tetanus toxoid as DPT or DT but the dose of diphtheria toxoid is no more than 2 Lf/dose, i.e. 1/5 of the dose in DPT/DT. This is done to reduce reactivity in persons who have been sensitized previously by vaccination or by natural infection.

This dose is sufficient to immunize non-sensitized (unvaccinated) individuals when given at 0, 1 and 6 months (TT is also given in the same schedule to previously unvaccinated individuals including adolescents and adults.)

In all individuals more than 7 years of age Td should be used and before this age DPT or DT can be used.

In previously unvaccinated individuals Td given at 0, 1 and 6 months will provide immunity against tetanus for 5 years and boosters are required after 5 years.

In pregnant women, TT or Td can be used and 2 doses should be given as early as possible but in a manner to provide the second dose at least 4 weeks before delivery.

The dose is 0.5 ml and is given intramuscularly.

Side effects: Common side effects are local swelling and pain. Serious side effects like neurologic and hypersensitivity reactions are rare.

SUGGESTED READING

1. Ballal M, Shivananda PG. Prevalence of rubella virus in suspected cases of congenital infections. Indian J Pediatr 1997;64:231-5.
2. Broor S, Kapil A, Kishore J, Seth P. Prevalence of rubella virus and cytomegalovirus infections in suspected cases of congenital infections. Indian J Pediatr 1991;58:75-8.
3. Eckstein M, Vijayalakshmi P, Killedar M, et al. Aetiology of childhood cataract in south India. Br J Ophthalmol 1996;80:628-32.
4. FDA Licenses New Vaccine for Prevention of Cervical Cancer and Other Diseases in Females Caused by Human Papillomavirus http://www.fda.gov/bbs/topics/NEWS/2006/NEW01385.html as accessed on 9 Nov 2006.
5. HPV in human cancer. Vaccine 24/S3 (2006) S3/1—S3/10.
6. Vaccines. Fourth Edition. SA Plotkins, WA Orenstien. Saunders, 2004.
7. Who Should Receive the New HPV Vaccine? http://www.medscape.com/viewarticle/542229?src=mp as accessed on 9 Nov 2006.
8. www.cdc.gov/mmrw
9. www.vaccine.org
10. www.who.int/vaccines

28 Leukorrhea and PID

Neeta Dhabhai, Roza Olayi

INTRODUCTION

Leukorrhea is a medical term for excessive secretion from the vagina, this excessive secretion plays an important role in maintaining a healthy vagina. The secretions are designed to flush out bacteria and other tiny organisms to prevent infection. Normal vaginal discharge is odourless with a clear or pale, milky color.

CLASSIFICATION

Leukorrhea can be classified into two types,

1. Physiological
2. Pathological

PHYSIOLOGICAL LEUKORRHEA

Occurs due to changes in levels of hormones like in conditions of pregnancy, ovulation, premenstrual phase of menstrual cycle and in puberty due to the increased vascularity of the genital tract which is a hormonal effect.

PATHOLOGICAL LEUKORRHEA

Is due to irritation, inflammation or infection of the cervix, vagina or vulva. The discharge is thick, lumpy, white, yellowish or greenish and foul smelling, can be blood stained and is associated with symptoms like:

1. Itching.
2. Burning and soreness.
3. Painful or burning urination with urgency.
4. Swelling of the vagina or vulva.
5. Pain in lower abdomen.

CAUSES

INFECTION

This is the most common cause of pathological Leukorrhea, common infections are due to *Candida albicans, Trichomonas vaginalis, Gardenella vaginalis (Bacterial vaginosis), others are STDs due to Chlamydia trachomatis, Neisseria gonorrhoea.*

IRRITATION

Synthetic underclothes, soaps and gels, usage of spermicidal jellies, creams, reactive inflammation due to pinworm infestation of anus.

MALIGNANCY

Rare in this age group, however carcinoma of the cervix is commoest followed by that of vagina and vulva.

DIAGNOSIS

HISTORY TAKING

Adolescents are reluctant patients and whatever may be her complaint, she should be promised complete confidentiality before taking history. Careful noting of duration of symptoms is important as there is late help seeking behavior. History taking should include details of color, consistency, quality, odor and duration of discharge should be noted along with symptoms of itching and burning. One should specifically ask for usage of or allergy to soaps, creams, associated symptoms, and sexual activity. It is important to ask if she is sexually active or not and a firm but gentle approach is sufficient to elicit the truth.

If there is a history of sexual contact then any history of pregnancy and abortion should be taken. History of fever, urgency, frequency or dysuria and menstrual symptoms are to be taken in detail.

Any history of past illness, medication like oral contraceptives should be noted.

An adolescent may not understand the female anatomy accurately, hence, one must explain in as simple terms as possible.

EXAMINATION

Visual inspection of the vulva and a per speculum examination of the vagina is important to note the characteristics of the discharge, and visualization of the cervix.

INVESTIGATIONS

1. **Wet Smear:** This is easily done with a drop of saline mixed with discharge and examined under the microscope for pus cells, clue cells(BV), and trichomonas, fungal hyphae seen in candidiasis (gram stain or 10% KOH can also be used)
2. **Whiff test (with KOH):** A fishy smell is characteristic of bacterial vaginosis
3. **Urine:** Routine examination
4. **Pap Smear:** (Specially in sexually active girls)

TREATMENT

REASSURANCE

Leukorrhea in adolescents can be unusually distressing for them and needs reassurance if none of the features of infecton exist.

EXPLAIN

About good hygienic measures and menstrual hygiene as fungal infections due to *Candida albicans* thrive in moist conditions.

CANDIDIASIS

Clotrimazole, miconazole pessaries for 1-14 days are sufficient. If recurrent candidiasis occurs then systemic reatment with oral fluconazole 50 mg for 1 week to eradicate gut reservoirs is needed. It is also important to look for signs of diabetes and oral pill intake in cases of recurrent candidiasis.

TRICHOMONIASIS

A single oral 2 gm dose of metronidazole is effective, in recurrent cases 400 mg bd for 7 days is recommended. .Treatment of the partner is important as *Trichomonas* is generally transmitted sexually.

BACTERIAL VAGINOSIS

A single 2 gm oral dose of metronidazole or clindamycin orally and vaginally is equally effective. BV is also considered a risk factor for development of PID.

PREVENTION

- Good genital hygiene and menstrual hygiene should be emphasized to the adolescents.'
- Simple precautions like washing the genital area from before backwards, changing under clothes frequently and sun drying of under clothes after washing are important.
- Pelvic inflammatory disease is the inflammation of the upper genital tract through the ascending spread of poly-microbial organisms from the cervix and vagina.
- The hallmark of PID is acute salpingitis, which is infrequently complicated by tubo-ovarian abscess, endometritis, periappendicitis, perihepatitis and peritonitis.

BIOLOGICAL VULNERABLITY

Adolescent susceptibility to PID and STDs reflects both their biologic and behavioral stages of development. The adolescent cervix is more susceptible to infection compared with the adult cervix because of the presence of cervical ectopy. The young female introitus is small and subject to more trauma and exchange of body fluids during intercourse. Adolescents who have not been sexually active for an extended period of time are less likely to have any partial protective immunity against *Chlamydia* from prior infections. Young adolescents' cognitive developmental stage may limit their ability to plan ahead for condom use.

CAUSES

- *N gonorrhoeae* and *C trachomatis* traditionally have been considered the etiologic agents of PID, alone or combined.
- Facultative anaerobes consistent with the endogenous vaginal and perineal flora have also been identified as potential etiologic agents in PID. These include the following flora:
  Gardnerella vaginalis, Streptococcus agalactiae, Peptostreptococcus species, Bacteroides species (other than Bacteroides fragilis), Genital Mycoplasma and Ureaplasma species, coliforms.
- Other nongenital pathogens, such as *Hemophilus influenzae* and *Hemophilus parainfluenzae,* may be the causes of some PID cases.
- Actinomyces species have been linked to some PID cases associated with intrauterine device (IUD) usage.
- In much less-developed countries, PID may be due to a granulomatous salpingitis caused by *Mycobacterium tuberculosis* and *Schistosoma* species
- Less commonly, direct spread from a nearby infection such as appendicitis or diverticulitis may occur. Hematogenous infection is rare except in cases of tuberculous PID.

GENITAL TUBERCULOSIS

It is very rampant in our country and is usually secondary to a primary focus elsewhere in the body. It is important to keep tuberculosis in mind specially when seeing virginal adolescents with pain abdomen or adnexal masses. Pelvic tuberculosis accounts for 0.75 to 1% of all gynecological admission. Tuberculosis causes a spectrum of menstrual disorders like menorrhagia/irregular periods/oligomenorrhea /amenorrhea with a history of low grade fever, loss of appetite and weight and lower abdominal pain with adnexal masses. A history of contact should be very carefully elicited.

PHYSICAL EXAMINATION

This includes looking for signs of chronic illness and systemic signs of pelvic sepsis. No single sign or symptom is pathognomonic for PID.

- Visual inspection of the vulva for evidence of inflammation or any local lesions and per speculum examination to visualize cervix and vagina
- PID should be diagnosed presumptively in any sexually active female with the following findings on pelvic or bi-manual examination when no other cause of illness is identified:
  Adnexal tenderness or uterine tenderness or cervical motion tenderness
- Pelvic examination provides a valuable opportunity to educate adolescents about their reproductive anatomy and to teach and reinforce preventive gynecologic health care practices that may prevent morbidity and mortality throughout life (Table 28.1).

Trusted primary care physicians are in the optimal position to provide this education. Although the examination engenders embarrassment and fear in some adolescents, this certainly does not justify not performing an important preventive health service.

Instead, we should focus on teaching health care professionals the communication and technical skills necessary to demonstrate respect and perform a comfortable examination.

BASELINE INVESTIGATIONS

- Urine pregnancy test.
- Urine or cervical DNA amplification tests for *N. gonorrhoeae* and *C. trachomatis.*
- Wet prep of vaginal secretions for the presence of WBCs and clue cells. The presence of clue cells, with an increased pH and positive whiff test, makes the diagnosis of bacterial vaginosis, which has been associated with PID.
- Urine analysis or urine dip stick and urine culture.
- Syphilis and HIV screen if STD suspected or detected.
- Consider CBC, ESR, and C-reactive protein.
- Ultrasound is useful only when diagnosis is in doubt or a mass is detected on bimanual examination.
- Mantoux test, X-ray chest, and PCR for *M.tuberculosis.*

Table 28.1: Diagnostic criteria for pelvic inflammatory disease

Minimum criteria

Uterine tenderness or
Adnexal tenderness or
Cervical motion tenderness

*Additional criteria**

Oral temperature >101° F (>38.3° C)
Abnormal cervical or vaginal mucopurulent discharge
Presence of increased white blood cells (WBC > epithelial cells) on saline microscopy of vaginal secretions
Increased erythrocyte sedimentation rate
Elevated C-reactive protein
Laboratory documentation of cervical infection with *Neisseria gonorrhoeae or Chlamydia trachomatis*

Definitive criteria

Endometrial biopsy with histopathologic evidence of endometritis.
Transvaginal ultrasonography or magnetic resonance imaging showing thickened, fluid-filled tubes with or without free pelvic fluid or tubo-ovarian complex (ultrasonography is not usually indicated, however).
Laparoscopic abnormalities consistent with pelvic inflammatory disease

*Although meeting any of the additional criteria is unnecessary for a diagnosis of pelvic inflammatory disease, doing so decreases the likelihood of a false-positive diagnosis.

DIFFERENTIAL DIAGNOSIS

- Ectopic pregnancy (most serious to exclude)
- Appendicitis (most serious to exclude)
- Urinary tract infection, pyelonephritis
- Constipation
- Gastroenteritis
- Rupture, bleeding, or torsion of an ovarian cyst
- Mittelschmertz pain
- Inflammatory bowel disease (rare)
- Renal colic (rare).

COUNSELING

Once you have diagnosed PID, encourage the patient to abstain from sexual intercourse until treatment is complete. Also stress the importance of complying with the treatment regimen and follow-up to prevent future problems in the reproductive organs, such as persistent pelvic pain. Talk to the adolescent about the importance of using barrier contraceptive methods and being screened regularly for STDs. Advise her not to douche, a common practice among teenagers that is not often addressed during routine visits. Recommend HIV testing. Syphilis testing should be routine, but remember that this test may be falsely negative if the patient was infected only recently. In addition, verify that she has been vaccinated against hepatitis B

PARTNER TREATMENT

To protect the patient from reinvention, her partner(s) need empiric treatment for gonorrhea and chlamydial infection, even if the patient's endocervical tests are negative. Stress to your patient the importance of this. Arrange for the partner(s) to come in for treatment. If your clinic is unable to provide treatment, provide the patient with a list of clinics where treatment can be obtained.

ANTIMICROBIAL REGIMENS

The CDC has outlined various treatment regimens for PID (Table 28.2). These regimens, as well as guidelines for the treatment of STDs, can be downloaded from the CDC Web site: www.cdc.gov/std/treatment/default.htm.

Table 28.2: Treatment of pelvic inflammatory disease

Outpatient

Regimen A: Ofloxacin 400 mg po bid for 14 days or levofloxacin 500 mg po OD for 14 days with or without metronidazole 500 mg po bid for 14 days

*Regimen B**:* Ceftriaxone 250 mg IM in a single dose or Other parenteral third-generation cephalosporin (such as ceftizoxime or cefotaxime) plus doxycycline 100 mg po bid for 14 days with or without metronidazole 500 mg po bid for 14 days

Inpatient

Regimen A: Cefoxitin 2 g IV every 6 hours plus doxycycline 100 mg po

*Regimen B**:* Clindamycin 900 mg IV every 8 hours plus gentamicin loading dose IV or IM (2 mg/kg of body weight) followed by a maintenance dose (1.5 mg/kg) every 8 hours. Single daily dosing may be substituted.

*Administer doxycycline orally whenever possible because of associated pain with IV infusion. Parenteral therapy can be discontinued 24 hours after the patient has improved. Administer doxycycline 100 mg po bid until completion of 14 days of treatment.

**Parenteral therapy can be discontinued 24 hours after the patient has improved clinically. Patient should continue on doxycycline 100 mg po bid or clindamycin 450 mg qid to complete 14 days of therapy.

Note that ofloxacin, levofloxacin, and doxycycline are contraindicated in pregnancy.

Adapted from Centres for Disease Control and Prevention.

For discussion on alternative regimens and special considerations in pregnancy and HIV patients, see the CDC guidelines: http://www.cdc.gov/std/treatment/default.htm

Generally treat PID with ceftriaxone plus doxycycline. Use ofloxacin if the patient has a documented allergy to cephalosporins, is unable to tolerate doxycycline, or has a concomitant urinary tract infection. If the speculum examination reveals bacterial vaginosis or trichomonis, we add to the PID treatment regimen a single 2 gm oral dose of metronidazole.

Although a single dose of azithromycin is appropriate for asymptomatic or symptomatic cervicitis, it should not be used to treat PID. Several patients test positive for *Chlamydia* who were treated with azithromycin and presented a few days later with lower abdominal pain and examination findings consistent with PID. Clearly, a single dose of azithromycin does not provide adequate treatment if the microorganism has already gained access to the upper genital tract.

FOLLOW-UP

Patients with PID should undergo a repeat history and bimanual examination 48 to 72 hours after beginning therapy to assess signs and symptoms. If the patient is getting better, see her about one week later and continue regular follow-up until she is well.

WHEN TO CONSIDER HOSPITALIZATION

CDC criteria for inpatient treatment are based on observational data and theoretical concerns and have not been well studied (CDC, 2006). They include the following situations:

- Surgical emergencies cannot be excluded
- Pregnancy.
- No clinical response to oral antibiotic therapy
- Inability to follow or tolerate an out-patient oral regimen.
- Severe illness, nausea, vomiting or high fever.
- Presence of a tubo-ovarian abscess—Treatment regimens for inpatients are available (CDC, 2006).

POTENTIAL SEQUELAE

- The most common long-term complications of PID include infertility, ectopic pregnancy, and chronic abdominal pain. The risk increases with each additional episode of PID.
- Infertility: Although antibiotic treatment has helped to significantly reduce the risk of infertility, approximately 10% of women develop infertility after one episode of PID,

and the percentages increase with subsequent episodes. Women less than 25 years of age have an overall better fertility prognosis than older women (Westrom and Eschenbach, 1998).

- 6 to 8 fold increased risk of ectopic pregnancy (Westrom and Eschenbach, 1998).
- Chronic pelvic pain is related to the number of PID episodes: 12% after 1 episode, 30% after 2, and 67% after 3 or more (Westrom and Eschenbach, 1998).

EDUCATION AND COUNSELING

- Avoid emphasizing the infertility issue, as adolescents may use this information to rationalize not using any contraception.
- Use the diagnosis of PID as a reason to advocate consistent use of barrier protection.
- Counsel on the importance of regular STI screening.
- Advise patients against vaginal douching.
- Emphasize the importance of partner testing

CONCLUSIONS

Leukorrhea in the adolescent age group generally needs reassurance after excluding any pathology.

PID in adolescents results in serious morbidity and prompt treatment is the key to avoid the morbid sequeale. Adolescents need nonjudgemental and confidential care, and should be encouraged to come for regular follow up. Acute PID in adolescents needs inpatient treatment. Counseling and sexual health education form an important part of the treatment and prevention strategy in adolescent care.

SUGGESTED READING

1. Centre for disease control and prevention 2006; Sexually transmitted disease treatment guidelines MMWR 2006.
2. Coping With Pelvic Inflammatory Disease in the Adolescent, April 1, 2004 By: Andrea T. Borot, MD, MPH, William L. Risser, MD, PhD, and Polly F Cromwell, RN, MSN, CPNP Contemporary Paediatrics
3. Diagnosis and management of Pelvic Inflamatory Disease in Adolescents Mona A.H. Eissa, MD, PhD, Polly F Cromwell, RN, MSN, CPNP. J Pediatr Health Care 2003;17(3);145-147, Mosby –Year Book.
4. GYNAECOLOGY Robert Shaw, W. Patrick Soutter, Stuart L. Stanton. J Pediatr Health Care 2003;17(3);145-147, Mosby –Year Book
5. Practical Approach to Reproductive Tract Infections in Adolescent Girls Dr Chitra Raghunandan, Professor OBGYN, LHMC and SSKH, New Delhi.

Section 10: Skin and Related Issues

29 Acne

Rajiv Joshi

INTRODUCTION

Acne is the most common skin condition to affect adolescents and it is estimated that almost 95% of all adolescents experience some form of acne during their adolescent years, usually from ages 12-20 years.

In most individuals, acne is a passing phase in their lives and does not require any special medical treatment, however, in a small percentage of adolescents, the disease is severe and requires medical treatment, both for prevention of acne as well as for the alleviation of disfiguring scars and blemishes caused by the disease.

Acne is an important cause of emotional disturbances in adolescents and may lead to embarrassment, inability to form meaningful relationships, depression and even lead to suicidal tendencies.

PATHOGENESIS OF ACNE

WHY DOES ACNE DEVELOP IN THE FIRST PLACE?

There are four steps in the pathogenesis of acne, namely:

1. Blockage of the follicular canal,
2. Increased sebum secretion with collection of sebaceous secretion in the blocked and distended follicular canal.
3. Proliferation of the lipophilic bacteria *Propionibacterium acnes,* and
4. Generation of inflammatory chemical components from the retained lipids due to the action of the proliferating bacteria.

Acne is a chronic affliction of pilosebaceous units that consist of the hair follicle and associated sebaceous (oil) glands.

- The sebaceous glands over the face, chest, upper back and upper outer arms are large and active and produce large quantities of sebum (oily secretion of sebaceous glands) and that is why acne lesions are mainly seen over these regions of the body.

The sebaceous glands and their secretion are under direct control of hormones, especially the androgens (male hormones) that are also secreted by females in small quantities. That is why acne develops in the pubertal period when profound hormonal changes are occurring and it often coincides with the development of the secondary sexual characters.

- In the male with the development of the terminal facial hair, i.e.beard and moustache, breaking of the voice and musculoskeletal development.
- In females with menstruation and development of the breasts along with a female type of fat distribution.

Acne is commoner and more severe in males as they produce much larger amounts of androgens (male sex hormones). Genetic factors are also implicated in the occurrence of acne and parents with acne tend to have children who go on to develop acne in their teens.

- The first step in the development of acne is the blockage of the pilosebaceous duct that causes accumulation of oily sebum within the distended follicular canal.
- The micro-comedo is the primary lesion in acne and develops due to changes in the pattern of keratinization of the follicular canal epithelium because of which the normally loose flaky keratin changes to a compact sticky keratin leading to blockage of the follicular canal and retention of the follicular and sebaceous secretions.
- The follicular keratinocytes tend to produce more DHT (dihydrotestosterone) due to high levels of the iso-enzyme 5 alpha-reductase.[1]
- The follicular canal is the home of certain lipophilic (fat loving) bacteria named *Propionibacterium acnes* and *P. granulosum* (both are anaerobic pleomorphic diptheroids) that tend to proliferate and grow on the accumulated sebaceous secretion. These bacteria produce lipases that break down triglycerides and long chain fatty acids and glycerol in the sebum into smaller chain free fatty acids that cause inflammation and hyperkeratosis of the follicular epithelium. In addition other enzymes like proteases, lecithinases, etc produce pro-inflammatory chemicals that leak out into the dermis causing chemotaxis of neutrophils that leads to inflammation. The accumulation of these inflammatory substances along with marked dilatation of the blocked hair follicle sometimes leads to rupture of the follicle with development of severe inflammation in the skin.

While hormonal changes are most important in the pathogenesis of acne other factors both local and systemic also contribute to the development of acne.

Local Factors

- The important ones include occlusion of the follicular pores due to sweat, dirt and oily substances like massage oils, medicated ointments and cosmetic products.
- Acne, therefore, often worsens in hot, humid and dusty environments.
- Occupations like motor mechanics who come in contact with mineral oils and greases are also more prone to develop acne.
- Oily skin is often an associated finding in acne.
- As is the presence of dandruff and seborrheic dermatitis.

Systemic Factors

- Drugs: especially oral steroids, antituberculosis drugs.
- Systemic occupational exposure to inhaled chlorine containing compounds.
- Stress is an important aggravating factor in acne and outbreaks of acne are often seen at times of stressful events like examinations.
- Premenstrual flare and worsening of acne is often described by female patients and may be related to the increased androgenic effects as well as increased hydration of the follicular epithelium.

CLINICAL FEATURES

Clinically the events described earlier correlate with different types of skin lesions that the dermatologist recognizes as follows:

1. ***Comedone:*** This is the earliest lesion in acne and is due to blockage of the pilo-sebaceous canal. It is a conical raised lesion with a plugged apex. The plug may be black (closed comedones or blackheads) or white (open comedones or whiteheads).
2. ***Inflammatory papules and pustules***: This stage is associated with inflammation in the skin and if the inflammation is severe then clinically one observes collection of pus at the mouths of the dilated follicular canals. (papulo-pustular acne)

3. ***Nodular-cystic acne:*** Severe inflammation of the skin leads to large nodular lesions that are difficult to treat and often heal with severe deep and irregular scarring.

CLINICAL GRADING

Clinical grading of acne is as follows:

Grade 1 (mild):	Comedones and occasional non-inflammatory papules.
Grade 2 (moderate):	Comedones, papules and pustules (inflammatory acne)
Grade 3 (severe):	Predominant pustules, nodules and fluctuant abscesses.
Grade 4 (cystic):	Mainly cysts, abscesses and widespread deep scarring with interconnected sinus tracts.(Acne conglobata)

SEQUELAE OF ACNE

Include pigmentary changes usually increased pigmentation and scarring in long standing and inflammatory lesions.

Various types of scars may develop including narrow deep icepick scars, shallow irregular scars to deep keloidal scars.

Self-picking of acne lesions is common in young, usually psychologically disturbed girls and tends to leave behind pigmentation and excoriation with later scarring.

TREATMENT OF ACNE

- Acne is influenced by various factors and thus various treatment modalities are used depending on the severity of the disease, the needs and expectations of the patient, response to treatment in past.
- Acne as a disease has a very wide variation in clinical presentations as well as great fluctuations in the natural course of the disease.
- The psychological effects of acne also need to be addressed as acne can produce profound social disability.

STEPS

Steps in the management of acne would include:
1. Diagnosis with grading of the disease, patient counseling and general measures.
2. Therapy appropriate for the severity of the disease: Topical treatment for grade 1, topical + systemic for more severe forms depending on the assessment of the physician.
3. Treatment of secondary changes like hyper-pigmentation, scars.

PATIENT COUNSELING

Patient counseling is of utmost importance in management of acne.

The patient should be made aware of the disease, its various manifestations, probable exacerbating factors and the physician in turn should be aware of the psychological impact that the disease has on his patient.

Appropriate counseling helps in optimizing treatment as an acceptable match between the possibilities of treatment outcomes and patients' desires and perceptions is achieved.

GENERAL MEASURES

General measures for acne include:
1. Avoid acnegenic agents like cosmetics, pomades, heavy oils, facial treatments, etc.
2. Measures to reduce stress.
3. Correct dietary imbalances.
4. Assess associated endocrine abnormalities if clinically suggestive (polycystic ovarian disease, etc)

MEDICAL TREATMENT

Medical treatment modalities in acne aim for one or more of the following:
1. Removal of follicular obstruction.
2. Reduce follicular bacterial population.
3. Reduce inflammation.
4. Decrease activity and secretion of sebaceous glands.

Treatment can be topical or systemic or a combination of both depending on the patient's need and assessment by the physician.

TOPICAL THERAPY IN ACNE

1. Cleansers.
2. Topical antibiotics (erythromycin, clindamycin, clarithromycin)
3. Benzoyl peroxide.
4. Retinoic acid and derivatives like adapalene and tazarotene.
5. Azelaic acid.

SYSTEMIC THERAPY IN ACNE

1. Oral antibiotics like tetracycline, doxycycline, minocycline, azithromycin, kincomycin, etc.
2. Estrogens and antiandrogens:
3. Oral retinoids (isotretinoin)

Most acne patients are well controlled with one or more of the above listed medications.

The duration of treatment in acne tends to be prolonged and some patients need to be on medications for several months.

MANAGEMENT OF SECONDARY EVENTS LIKE SCARRING

Can be achieved by using various modalities like chemical peeling, dermabrasion of the affected skin, surgical measures like scar subcision, scar revision or even use of lasers for resurfacing of the scarred skin.

PRACTICAL ASPECTS OF ACNE MANAGEMENT

FACIAL CLEANSING

- Acne is invariably associated with oily skin and regular and frequent cleaning of the face helps in removing the accumulated sebaceous secretions, dust and dirt that accumulates on the skin as well as cosmetics and other facial products that the person applies. It also helps open the pores and allows the skin to 'breathe'.
- Although the facial skin is more greasy than usual, the distribution of oiliness of the skin is not uniform and is most often seen in the T zone that comprised the forehead and the nose. Therefore, while vigorous cleaning of this area is useful the rest of the facial skin that is normal or even dry in nature may develop further dryness and lead to facial irritation and sensitive skin.
- Proprietary facial cleansers may be used but with caution. The best still remains luke warm water alone or with a mild soap once or twice daily.
- Salicylic acid and sulphur containing preparation help if there is excessive oiliness.

USE OF COSMETICS ON THE FACE

- In acne prone skin use of facial cosmetics is best avoided, especially cosmetics with heavy bases and chemical contents as they tend to obstruct pores especially in hot and humid climatic conditions and often worsen acne.
- Additionally most acne treatments cause facial sensitivity and irritation and cosmetics may worsen the irritability of skin and even predispose to development of contact (cosmetic) allergy.

MILD, MAINLY COMEDONAL ACNE

- Is usually treated with a nightly application of a retinoid preparation like isotretinoin or adapalene.
- Retinoids may cause severe reactions on sun exposure and therefore, should be applied only at bedtime.
- Further more retinoids cause drying of the skin and marked irritation may occur especially in winters or in areas with cold dry climates.
- Use of retinoid should therefore be started in a gradual manner with initial use for only about 30 min to 1 hour to assess its irritant effects before using it overnight.

IN MODERATE ACNE

- Especially when inflammatory lesions are present it is best to avoid self-medication and seek advice from a dermatologist.
- A combination of a retinoid preparation applied at night and either a topical antibiotic

like clindamycin or benzoyl peroxide during the day or an oral antibiotic may be started. Knowledge of the possible side-effects of all medications should be clearly understood and if such do occur the medication should be discontinued forthwith and the physician consulted.

IN SEVERE NODULAR AND NODULOCYSTIC ACNE

- Oral retinoid form the mainstay of treatment and a typical course of treatment extends to 16-20 weeks.
- Oral retinoids are associated with several side effects most of which are minor like drying of the skin and nasal mucosa and can be dealt with by proper use of moisturizing creams and lotions.
- However, more severe side effects like rise in serum triglycerides and hepatic damage may occur.
- Retinoid are teratogenic, i.e. damage the growing fetus and are absolutely contraindicated in pregnant women or women desirous of having a baby.
- If the woman is on oral retinoids then effective contraception is most mandatory and the person should not conceive for at least 2 months, preferable 6 months after complete discontinuation of the retinoids (isotretinoin).

COMBINATION THERAPIES AND HORMONAL THERAPIES

These must be taken under proper supervision of the physician and there is absolutely no place for self-medication.

OVER THE COUNTER THERAPIES

Colorful light therapies and other pathies for treatment of acne must be properly evaluated before using them.

SURGICAL METHODS

For improving facial acne scars need proper counseling for a proper match between the results of surgery/laser treatments and the expectations of the patient.

SUGGESTED READING

1. Acne net sponsored by the American Academy of Dermatology is a comprehensive online acne information resource available at www.skincarephysicians.com.
2. Andrew's Textbook of Dermatology: 2005 (edn). WB Saunders publishers.
3. Handbook of Skin Diseases by Dr. Uday Khopkar. Bhalani Publications.
4. Rook's Textbook of Dermatology: 2005 (edn). Blackwell publishers.

30 Hirsutism

Nina Madnani

INTRODUCTION

Hirsutism is defined as the presence of terminal hairs in a female in the androgen-dependent areas. The areas include the upper lip, chin, periareolar, abdomen, upper back, upper arms, and upper thighs.

Ferriman and Gallway devised a scoring system based on the above sites. The practical application of this system is questionable today.

Hirsutism has existed throughout the ages. The earliest report was ascribed to Hippocrates (Medvei 1982) describing two women who became generally hairy and whose bodies "assumed a masculine appearance". They both became amenorrheic and died soon afterwords. The most famous art representation of hirsutism is in "The Woman with Two Beards" by William Keys (1520-1550). Today, the degree of social acceptability of a hirsute woman would depend on racial and cultural factors.

Majority of cases are caused by either excessive circulating androgens, or by end-organ hypersensitivity. Androgen production may be from the adrenals, the ovaries, or by exaggerated stimulation from the pituitary. Androgens have to be first converted in the skin to testosterone or androstenedione to exert their effects. Most of the testosterone circulates in the blood bound to sex hormone binding globulin (SHBG). A small proportion circulates free. It is this unbound testosterone which exerts its effect on the hair follicles, where it is converted by an enzyme 5 alfa-reductase type 1 to highly active dehydrotestosterone. This in turn stimulates an enzyme ornithine decarboxylase to synthesize polyamines which cause proliferation of the hair matrix cells, and hair growth.

CLASSIFICATION

Hirsutism may be classified as:

1. Androgen-induced (hyperandrogenism).
2. Non-androgen induced (idiopathic and familial).
3. Drug-induced.

1. Androgen-induced: The source of androgens may be ovarian or adrenal.

Ovarian causes:

1. Polycystic ovary syndrome (PCOS)
2. Ovarian hyperthecosis in post-menopausal women
3. Ovarian tumors.

Adrenal causes:

1. Late-onset adrenal hyperplasia (LOAH).
2. Congenital adrenal hyperplasia (CAH).
3. Cushing's syndrome.
4. Pituitary adenomas that produce excess corticotrophin or prolactin.
5. Acromegaly.

6. 21-hydroxylase deficiency, 3-beta 11-hydroxysteroid dehydrogenase deficiency.

2. Non-androgen induced:
1. Idiopathic: Patients with no underlying endocrine disorder.
2. Familial: Familial clustering of hirsutism with no underlying cause is well documented. Many underlying disorders like PCOS and CAH have a familial basis.

3. Drug-induced:
- Drugs such as phenytoin, diazoxide, acetazolamide, hydrochlorthiazide, psoralens, minoxidil, cyclosporine, and penicillamine, can induce hirsutism with a non-androgenic activity.
- Others like testosterone, danazol, corticotropin, high-dose corticosteroids, anabolic steroids, androgenic progestins, stimulate by virtue of their androgenic activity.

CHARACTERISTIC CLINICAL PRESENTATIONS FOR EACH SYNDROME

Cushing's Syndrome

Children tend to be obese with striae, and slow growth rates. Upper-body obesity, a moon-face, buffalo-hump, and thin arms and legs are common. Hirsutism is present. Fasting cortisol levels are raised.

Polycystic Ovary Syndrome (PCOS)

PCOS is a common clinical condition that manifests during adolescence. 70-80% of hirsute women have PCOS. Hirsutism, menstrual irregularities, acne, obesity, acanthosis nigricans, alopecia, and infertility may be the presenting complaints. Such women may be hypertensive with insulin-resistant diabetes, have hyperinsulinemia, dyslipidemia, and have risk factors for cardiac disease, endometrial carcinomas and infertility. Transvaginal /pelvic sonography may reveal the polycystic ovaries. A reversal of the FSH/LH ratio may be present.

Congenital Adrenal Hyperplasia

Females at birth may have masculine-appearing external genitals with female internal sex organs. Males with classical CAH may appear normal at birth. Patients may present with dehydration at birth, and have trouble retaining salt. The late-onset CAH may present with precocious puberty, hirsutism, and clitoromegally.

Tumors

Patients with adrenal or ovarian neoplasms have a very rapid onset of hirsutism. Scans of the brain, pelvis and abdomen are required to identify the neoplasm.

HAIR-AN Syndrome (Hyperandrogenism, Acanthosis Nigricans, and Insulin Resistance)

"Diabetes of the bearded women" has been recognized since several years where the disordered carbohydrate metabolism is due to insulin resistance. Acanthosis nigricans and insulin resistance occurs in 5% of women with hyperandrogenism. Women with HAIR-AN may have a masculine physique, acne, alopecia and hidradenitis suppurativa in addition to insulin resistance, hirsutism and acanthosis nigricans.

PRESENTING COMPLAINTS

The hirsute patient could seek medical help from a dermatologist, endocrinologist, pediatrician or gynecologist, depending on her main complaint. This could be one or more of the following:
1. Excessive facial and body hair.
2. Greasy skin and hair (seborrhea).
3. Acne.
4. Obesity.
5. Irregular or scanty periods.
6. Alopecia.
7. Hyperinsulinemia.
8. Acanthosis nigricans.

HISTORY TAKING

A good history and clinical examination is often enough to determine the source of androgen-production. It should include the following questions:

1. What age did the hirsutism start?
2. Was the onset sudden or gradual?
3. Was the hirsutism noticed before or after puberty?
4. How irregular is your menstrual cycle?
5. Are your periods scanty or painful?
6. Do you have greasy skin/acne?
7. Have you suffered from hair fall/baldness?
8. Do you have diabetes, high cholesterol or any cardiac problems?
9. Do you have any problems conceiving ?
10. Have you had any abortions?
11. Do you practice any birth-control methods?
12. Do you have a family history of diabetes, heart disease, cancers or hyperlipidemia?

CLINICAL EXAMINATION

Clinical examination should include:

- Height and weight with body mass index (BMI).
- Evidence of acne and seborrhea.
- Mapping and grading of hirsutism.
- Evidence of alopecia with hair-pull test.
- Look for evidence of cushingoid features, i.e moon face, buffalo hump, striae.
- Check for clitoromegaly.
- Observe the body contours, voice tone and muscle bulk.

INVESTIGATIONS

Investigations have to be tailored to each patient and may include one or more of the following:

BASELINE INVESTIGATIONS

1. Testosterone free and total.
2. Dehydroepiandrosterone-sulfate (DHEAS)
3. Androstenedione
4. TSH
5. Blood sugars
6. Lipid profile.

FURTHER SPECIAL INVESTIGATIONS

1. FSH/LH ratios
2. Prolactin level
3. Cortisol levels
4. Insulin levels
5. Estradiol levels
6. Dexamethasone suppression test
7. 17-alfa-hydroxyprogesterone
8. 3-beta 11-hydroxysteroid
9. Transvaginal/abdominal/pelvic sonography
10. CT scans of skull, abdomen and pelvis
11. Selective venous catheterization
12. Radioisotope studies.

Hormonal tests should preferably be carried out between the 3rd and 5th day of the cycle.

INVESTIGATIVE APPROACH FOR VARIOUS SYNDROMES

Polycystic Ovary Syndrome

FSH/LH ratio, prolactin levels, blood sugars, lipid profile, ultrasound of abdomen and pelvis.

Congenital/Late-onset Congenital Adrenal Hyperplasia

Testosterone free and total, DHEAS, SHBG, 17-alfa-hydroxyprogesterone.

Cushings Syndrome

Serum cortisol or 24 hr urinary free cortisol.

Tumors

Pelvic MRIs or CT scans, pituitary scans.

Adrenal Pathology

Dexamethasone - suppression test.

Pituitary Pathology

Pituitary fossa CT scan or MRI.

INTERPRETATION OF TESTS

- The LH/FSH ratio is normally less than 2. A reversal of ratio is normally seen in PCOS, where the LH value can be 4 times the FSH. A normal ratio will rule out other causes of oligomenorrhea such as hypothalamic amenorrhea and ovarian failure. Testosterone, androstenedione or LH, either alone or in combination are most sensitive for diagnosing PCOS.
- Consider an androgen-secreting tumor if total testosterone levels are greater than 200 ng/ml.
- Prolactin levels are raised in PCOS, hyperprolactinemia, and hypothyroidism.
- Androstenedione is raised in 21-hydroxylase deficiency.
- DHEAS may be normal or moderately elevated in PCOS. Cosider an adrenal tumor if levels exceed 500-700 µg/ml.
- In the dexamethasone-suppression test, a clear suppression of testosterone rules out a neoplastic cause.

TREATMENT

1. Medical management
2. Cosmetic relief.

MEDICAL MANAGEMENT

Medical management is directed towards androgen suppression.

The drugs useful are:

Oral Contraceptives

Usually a combination of an estrogen (ethinyl estradiol) and a progestogen with low androgenic potential (norgestimate, desogestrol, ethynodiol diacetate, gestodene) is given cyclically from the 5th day of the cycle. A minimum of 6 cycles are given. They may also be combined with an anti-androgen in a single pill. Recently a low-dose ethinyl estradiol has been combined with a spironolactone derivative, drosperidone, in a pill form (Yasmin), with lower water- retention.

OCs are contraindicated in women with a history of thromboembolic disease, carcinoma of the breast or uterus, and used carefully in those with hypertension. Breast tenderness, mood changes, flushing, water retention, nausea, liver dysfunction and break-through bleeding are the side-effects expected.

Spironolactone

A dose of 50-200 mg/day is given for minimum 6 months. Side effects include menstrual irregularity, headache, nausea, diarrhea, decreased libido, hypercalcemia and increased creatinine levels. It is usually combined with an OC pill.

Flutamide

A dose of 250-375 mg/day is administered for 6-24 months.Doses of 500 mg or more per day are poorly tolerated and may cause toxic hepatitis.

Cyproterone Acetate

This is a potent progestogen and is usually combined with an estrogen. Side effects include headache, nausea, mastodynia, depression, and elevation of blood pressure.

Finasteride

As a potent inhibitor of 5 alfa-reductase type 2, it is usually given in a dose of 2.5 mg per day in combination with OCs. It can cause feminization of the male fetus, and hence, caution exercised when administering to women of child-bearing age.

Corticosteroids

This is the treatment of choice in CAH. Prednisolone in a dose of 7.5 mg/day tapered to 2.5 mg per day over 4 months.

Antagonists of gonadotrophin-releasing hormone: Nafarelin, leuprolide, and triptorelin are some of the drugs in this category.

Metformin

Admisitered in a dose of 500 mg to 2 g per day, in cases of PCOS to increase insulin sensitivity.

Gastrointestinal disturbances, alpecia, Vitamin B_{12} deficiencies and anemia have to be looked out for.

COSMETIC PROCEDURES

As the drugs for reducing hirsutism work slowly, advice on hair removal/lightening have to be discussed in depth with the patient. These include:

Plucking, Tweezing

Hair is individually pulled out from the root by a forceps-like tweezer. This is applicable when dealing with a few hairs. Although the hair comes out from the root, regrowth occurs.

Threading

In this procedure, large groups of hairs are pulled out rapidly by running a coil of thread over the skin. This is a temporary method commonly used for the eyebrows and upper lip.

Shaving

The hair is cut at the hair surface with a razor. Studies have shown that shaving does not make the regrowth thicker.

Waxing

A special sticky paste is applied to the hairy area. A cloth or synthetic strip is placed over the wax, and then pulled rapidly against the direction of growth. This is a painful method popular for large hairy areas. Post-procedure, folliculitis is quite common. Regrowth occurs after a couple of weeks.

Depilatory Creams

These sulfur-containing thioglycollates on contact, dissolve the hair shaft. Irritant dermatitis and allergic contact dermatitis has been reported with it's use. A patch test is useful to screen those allergic to it.

Electrolysis/electroepilation

Both these methods require a fine needle to be inserted into individual hair follicles for the treatment. It is a painful and time-consuming procedure. Scarring is a possibility with an untrained technician. It is useful for treating vellous or white hairs.

Lasers

Laser epilation is useful for pigmented hairs as it selectively targets the melanin in the hair bulb. The diode, Nd:YAG, and Alexandrite are commonly used. Results with all are comparable. The IPL, a light system is also useful. Laser sittings need to be repeated at least 6 times. The end result is the conversion of the terminal hairs to vellus or lightly pigmented ones. Maintenance sessions may be required. Post-inflammatory pigmentation is a possibility in dark skins. Laser works best on light skins with dark hairs.

Eflornithine

Recently a topical FDA-approved cream, eflornithine, has hit the market for use in hirsutism. It is the first topical treatment effective in reducing the growth and thickness of hairs. Efficacy is noted after 8 weeks of use when applied twice a day. It works at the matrix level to inhibit the multiplication of the matrix cells, thus inhibiting hair growth. Eflornithine can be successfully combined with lasers, and anti-androgen therapies for quicker and more effective results.

CONCLUSIONS

Managing a hirsute patient can be frustrating, as often, it is difficult to categorize a patient into any specific syndrome.

Reponse to therapy is usually slow, and a lot of counseling and hand-holding is required from the treating physician to improve compliance.

A combined consultation with a dermatologist, gynecologist and endocrinologist, can maximize success.

Regular hormonal investigations are required to assess response to therapy.

Lasers and topical eflornithine have given new hope in the management of hirsute patients (Figs 30.1 and 30.2, Plate 3).

SUGGESTED READING

1. Kaplan B. Desogestrel, norgestimate, and gestodene: the newer progestins. Ann Pharmacother 1995;29(7-8):736-42.
2. Mueller A, et al. Endocrinological Markers For Assessment of Hyperandrogenemia in Hirsute Women. Horm Res 2006;67(1):35-41.
3. Ojanieme M, Pugeat M. An adolescent with polycystic ovary syndrome. Eur J Endocrinol. 2006;155 Suppl 1:S149-52.
4. Robinson S, et al. Which hormone tests for the diagnosis of polycystic ovary syndrome? Br J Obstet Gynaecol 1992;99(3):232-38.
5. Sarac F, et al. Assessment of Insulin Resistance in the Idiopathic Hirsutism. Gynecol Obstet Invest 2006;63(3):126-31.
6. Smith SR, et al. Eflornithine cream combined with laser therapy in the management of unwanted facial hair growth in women: A randomized trial. Dermatol Surg. 2006;32(10):1237-43.

31 Cosmetics: Use and Abuse

Nina Madnani

INTRODUCTION

Cosmetics are defined as products used for the purposes of cleansing, beautifying, promoting attractiveness, or altering one's appearance.

Cosmetics have been in use from time immemorial, and face painting has been historically mentioned in the Old Testament (Ezekiel 23:40). Cosmetics in ancient times were indigenously devised from fragrant plants, herbs, oils, natural dyes, etc. and used to anoint, enhance, and protect from various evil spirits. In India, cosmetics were originally used for religious purposes and by older individuals, or the economically fortunate ones. Today, the use of cosmetics has invaded a large chunk of our population, permeating down to the adolescent and pre-adolescent youth. The media blitz has revolutionized the way in which cosmetics are perceived. Today, they seem to be an essential component of skin, hair and nail care.

THE ADOLESCENT SKIN

Prepuberty, the skin undergoes modifications in its structure and physiology. The early hormonal surge begins to modify the activity of the pilosebaceous follicles. The skin becomes greasy around the nose, forehead and chin. As puberty sets in, the seborrhea increases, and the apocrine and eccrine glands increase their secretary activities. There is evidence of excessive sweating and body odour resulting from the action of bacteria on the apocrine secretions. Although the majority of adolescents will complain of greasy skins, a proportion will continue to have dry, sensitive skins, or combination skins.

RECOGNIZING THE SKIN TYPE

It is essential to categorize the skin type in order to be able to understand and advise the correct cosmetic usage.

Greasy skin: This type is characterized by large pores, thick skin, and an oily shine especially on the centrofacial areas.

Dry skin: A dull look usually characterizes this type. The pores are barely visible, and there may or may not be visible scaling. There may be perioral and periorbital hyperpigmentation. P. alba is common in this skin-type.

Combination skin: This type is oily around the nose, forehead and chin, and dry on the cheeks, around the eyes, and mouth.

Sensitive skin: Although often not clinically evident, such patients will complain of intolerance to most of the face products.

COSMETICS IN COMMON USE

Skin products: Soaps, syndets, face washes, cleansers, moisturizers, cold creams, powders, foundation creams, blushers, sunscreens, bleaching agents, deodorants.

Eye products: Like eye-liners, eye pencils, eye shadows, mascara, under-eye lightening creams and concealers.

Hair products: Like shampoos, conditioners, gels, serum, henna, color tints, rinses and dyes.

SKIN PRODUCTS

Cleansing agents: Cleansing of the skin is required to remove surface lipids, bacteria and sweat, for good hygiene.

Soaps: These are sodium fatty acid salts. They emulsify the skin lipids and facilitate their removal during washing. As they are alkaline, they raise the pH of the skin for up to 2 hours.

Abuse of soap by repeated use may strip the skin of its protective lipid layer, leading to irritation. Patients with acne try to get rid of their problem by excessive washing with medicated soaps, leaving their skins dry, irritated, and intolerant to anti - acne topicals.

Syndets: These contain synthetic surfactants and do not alter the skin pH. Their use is recommended instead of soap.

Mild non-soap cleansers: These are useful for dry and sensitive skins, and for those undergoing acne treatment.

Cleansing lotions: Specially formulated for dry and sensitive skins. They are effective in removing dirt, grime, and make up. A cleansing lotion or cream is to be applied to dry skin and wiped off with cotton; the final residue removed with a toner or rinsed off with water. Cold cream is a very good cleanser.

Cleansers for oily skins: These have efficient decreasing-surfactants and oil-absorbing ingredients like bentonite. Some newer cleansers make the skin lipophobic, and hence visibly less oily. Cleansers with benzoyl peroxide or salicylic acid are specialized for acne-prone skin.

Toners/astringents: These are used as a second step in the cleansing routine. They usually contain botanical extracts with or without alcohol. Their use is recommended mainly in acne-prone or very oily skin.

Excessive and repeated use of astringents may dehydrate the skin and cause a contact dermatitis.

Moisturizers: These are key components in any skin care regime. Besides trapping moisture, the newer formulations provide superior skin-conditioning and barrier repair properties. They may be simple oil-in-water (for oily skins) or water-in-oil (for dry skins) emulsions or have specialized ingredients like vitamins, sunscreens, etc, incorporated into them. Glycerin and rose water is a natural moisturizer. Moisturizers are applied immediately after washing. Cold creams are useful for dry skins.

Some moisturizers have comedogenic ingredients like isopropyl myristate, and irritate the pilosebaceous follicles when massaged into the skin. Patients with acne, should choose their products carefully.

Face packs/masks: These are popular as quick-fix skin smootheners, for removal of sebum, for a refreshed feeling, or to unclog pores. They may be clay-based for oily skins, or may have certain medications or ingredients and function as delivery systems. Specialized masks may be wax-based, vinyl or rubber-based, or hydrocolloid-based. Masks containing sulfur are especially useful for acne-prone skin. They are recommended to be applied once a week to cleansed skin, allowed to dry or set, and then rubbed, washed, or peeled off. Home-made masks usually incorporate gram flour, turmeric, lemon juice, yoghurt, egg yolk, rice flour, sandalwood, or various mashed fruits, etc.

Frequent use of face packs to give the skin a "glow" may leave the skin dry and irritated.

Pore-cleansing strips: These strips contain an acrylate, which when placed on the nose, pressed, and then peeled off, is capable of removing follicular debris and tiny hairs—so called "blackhead removal". As the debris and hairs recur within a week, there is a tendency to overuse.

Young and sensitive skins, may develop erythema and contact irritant dermatitis post-use of the pore-cleanser tape.

Facial foundations: They can cover blemishes, smooth surfaces, and add color to the skin. Girls with acne use a foundation to cover and camoflague pimples to avoid embarrassment.

Those foundations containing comedogenic ingredients can clog the pilo-sebaceous openings and aggravate or initiate the acne process. Teens should avoid oily foundations.

Powders: Oily skins do well with the use of dusting powder which absorbs the surface grease.

Dry skins should avoid their usage.

Skin lighteners/bleaches: The quest for a fairer skin is obsessive amongst Indians. Several products which contain various lightening agents like kojic acid, arbutin, hydroquinone, ammoniated mercury, botanical extracts etc are available as OTC products in soaps, creams, lotions, masks, etc. They are applied daily. Some have been using them for several years.

Excessive and prolonged use of skin-lighteners or bleaches may cause exogenous ochronosis. The skin instead of lightening gets darker. Allergic contact dermatitis is also common (Fig. 31.1, Plate 3)

Sunscreens: Although sunscreens are useful to protect against sunburn, Indians use it to prevent tanning. This will be possible only if they are totally opaque. Sunscreens are also incorporated into moisturizers and make-up.

Blusher: It is a cosmetic used to impart a rosy glow to the skin. Some blushes contain light-reflective particles. A blusher is usually applied to the malar eminences.

Abrasive products in blushers and eyeshadows can irritate the skin. Fragrances can initiate a photocontact dermatitis resulting in unwanted pigmentation.

Eye shadow: Usually available in various colors, frosted or non-frosted, cream or powder-based, to be applied to the upper eyelids with the finger or brush applicator. Eye shadows sometimes double-up as a blusher.

The frosted ones contain rough particles of mica, silica which are abrasive to the delicate skin.

Eyeliners and eye pencils/crayons: These are liquid or wax-based, used to outline the eye contour. Although sterile when unopened, they rapidly pick up bacteria from the skin surface.

They have a short shelf life, and have to be discarded after the recommended period.

Sharing of eye makeup with friends or siblings is not recommended for fear of transferring eye infections.

Lipsticks: A lipstick is formulated from waxes, fats, blend of oils and pigments. It may be matt or dull-finished or glossy. Teens prefer lip glosses which are formulated with more oil and lower wax content, and impart a transparent shine to the lips. Lip liners are used to define the lip shape. They have higher melting-point waxes.

Lipsticks and lip glosses are commonly shared, and are capable of transferring viral infections (herpes) and bacterial infections from one user to another.

Contact cheilitis is common especially with the darker shades.

Lip glosses can cause or intensify perioral dermatitis, or cause vermillian border comedones.

Perfumes, Eau-de-cologne, colognes are usually sprayed or dabbed onto the skin or clothes. They are a complex mix of various fragrances, and used by both sexes.

The tendency to use "natural" aroma oils and herbal oils on the skin needs to be discouraged, especially for those with outdoor activities.

Fragrances are the commonest cause of allergic and photocontact dermatitis.

Deodorants: These are available as sprays, roll-ons, or sticks, to be applied to the underarms. They mask body odor. Most contain triclosan, and fragrances.

Anti-perspirants: usually contain aluminium and aluminium-zirconium salts.

Irritant reactions to antiperspirants are common. This is common with the sprays which have propellants.

Granulomas have been reported with those containing zirconium salts.

Temporary tattoos; If pure henna is used it is safe.

But to impart a deeper color henna is being incorporated with dye components (PPD-para-phenylene-diamine) or pigments to impart a deeper color.

Herbal tattoos with PPD can cause severe allergic contact dermatitis (Fig. 31.2, Plate 3).

Natural tattoos are not as innocent as projected. A spot test is recommended in those contemplating henna tattoos at beaches and holiday resorts.

PERMANENT TATTOOS

Teenagers should be warned that they should avoid tattooing and if they are very keen ensure that it is done at a safe well reputed clinic and only disposable piercing equipment should be used .Tattoo stikers that can be used temporality are much better alternative to having permanent tattoos

In addition to the chemical toxins tattooing process has a high risk of transmitting blood borne infections like hepatitis B, C and HIV specially if sterile and disposable equipment is not used.

HAIR COSMETICS

Shampoos: Shampoos are cleansers specially formulated for the hair. They are designed to remove dirt, sebum, sweat, skin scales, and styling products. In addition, shampoos are expected to soften, smoothen and impart shine to the hairs. Demanding consumers expect growth stimulating effects too. The frequency of shampooing varies depending upon the condition of the scalp, sweating, and environmental pollutants, and can vary from daily to once a week.

Daily shampooing of dry hair can damage the hair shaft, and make it very brittle and uncombable.

Conditioners: Use of hair conditioners forms the second step of hair cleansing. They make the hairs soft, glossy, and easily combed. The newer specialized conditioners also repair damaged hairs and protect colored hair. Application of vegetable oils prior to shampooing is a way of natural hair - conditioning.

Hair gels and mousse: These are applied to dry or wet hairs for setting or styling.

Regular shampooing is recommended to remove the residue after use.

Hair gels, oils, and mousses can cause acneiform eruptions on the face.

Hair dyes: The adolescent population has started using hair dyes to lighten, darken, or "highlight" their natural hair color. Although temporary or semi - permanent dyes are used, some resort to the permanent ones. Henna, a natural dye, is used in a paste form to give a reddish hue, or to color stray gray hairs.

Permanent hair dye usage can expose and sensitize young individuals to PPD at an early age.

Cross-sensitivity to latex and benzocaine can also occur.

Use of hair colors should be discouraged.

Severe allergic contact dermatitis to PPD is known.

Frequent hair lightening or coloring, can lead to dryness, brittleness, and dullness due to irreversible damage to the hair shaft.

Cosmetic alopecia may follow.

Teens should avoid early chemical manipulation to prevent cumulative chemical damage.

NAIL COSMETICS

Nail polish: This is a tinted liquid which is applied to the surface of the nail. It is available in various colors and dries quickly on contact. It may be applied on a transparent base coat and below a transparent top coat.

Prolonged usage of nail varnish can lead to nail staining. Avoidance of repeated application and removal should be encouraged.

Nail polish remover: Nail polish can be removed from the nail with a remover which may contain, acetone, ethyl alcohol, ethyl acetate, or butyl acetate.

Frequent use of nail polish removers can irritate the nail fold and cause paronychia.

Use of acetone-based nail polish removers can dehydrate the nail plate.

Nail hardeners: These contain formaldehyde, nitrocellulose, acrylic, polyamide resins, acetates or toluene to reinforce the nail plate and correct brittleness.

Artificial nails: Preformed nails are available, which can be stuck onto the existing nails with special glue. These can cover damaged nails, or elongate the existing nail.

Glues used to fix artificial nails can damage the nail matrix. Onycholysis (nail separation) may be temporary or permanent.

Forceful removal of artificial nails can lead to nail pitting, splitting, or nail separation.

CONCLUSIONS

Cumulative damage to skin, hair, and nails is to be expected with uncontrolled and un-supervised use. Lightening, coloring, straightening, or perming of hairs is done from an early age. Patients even as young as 12 years of age, are resorting to these methods. Cosmetics serve as double-edged weapons—used properly, the results are sensational, but abuse may be disastrous.

SUGGESTED READING

1. Atlas of Cosmetic Dermatology. Draelos. 2004. Churchill Livingstone.
2. Adams RM, Maibach HI, Wilson D. A five-year study of cosmetic reactions. J Am Acad Dermatol 1985; 13:1062-9.
3. Amin S, Maibach HI. Cosmetic intolerance syndrome. Pathophysiology and management. Cosmet Dermatol 1996;9(1):34-42.
4. Fisher AA. Adverse nail reactions and paraesthesia from photobonded acrylate sculptured nails. Cutis 1990;45:293-4.
5. Jass HE. Rationale of formulations of deodorants and antiperspirants. In: Frost P, Horwitz SN (Eds.). Principals of Cosmetics for the Dermatologist. St Louis, MO:CV Mosby, 1982;89).
6. Nortan LA. Common and uncommon reactions to formaldehyde-containing nail hardeners. Semin Dermatol 1991; 10: 29-33.
7. Pasricha IS, Gupta R, Panjwani S. Contact dermatitis to henna (Lawsonia). Contact Dermatitis 1980;6:288-9.

Section 11: Sexual Abuse

32 Sexual Abuse in Adolescent

Nikhil D Datar

"Fear makes me tremble in my shoes
Fear is touching stillness and makes trembling noises
Fear makes me taste something about me
Fear makes my ears hear stuff that isn't there
That is FEAR"
— Joel Fazone age 10 years (victim of sexual abuse)

INTRODUCTION

Women who have been sexually assaulted experience threat of physical injury and death, threat to sexual integrity, their personal control, their worthiness as human being and to the confidence and trust in others.[1]

The children and adolescents are vulnerable to sexual assaults as:

1. In 25-40% cases the perpetrator of child sex abuse is a family member or relative. The child or adolescent places its unquestioned trust in the family. Thus, the sexual abuse by the relative is the abuse of this trust over and above the agony of the act itself.
2. The children and adolescents may not have knowledge or may not even know the words to express the exact incidence.
3. The children may not have capacity to comprehend and understand the consequences of the act.
4. The children and adolescent may feel guilty or even may be under severe threat and may not express.
5. The physical capacity to resist is obviously limited.

These factors make them easy targets for the sexual assaults. The sexual abuse devastates the victim mentally, socially and psychologically more than physical assault and has long term effects.

"We see what we look for, we look for what we know."

The physician must have thorough knowledge of the law and medicine both when presented with a case of sexual abuse.

This article deals with legal and medical aspects of child and adolescent sex abuse with special emphasis on examination of the victim of sexual assault especially rape.

RARELY REPORTED BUT COMMON

We Indians believe that our children are well protected in the close knit families and are far from sexual abuse. In fact there is severe under reporting of cases of child abuse due to various reasons. "Of all the cases of rape reported in 1999, children alone accounted for 20.4%. An increase of 13% was noted in cases of sexual abuse in children." Studies among adolescents report significant numbers of non-consensual sexual activity in both sexes. Mumbai has been reporting alarmingly high incidence of sexual abuse.

LEGAL PRINCIPLES THAT PHYSICIAN MUST KNOW

The word "sexual abuse" connotes a very vast meaning contrary to popular belief. Sexual intercourse forms only a part of the concept. It was in 1997 in Vishaka vs State of Rajasthan and others, sexual harassment had been explicitly-legally defined as an unwelcome sexual gesture or behavior whether directly or indirectly as:

1. Sexually colored remarks
2. Physical contact and advances
3. Showing pornography
4. A demand or request for sexual favours
5. Any other unwelcome physical, verbal/non-verbal conduct being sexual in nature.

The sexual violence against children and adolescents includes both sexual abuse and sexual exploitation. Schechter and Roberg (1976) defined child sexual abuse as the involvement of dependent, developmentally immature children and adolescents in sexual activities they do not truly comprehend to which they are unable to give informed consent or that violate the social taboos of family roles.

LAWS OF THE LAND

It is very unfortunate that there is no comprehensive law dealing with child or adolescent sex abuse. The offences against children are covered under:

- Indian Penal Code
- Criminal Procedure Code
- Immoral Traffic Prevention Act
- Juvenile Justice Act (Care and Prevention of children 2000).

Acts such as Cinematography Act 1952, Young Persons Harmful Publication Act, Indecent Representation of Women (prohibition) Act 1986, Press Council Act have provisions related to the subject matter.

Detailed discussion of all the laws is out of the scope of this article. The offence of rape which is most relevant to physicians is being discussed hereunder.

DEFINITION OF RAPE (SECTION 375 OF INDIAN PENAL CODE)

A man is said to commit rape who has a sexual intercourse with a woman under following circumstances:

1. Against her will.
2. Without her consent.
3. With her consent, when her consent has been obtained by putting her or any person in whom she is interested in fear of death or hurt.
4. With her consent, when the man knows that he is not her husband and her consent is given because she believes that he is a man to whom she is or believes herself to be lawfully married.
5. With her consent when at the time of giving consent by reason of unsoundness of mind or intoxication or the administration by him personally or through another of any stupefying or any unwholesome substance, she is unable to understand the nature and consequences of that to which she gives consent.
6. With or without her consent when she is under 16 years of age.

Explanation

Penetration is sufficient to constitute this offence.

Exception

Sexual intercourse by a man with his own wife, the wife not being under fifteen years of age is not a rape.

INGREDIENTS OF THE OFFENCE

1. *Unlawful:* To constitute the offence of rape the intercourse has to be unlawful. This further means that there can be a lawful forced intercourse not amounting to rape. The forced intercourse by a husband on his wife without her consent does not amount to rape. The law considers that the woman cannot retract the consent for intercourse given by her at the time of marriage.

However, if a man has a sexual intercourse with his wife who is willing or otherwise and if the wife is below the age of 15 years, it is considered as rape.

2. *Sexual Intercourse:* The term sexual intercourse means slightest penetration of the vulva by the penis.[8] It is immaterial whether ejaculation takes place or no.
3. *By a Man:* Law does not presume any age bar under which a boy is considered incapable of sexual offence.
4. *Of a Woman:* The offence of rape can be committed only upon a woman. Thus, a woman cannot rape a man.
   Similarly a man cannot be raped by a man and animal cannot be raped. These sexual offences are classified as "unnatural sexual offences."
5. *Against her Will:* The intercourse must take place against the wish of a woman to constitute the offence.
   The question whether woman consented or no is a question of facts. The consent must be free, voluntary and while she is in full senses.
   Hence, consent obtained by misrepresentation, fraud or under threat is not valid consent.

CAPABILITY TO CONSENT

- Unsound mind: A woman who is mentally deranged and cannot appreciate the nature of act and consequences hence, can not consent.
- A woman who is unconscious or under the effect of intoxicating substances cannot consent.
- A woman who is under threat of life of her own or of some one in whom she is interested can not give valid consent
- In India, a woman above the age of 16 years has a capacity to consent for sexual intercourse. Thus, a woman below the age of 16 years even if willfully allows an intercourse, it will be considered as rape.

6. *By force:* Normally, a woman would resist the unwanted intercourse. Hence, the evidence of resistance shown by the victim must be recorded to book the accused.
   However, a woman may be unable to resist due to terror, feeling of helplessness, or fear of risk to her life or life of others.
   This is very relevant in child and adolescent sex abuse.

ROLE OF THE DOCTOR

Physician has three well-defined roles to play in cases of sexual assault. Firstly, physician can provide important evidence of the crime and help judges to understand the physical and mental condition of the victim. Secondly, the reports can serve to corroborate the victim's story. In fact the sympathetic and kind approach of the doctor may comfort the adolescent and allow her to record correct statement. Most importantly physician must offer treatment, primary level counseling and referral for the physical and psychological sequele of the assault.

Clinical settings in which the adolescent may present to the physician:

1. The adolescent may be brought by the police or the relatives with history of sexual assault.
2. The adolescent may present with pregnancy or gynecological complaints.
3. The adolescent may come with symptoms of nonspecific nature, not corresponding with signs.

The parents may give history of behavioral changes without any apparent cause. The common behavioral changes seen are:

- Depression
- Withdrawal from family and friends
- Sleep disturbances
- Excessive bathing and poor hygine
- Self-destructive behavior
- Low self-esteem
- Fear and dislike for certain people or places
- Lack of concentration.

The physician must exhibit high degree of suspicion while taking history and examination of the patient.

IS DOCTOR RESPONSIBLE TO REPORT OFFENCE?

Rape is a cognizable offence. As a citizen of the country a doctor is duty bound to inform to the police when he is aware of this grave offence. Additionally, examination of the rape victim or doing MTP for rape victim may amount to tampering of evidence, if the same is carried out without informing the police. Hence, a doctor who is aware of such an incidence must report to police.

The question whether the patient or the parents wish to inform the police or not, does not arise in such situations.

EXAMINATION OF VICTIM/PATIENT

The word patient has been used only to show that the mind set of the doctor should be no different while examining these cases. The approach of concern and empathy is important. It must be noted that when the physician is collecting the evidences of offence under the order of State, NO doctor–patient relationship gets established.

THE OBJECTIVE OF THE EXAMINATION OF THE PATIENT IS TO ESTABLISH THE FOLLOWING

1. *A sexual act has been attempted or completed:* Apart from penetration of penis other sexual acts such as touching genitals, anal, oral penetration, penetration by fingers, objects also constitute the sexual acts and evidence of the same must be looked for.
2. *The woman has not given consent:* This can be established from history, evidences of struggle such as injuries inflicted.
3. *The victim was not capable of giving valid consent:* This can be established from influence of alcohol and drugs, unsoundness of mind. She may be minor.
4. *Verification of identity and age.*
5. *Providing treatment, care and appropriate referrals.*

WHO CAN EXAMINE THE VICTIM?

- Usually, this examination is conducted by forensic specialist or police surgeon and/or physician (gynecologist) from public health sector.
- Technically any medical graduate is eligible to carry out the examination. It is unfortunate that the medical graduates are not adequately trained during curriculum to carry out such examinations.
- A private practitioner can also examine the patient.

WHO CAN REQUEST FOR EXAMINATION?

Any of the following can request for examination.
- The victim
- Her relative or guardian
- Law enforcement agencies.

Thus, it must be noted that it is not mandatory that the request must be initiated by the police only. Similarly, it is not mandatory that the police complaint must precede the examination.

CARE THAT THE EXAMINER NEEDS TO TAKE WHILE EXAMINING

The examiner should ensure that the persons belonging to offender's group should not be present at the time of examination. Similarly, the police should not be present in the examination room.

A female medical attendant must be present through out the examination. In case of minor girl, victim's mother and female attendant both should be present. It is not mandatory that only female doctor must examine .

The procedure of examination must be explained to the survivor. It must be clarified that she may ask the doctor to stop the examination at any juncture of time.

TIMING OF EXAMINATION

Spermatozoa, usually, remain motile for 2-3 hours in the vagina. The non-motile sperms can be found up to for 24 hours. Intact spermatozoa are rarely found in the vagina beyond 72 hours. It is obvious that undue delay must be avoided.

SYSTEMATIC EXAMINATION OF A FEMALE VICTIM CAN BE DISCUSSED UNDER FOLLOWING HEADS

1. Preliminary data.
2. Consent.
3. Medical history.
4. Sexual assault history.
5. Collecting the evidence from clothing etc.
6. General examination and sample collection
7. Genital examination and sample collection.
8. Age estimation
9. Inference.

Preliminary Data

Following must be noted:

1. Who has requested examination?
2. Name of victim.
3. Parent's name.
4. Address.
5. Occupation.
6. Caste.
7. Marital status.
8. Age.
9. Person accompanying.
10. Time and place of examination.
11. Identification marks.
12. Name of female attendant.

Consent

Written consent is mandatory prior to examination.

If the victim is above the age of 12 years, then her consent is taken.

If she is below 12 years, or of unsound mind the consent of parents or guardians must be obtained.

The consent must be obtained in presence of a witness.

Age and capacity to consent: Under the civil law, the age at which person becomes competent to consent is considered as 18 years. The law considers that at the age of 16 years a woman is capable to consent for sexual intercourse. Section 90 of Indian Penal Code states that consent is not a true consent if given by a person under twelve years.

Consent of the patient to be taken for:

- For examination and treatment for effects of the assault
- For collection of the evidence.

Medical History

Personal details and medical history including menstrual history and details of pregnancy (if any), medical, surgical history are recorded.

Sexual Assault History

Patient's narration of the assault should be recorded verbatim. The examiner must be tactful and may put direct questions to bring out relevant details such as:

1. The place and time of incidence.
2. Number of assailants.
3. The amount of violence.
4. Position.
5. Resistance offered.
6. Pain, hemorrhage, sensation of penetration and emission.
7. H/o loss of consciousness
8. Clothes which victim worn.

The statement must include whether the victim has changed clothes, urinated or douched her vagina or taken bath after the assault.

History of the assault as told to the physician may be the first opportunity for the patient to tell her story in a relatively secure setting.

In case of minor children, illustrative books or a doll can be used if available, to elicit the history of the assault.

Collecting and Storing the Clothing Evidence

The clothes should be looked for the corroborative evidence. Thus, it is important to examine the victim before changing the clothes. The collection of specimens of foreign material, e.g. grass, mud, hair, etc. which may have been left on her person from the site of assault or from the assailant must be done carefully. It is a very good idea to make the victim stand on large sheet of paper and then made to change. The samples of foreign material thus will get collected on the paper preventing the loss of such evidence.

The clothing should be retained, labeled and sent for examination. A set of spare clothing can be requested from the patient's relatives.

General Examination

A doctor should ascertain the general condition of the victim and the vital parameters.

Injuries and hemorrhage may put the victim's life at risk and if so, treatment must be initiated immediately. The medical needs must be prioritized over evidence collection.

Examination of injuries

The whole body must be examined for marks of violence such as bruises, scratches, bites and other injuries. The victim should be requested to undress herself. In cases of sexual assault it is common to find marks on the face, neck, shoulders, breast, upper arms, buttocks and thighs.

All the injuries must be described in terms of nature, location, severity and should be diagrammatically represented.

Following injuries are common:

- Head: Blow on head or head injury due to fall.
- Neck: Gripping of throat.
- Injuries on cheeks, lips, breast, and chest are common.
- Generalised bruises, lacerations, contusions, bite marks, nail marks.
- The marks of rope knots on the wrists and ankles.

Examination of nails:

Scraping from the nail beds can be collected by thin swab stick or blunt knife. Tags of epithelium, hair, fibers of clothing, blood stains are important evidences.

Gait: The patient's gait must be made a note of. An assessment of the emotional and mental state of the patient should be made and documented. A second examination after 48 hours may reveal deep bruises, which may not be evident at the first examination.

Collections of samples:

- Moistened swabs can be used to collect smears from the oral cavity, blood stains on the body, foreign material on the body surfaces, seminal stains on the skin surfaces.
- The head hair of the patient should be combed for specimens of any loose hair or debris if present.
- A sample of 5-10 scalp hair should be cut and preserved in an envelope for the purpose of comparison or to serve as control sample.
- The 7 ml venous blood should be collected with the sterile syringe and needle. About 2ml in EDTA bulb for grouping and for DNA analysis when required. The remaining 5 ml can be collected in a bulb containing 5 mg sodium flouride + 50 mg potassium oxalate in solid state. The second sample will be used for assessing alcohol levels and drugs.

Examination of Genitals

A gynecological examination should be conducted in lithotomy position and in good light. The history of last menstrual period must be asked for to differentiate menstruation from bleeding due injuries.

A systematic examination of perineum, vulva, labia, vagina and hymen must be done to ascertain injuries.

- *Hymen*: It is significant if the victim is not sexually active. Bleeding, redness, edema, ragged fresh edges suggest recent injury.
- Examination of external genitalia.
- Examination of vulva, labia, paraurethral area, fourchete must be examinaed for tears and lacerations. Bleeding, blunt injuries, edema must be noted.

- Examination of vagina.
- *Distensibility of vagina*: The distensibility should be noted in relation to number of fingers it admits.
- The vagina, fornices must be examined for lacerations, tears, bleeding by using sterile speculum in good illumination.

Lacerations of posterior forchette are very commonly associated with forceful intercourse especially with a virgin.

Indecent assault with finger penetration may lead to lateral vaginal wall tears.

Collection of samples:

- The pubic hair matted due to blood stains, seminal stains or secretions should be cut and preserved.
- Pubic hair should be combed for specimens of the offender's pubic hair. If pubic hair are shaved then it must be specifically mentioned.
- As the examination proceeds, separate swabs are taken from the vulva, vagina and anal opening

Collection of vaginal secretions:

- Instillation of 15 ml of normal saline in posterior fornix and aspiration of contents can be collected and examined.
- A wet preparation when studied under microscope may reveal motile or non motile spermatozoa. Absence of spermatozoon does not mean absence of intercourse.
- Ziehl Neelson's staining of another slide may reveal acid fast, rod shaped organisms, which are smegma bacilli.

Evidence of venereal disease: The examiner should keep in mind signs of various veneral diseases such as syphilis, gonorrhea, chanchroid, etc.

Assessment of the Age

The patient can be asked for the age proof such as school leaving certificate, etc. Tanner's charts can be used for this purpose. Secondary sex characteristics, dentition and, in selected cases, ossification tests by radiography are used to estimate age. These tests should be done only when in doubt about the age.

Inference

The job of the examiner is not to give verdict. The medical examiner should concentrate on:

- Finding an evidence of intercourse.
- Finding an evidence of resistance.

Special attention should be given to following:

1. All injuries are to be noted preferably in diagrammatic form.
2. Always ensure that the samples are air dried before storing them in their respective containers.
3. Always ensure that all the envelopes containing the samples are labeled (Type of Sample/ Name and Initials of the Examining Doctor/Crime Registration/MLC No./Time/ Date) and sealed appropriately before handing them over to the concerned authority (Police/ Laboratory).
4. It is the duty of physician to maintain secrecy about the identity of the victim.
5. The examination may have to be performed under general anesthesia.
6. The physician must write the notes very clearly. Clearly written notes are particularly useful when they are referred to after few years when the case comes up for hearing in the courts.

TREATMENT GUIDELINES

PREVENTION OF INFECTIONS

1. Empirically, azithromycin 1gm single dose or doxycycline and metronidazole can be given.
2. All children with gonococcal infection should be treated for presumptive *C. trachomatis* infection and vice versa. These patients should also be evaluated for concurrent syphilis, hepatitis B and HIV. The drugs of choice for uncomplicated vulvo-vaginitis or prophylaxis for gonococcal and clamydial infection are ceftriaxone plus erythromycin/ doxycycline/azithromycin.

3. *Hepatitis B prophylaxis:* A sample of blood for HBsAg should be collected and simultaneously immunoglobulin should be administered immediately (up to 72 hours after sexual act) in dose of 0.06 ml/kg body weight.
4. *Post Exposure Prophylaxis (PEP) for HIV:* The patient should be treated in the same way as that for needle stick injuries. If no injuries are present then the treatment should proceed depending upon mucosal integrity.

TREATMENT OF INJURIES

The wounds should be cleaned with antiseptic solutions, sutured if required and dressed. The physician should check on tetanus immunization.

PREVENTING UNWANTED PREGNANCY

The preferred choice of treatment is 2 tablets of Levonorgestrel 750 µg within 72 hours. If vomiting occurs, within 3 hours repeat.

TERMINATION OF PREGNANCY

Medical or surgical abortion should be considered depending on the weeks of gestation.

If any patient presents for termination of pregnancy with the history of sexual assault, the police should be notified about the same.

COUNSELING

The immediate and primary counseling can be done by physician.

It is important to reassure that the abuse shall not leave a permanent detriment on the body of the survivor.

Patient can be referred to rape crisis center if such is available.

Alternatively one can refer to psychologist, psychiatrist or counselor .

FOLLOW-UP

- Within 72 hours after initial assessment to record developing bruises
- Repeat test for gonorrhea if possible.
- Test for pregnancy.
- Repeat after six weeks for VDRL.
- Assess for psychological sequelae.

CONCLUSIONS

The examination of the survivors of alleged sexual offence is a very difficult task.

There is a danger that the criminal may get acquitted as well as a possibility of wrong conviction. This puts a great responsibility on the medical examiner to give exact and correct inputs.

The offence itself has medical, psychological, social, emotional attributes. All over the world the assault was only viewed from criminal justice point of view. It is a need of the hour that the society recognizes it as issue of human rights and health.

There is a severe paucity of knowledge of law related to the issue amongst the doctors.

There is a great need to standardize the examination protocol so that no piece of evidence is left out.

THE SAFE Kit

The prominent NGO "CEHAT" (Center of enquiry into health and allied themes) has come out with a unique kit called "SAFE Kit" (Sexual Assault Forensic Evidence Kit).

This kit comprises of manual, forms and all the accessories required for the collection and preservation of forensic evidence. Use of such protocols will go long way in delivering justice to victims of both sexual assault and false allegations.

SUGGESTED READING

1. "A Guide Book for the Media on Sexual Violence against Children." National Human Rights Commission Prasar Bharati p. 12
2. "Care And Rehabilitation Of Rape, Torture and Other Severe Traumas of War In The Republic Of Ex Yugoslavia." Dahl Soherg 1993.
3. "Child Sex Abuse—A Clinician Dilemma" Parul Kotdawal Adolescent Girl: An Update FOGSI Publication, p. 226.

4. Dr Lalitha D Souza. Sexual Assault of Women and Girl Children: A Manual For The Examining Physicians Published By CEHAT Updated In Nov 2004; p. 10.
5. Modi's Medical Jurisprudence and Toxicology (22nd edn) p. 501.
6. Modi's Medical Jurisprudence and Toxicology, 22nd Edition, p. 494.
7. National Crime Records Bereau .Ministry of Home Affairs. Govt. of India 2001; p. 218
8. "Non-consensual Sexual Experiences of Young People: A Review of the Evidence from Developing Countries," Jejeebhoy S, Bott S, Population Council Of India, New Delhi, India 2003.
9. Ratanlal and Dhirajlal's The Indian Penal Code Twenty Eight, Edition Reprint, 2002; p. 102-103
10. Ratanlal and Dhirajlal's The Indian Penal Code, Twenty Eight, Edition Reprint, 2002; p. 512.

33 Psychological Aspects of Sexual Abuse

Jitendra Nagpal, Swati Y Bhave

INTRODUCTION

Sexual abuse is very common in the adolescent age group. Adolescents are exposed to aduts who have control and authority in their life and they will find it difficult to resist or report this behaviors. The perpeters can be parents, family members, family friends, teachers, tutors for extra coaching like music and other activities, sports coaches

One important aspect of sexuality education in schools is making children and adolescents aware of what is sexual abuse and empower them with life skills to protect themselves.

Increasing awareness in the community regarding sexual abuse will lead to more protections of potential victims and lesser incidence of sexual abuse which is unfortuantley on the rise in todays society.

THE EFFECTS OF SEXUAL ABUSE ARE VERY COMPLEX

Adolescscents can be both victims and preceptors of sexual abuse specially if they have been molested as children

When we talk of sexual abuse in adolescents it may:

- Recent, i.e. which has occurred in the adolescent age
- Chronic, i.e. going on since child hood this is specially true of incest and sexual abuse by family members or known family friends.
- Sexual abuse occurred in childhood but the psychological trauma is persisting in adolescence.

The adverse impact of sexual abuse SA depends on:

- The age and developmental stage (or stages) at which the SA occurred.
- The age when SA ended.
- The frequency of sexual acts.
- Whether or not penetration occurred.
- The relationship of the perpetrator to the victim (how much betrayal of trust occurred).
- The presence or absence of parental support.
- The nature of the family context.
  - Chaotic family context
  - Co-occurring forms of maltreatment.

SEXUAL ABUSE

- **Can be a one-time episode** (most common when perpetrator is a stranger) **Or**
- **It can be a repeated event**—Regularly over many years (most common when perpetrator is a family member or other person with regular sanctioned contact).

Sexual abuser may be:

- **A Situational** molester does not have a sole preference for sex with children and adolescents but exploits others as well.

- The **Preferential** (Pedophile), prefers sexual activity with children and often uses coercion, threat, intimidation, seduction, bribery and manipulation.

THE PROFILE OF A FEMALE SEXUAL OFFENDERS

- Predisposed or intergenerational offender—Likely to have deviant sexual fantasies that she considers shameful.
- Male-coerced offender—Extremely dependent on males, has low self-esteem and feels powerless in relationships.
- Teacher-lover molester—sees the child or adolescent as her equal.

Very often sexual abuse is a continuum from child to adolescent stage

In clinically referred maltreated children, the reported incidence rates of PTSD resulting from sexual abuse range from 42 to 90% (Dubner and Motta, 1999; Lipschitz et al, 1999; McLeer et al, 1994).

Recently, a prevalence rate of PTSD of 36.3% in non-clinically referred sexually abused children, 60 days immediately following sexual abuse disclosure was reported (McLeer et al 1998). Thus, PTSD is commonly seen in maltreated children, especially during the period immediately following maltreatment disclosure.

PSYCHOLOGICAL IMPACT OF CHILD/ ADOLESCENT SEXUAL ABUSE

- Anxiety disorders—Sexually abuse causes psychological impairment consisting of anxiety that involves symptoms such as chronic tension, sleep disturbances, nightmares and somatic complaints.
- If there is stigmatization it results in shame, guilt, low self-esteem and depression.
- They can exhibit affective disregulation, impulsivity and dissociative defenses.
- There is higher incidence of suicidal attempts.
- Phobic reactions are also found to be present.
- Increased aggression—Angry reactions and poor impulse control has also been noted.
- Impaired peer relationships have been frequently reported.
- Inadequate social skills, difficulties in personal relationships and social withdrawal are also been found.
- Poor school performance, difficulties in intellectual, physical and social development, angry reactions and poor impulse control are the other reported symptoms.
- This is adverse impact on psychosocial development, gender identity and future capacity for sexual intimacy.
- Victims are unable to differentiate affectionate from sexual relationships.
- Borderline personality disorder has been frequently observed in adult female survivors of sexual abuse.
- Memories of victimization become integrated in the total organization and become ego syntonic.
- Women survivors of child sexual abuse appear to be vulnerable to revictimization later in life.
- Post-traumatic stress disorder syndrome may be seen in about 30 to 40% of sexual abuse cases.

LONG-TERM EFFECTS

- Depression
- Anxiety disorders
- Dissociative and PTSD
- Specific phobias
- Personality disorders
- Medical illness (increased rates of IBS, chronic pelvic pain, genitourinary complaints, autoimmune disorders)
- Children who appear to be asymptomatic immediately postabuse may show ADHD in later childhood.

MEDICAL ADVERSE EFFECTS OF SEXUAL ABUSE

Postpubertal girls need to be tested for preganancy and it has to be dealt with sexually transmitted diseases have to be looked for and treated. Prophylactic vaccines like hepatitis B and HPV need to be given.

If there are medical adverse effects, it will further add to the psychological trauma.

Management of psychological manifestations of sexual abuse:

- Antidepressant, mood stabilizers or anxiolytic medications.
- Psychotherapy
- Group therapy
- Self-help groups
- Must involve the family.

VARIOUS STAGES OF PSYCHOLOGICAL TREATMENT FOR ADOLESCENT SEXUAL ABUSE

It involves the following stages:

SKILL BUILDING COMPONENTS

Affective modulation: Encourage appropriate feeling identification and expression, including "negative" emotions.

STRESS INOCULATION SKILLS

Focused breathing, progressive muscle relaxation, positive imagery, thought stopping.

COGNITIVE COPING SKILLS

Learning about the connections between thoughts, feelings and behaviors (not only abuse related, but also in the context of normal life) and how examining and changing a the thoughts can lead to less distress and more adaptive behaviors.

SAFETY SKILLS

Optimize adolescent's decision making ability in a variety of potentially dangerous situations.

CREATING THE TRAUMA NARRATIVE

"Gradual exposure" and cognitive processing of traumatic events gradually by encouraging the adolescent to create a narrative (written or otherwise) of the abuse. This includes retelling the "worst moment." Greater details are revealed during each subsequent session to help the adolescent identify traumatic reminders, identify cognitive distortions (blame, responsibility, shame and what it means) and to help the him/her to fit the traumatic experiences into a larger context of the his/her whole life.

PSYCHOEDUCATION

For example, to provide information about sexual abuse (i.e., how commonly it occurs, why people abuse kids, common responses to abuse, why people often don't tell right away, potential for long-term positive outcome with treatment).

PARENT COMPONENTS

Parallel the above, in addition, to provide parenting skills such as positive praise, active ignoring, time out and contingency reinforcement programs to manage behavioral problems including sexually inappropriate behaviors.

JOINT PARENT—CHILD SESSIONS

To optimize parent—Child communication about the abuse and the adolescent's response to it, to foster parent child trust and communication, to model positive parenting strategies for parent, and to optimize the successful sharing of the child's trauma narrative with the parents in such a way that the parent will not be traumatized but be encouraged to support their child.

SUMMARY

Sexuality education given in a age appropriate manner will make children and adolescents aware of what is sexual abuse and how to prevent it. Sexual abuse may be a continuum from child hood to adolescence. Adolescents with low self-esteem are more vulnerable to sexual exploitation.

SUGGESTED READING

1. Cohen JA, Mannarino AP. A treatment model for sexually abused preschool children. J Interpers Violence, 1996; 8:115-31
2. Deblinger E, Heflin AH. Treating sexually Abused Children and their Nonoffending Parents: A Cognitive Behavioural Approach. Thousand Oakes, CA, Sage 1996a.
3. Dubner AE, Motta RW. Sexually and physically abused foster care children and post-traumatic stress disorder. J Consult Clin Psychol, 1999; 67: 367-73
4. Lipschitz Ds, Winegr RK, Hartnick E., Foote B, Southwick SM. Post traumatic stress disorder in hospitalized adolescents: Psychiatric comorbidity and clinical correlates. J Am Acad Child Adoles Psychiatry 1999;38:385-92.
5. McLeer SV, Dixon JF, Henry D, Ruggiero K, Niedda T, et al. Psychopathology in non-clinically referred sexually abused children. J Am Acad Child Adolesc Psychiatry, 1998;37:1326-33.

Section 12: Psychiatric Problems

34 Anxiety Disorders

Swati Y Bhave

INTRODUCTION

Due to the turmoil of the transition phase of adolescence they are more prone to stress and this increases the likely hood of anxiety disorders and depression. An adolescent who is mentally not at peace will look for sources of relief and is more likely to experiment with early sex and indulge in drug abuse and also become victims or perpeters of sexual abuse and violence. An early diagnosis and treatment will restore positive mental balance and have a reduction of ARSH related problems.

Brief anxiety caused by a stressful activity like appearing for a exam going to a new school or college, appearing for an interview is a normal part of adolescent life But when anxiety fills life and starts affecting performance and day to day life activity, it becomes a anxiety disorder

As clinicians working with adolescents we need to be familiar with these disorders as they first present to us in various forms, very often as physical illness and we have to learn to diagnose them so that we do not subject the adolescent to unnecessary investigations and also understand when they require referral to mental health professionals.

TYPES

Anxiety disorders are of various types:

- Separation anxiety disorder (SAD)
- Generalized anxiety disorder (GAD)
- Panic disorders or attacks
- Obsessive compulsive disorder (OCD)
- Phobias
- Post-traumatic stress disorder (PTSD).

MANIFESTATION OF ANXIETY DISORDERS IN ADOLESCENTS

- Irrational fears
- Physical symptoms palpitations, sweating, trembling, stomachache, or headache.
- Always feeling on being on edge and irritable
- Avoidance of situations that cause anxiety leading to social withdrwal
- Excessive worry about ordinary daily activities
- Insomnia and sleep disturbances.

SEPARATION ANXIETY DISORDER (SAD)

Generally seen in childhood, as school refusal it, may sometimes be also seen in adolescents, e.g. avoidance of situations involving separation like going for long trips or vacations or going away to school or college. They get a variety of physical symptoms and emotional distress when they have to be separated from parents or any "attachment figure " in their life. They feel afraid that the parents may be victims of violence or die while they are separated.

GENERALIZED ANXIETY DISORDER (GAD)

This disorder is exaggerated worry and tension over everyday normal activites and decision making. Adolescents with such disorder are always worrying about everything in life and fear the worst in every small event or action. These are accompanies by a variety of Psychosomatic manifestations like vague aches and pains, fatigue, breathing difficulty, sleep disorders nausea, frequent urination, etc. They may not have social withdrawal but are always distressed about facing situations.

PANIC DISORDER

This is more distressing and serious than GAD Onset most often begins during late adolescence. Panic attacks are more common among females. There is sudden feeling of extreme fear and symptoms will be as a result of.

Since they cannot predict when and how often these attack will come they live in constant dread. An attack generally peaks within 10 minutes, but some symptoms may last much longer.

The symptoms can mimic a heart attack or feeling of impending death or mental disorientation and are extremely distressing risk is increased with positive family history depression, drug abuse, or alcoholism. Avoidance of places and situation where attack has occurred makes life extremely restricted often resulting in making them house bound in severe cases called *agoraphobia*.

OBSESSIVE-COMPULSIVE DISORDER

The adolescent keeps getting unwanted, repetitive thoughts which keep intruding the mind and are very distressing called *obsessions*, e.g. contamination of hands by germs and to get relief from these thoughts he/she is forced to perform rituals which are called *compulsions*, e.g repeated hand washing Rituals give very temporary relief. Neither the thoughts nor rituals are under his/her control which can lead to total disruption of life and mental peace and his her actions are perceived by society as weird or abnormal many adolescents do not realize their behavior is abnormal and suffer intensely by peer rejection or ridicule which can be very cruel.

OCD may be more severe when it involves thoughts of harming people, performing repugnant sexual acts, etc. Hyper-religiosity may also be seen in cases of OCD, bt.

Many normal people have some obsessive rituals like repeatedly checking door locks at night or switching of gas, etc. But when they consume more than an hour a day and casue a lot of distress including interfering with daily life, they fall under the category of disorder. The symptoms may gradually worsen or may also improve over time.

OCD may be familial, it may coexist or be aggravated by eating disorders, depression and other anxiety disorders. Patients may try to find relief in drugs and alcohol which in turns can lead to high-risk sexual behavior and lead to ARSH problems.

POST-TRAUMATIC STRESS DISORDER (PTSD)

PTSD is a debilitating condition that can occur after exposure to a terrifying event (catastrophic or psychiatric trauma).

A adolescent who has been a victim of sexual abuse can present to the clinic with symptoms of PTSD and it requires a astute clinical to diagnose the problem. Rape, sexual violence and severe ragging can all lead to PTSD symptoms may present as acute, i.e. within 3 to 6 months after the traumatizing event or chronic persisting for more than 6 months. The terrifying event keeps haunting the patient by frightening, intrusive memories. It is associated with hyper vigilance and can present with a wide variety of somatic and psychological complains

PHOBIAS ARE IRRATIONAL FEARS

Specific Phobia

Specific phobia like a fear of an object or situation, e.g. pets or animals flying, heights, etc.

Social Phobias

Adolescent in their growing up phase are very self-conscious, have low self-esteem and often have body dissatisfaction. If in addition they have social phobia which means fear of facing people and social situations, it can be seriously debilitating. They not only are distressed during the social event, but worry days before in anticipation and days afterwards, regarding their behaviors and social criticism. Social phobia also may be limited to one aspect only like performing on stage or eating in front of others.

Physical symptoms often accompany the intense anxiety of social phobia and include blushing, profuse sweating, trembling, nausea, and difficulty talking. If the adolescent suffers from social phobia, he or she may be painfully embarrassed by these symptoms and feel as though all eyes are focused on him/her. The adolescent may also be afraid of being with people other than his or her family. In social phobia there may be physical symptoms like blushing, sweating, stammering, etc.

EVALUATION

If a clinician suspects an anxiety disorder careful psychosocial history should be taken which will help to analyze whether there is a anxiety disorder and what type is likely to be present. There are objective assessment tools which can be used in a clinicians office or the adolescent can be referred for evaluation to a clinical psychologists

MANAGEMENT

If the disorders are mild simple reassurance and making the adolescent aware of the problem will help in improvement. More advanced disorders require referral to clinical psychologists for behavioral therapy and to Psychiatrists for medications and to rule out co-morbid conditions that often exist.

Timely referral will prevent the adolescence of anxiety disorder from finding solace in alcohol, substance abuse and high risk sexual behavior.

High-risk sexual behaviors, in turn can also give rise to anxiety disorders and has to be dealt with in management

Mild anxiyolytic medications can be given to establish therapeutic effect but the clinician has to be careful to know everything about the prescribed drug and not land the adolescent into drug dependence or addictions.

SUGGESTED READING

1. Bernstein GA, Rapoport JL, Leonard HL. Sepa-ra-tion anxiety and generalized anxiety disorders IN Weiner JM: Textbook of Child and Adolescent Psychiatry, 2nd ed., pp 467-490. Washington, DC: American Psychiatric Press 1997.
2. Bhave Swati Y Jitendra Nagpal Divya s Prasad Post-traumatic stress syndrome. General features and principles of management in Bhaves Textbook of Adolescent Medicine 1st edn, New Delhi: Jaypee Publishers. Chapter 2006;26.5: 979-983.
3. Bhave SY, Nagpal J, Anxiety and Depressive Disorders in College youth; Pediatr Clin N Am PCNA 2005; 52: 97-134.
4. Black B, Leonard HL, Rapoport JL: Specific phobia, panic disorder, social phobia and selective mutism. IN Weiner JM: Textbook of Child and Adolescent Psychiatry, 2nd edn., pp 491-503. Washington, DC: American Psychiatric Press 1997
5. Hayward C, Killen JD, Kraemer HC: Predictors of panic attacks in adolescents. Journal of the American Academy of Child and Adolescent Psychiatry 2000; 39(2): 207-14.
6. National Institute of Mental Health: Facts about Generalized Anxiety Disorder. Bethesda, MD: Author. 1999. Publication No. OM-99 4153, 1999. Updated: December 07, 2000.
7. Pratt H, Sovani. A. Anxiety orders in adolescents in Bhaves' Textbook of Adolescent Medicine 1st edn 2006, New Delhi: · Jaypee Publishers. Chapter 23.3:pp757-63.

35 Depression Related to ARSH

Swati Y Bhave

INTRODUCTION

Till 1930's the psychoanalytic school of thought that adolescents are basically incapable of experiencing major depressive episodes adolescent depression was officially recognized in US in the NIMH Conference on depression in adolescents in 1975.

WHO in 2001 recognized that amongst many disorders commonly in adults, depression is being increasingly identified among adolescent.

Adolescents in India under lot of pressure. In school there is a rigid system where they are not allowed to grow as individuals. There is severe academic pressures to excel. Children and adolescents are expected to fulfill their parents unrealistic dreams and used as trophies. They have no time to relax and have fun. After school hours they are again roped into competitive activities. There are conflicting issues of morality: what is taught at home and what is seen in media and society.

Depression can have serious consequences and it needs to be identified early. Clinicians dealing with adolescents should have a high alertness when dealing with adolescents. Most adolescents and families are often reluctant to go to a psychiatrist. Clinicians need to decide when there is of severe depression and suicide risk and help the family accept the referral to the psychiatrist.

HOW IS DEPRESSION RELATED TO ARSH ISSUES?

A variety of ARSH related issues can cause depression in a adolescent. Conversely depression can lead to high risk behavior and cause ARSH issues.

Awareness of depression is very important for clinicians dealing with adolescent and ARSH issues as they are closely interlinked and management on both is equally vital. Timely recognition of severe depression and referral can mean saving a life from suicide.

Depression can result from:

- Body dissatisfaction and negative body image, even a minor matter like acne
- Failure to attract the opposite sex
- Rejection or neglect by opposite sex
- Different sexual orientation
- PCOS or menstrual problems
- Masturbation
- Alcohol or substance abuse
- Premarital sex
- Sexually transmitted diseases including HIV/AIDS
- Unwanted pregnancy.

SPECIAL ISSUES OF ADOLESCENT DEPRESSION

ADOLESCENT DEPRESSION CAN BE MISSED

They can appear to be normal and happy or even aggressive, hostile, defiant, disobedient.

So one has to look for subtle or gross changes in.

- Appetite and weight
- Scholastic performance
- Friends
- Behavior
- Loss of interest in previous activity.

They may also come with:

- Unexplained physical complaints, headaches, or stomachaches
- Degrees of disability are in excess of any clear medical cause
- Hyperactive, impulsive, motor-driven tear up the world around them,
- Often with severe aggression and deny all along that anything is wrong (bipolar)
- May occur in a 'masked' form, expressed through symptoms - delinquency or phobias, etc.

DILEMMAS IN DIAGNOSIS

- Adolescents feel things deeply and marked mood swings are common.
- Parents are better informants on overt behavioral difficulties but may not notice depression in their children or be aware of suicidal ideas or even attempts.
- DSM-IV criteria and structured interviews: may be overinclusive and some adolescents who meet the criteria for major depression remit within a few weeks.
- Depression questionnaires have low specificity for depressive disorders. Many young people with high scores on the screening questionnaire will turn out not to have a depressive disorder at interview.

Hence, a very careful history taking is important to enquire about the:

- Impact of symptoms on every day functioning
- About the presence of symptoms of unequivocal psychopathological significance such as *suicidal planning* or *marked weight loss*
- Best indicator **is the** duration of the problem: Polysymptomatic depressive states that persist *for more than 6 weeks* usually require intervention
- Symptom-oriented, personal interviews are important for recognition of depression.

Additional questions *in history taking are very important to determine* degree of depression and find out the risk of suicide.

Physical examination: It is necessary to rule out medical causes of depression (Table 35.1). As clinicians we must always rule of the medical causes of depression and do the necessary tests.

Table 35.1: Medical causes of depression

- Infections: Infectious mononucleosis, influenza, hepatitis, AIDS,
- Endocrine: Cushing's, hypothyroidism, hyperparathyroid
- Metabolic: Porphyria, uremia
- Electrolyte dysfunction
- Drugs B-blockers, cimetidine, corticosteroids
- Substance abuse
- Neurological disorders
- Misc

DEPRESSIVE DISORDERS BY DSM IV CLASSIFICATION

1. Major depressive disorder (MDD),
2. Dysthymia, cyclothymia,
3. Depressive disorder not otherwise specified,
4. Bi-polar disorder (BPD),
5. Bipolar disorder not otherwise specified.

Those with BPD have an increased risk of a psychotic episode, most often mania.

Prominent and Persistent Features of Depression

Lowering of mood *(dysphoria)* and lack of pleasure in life *(anhedonia).*

Symptoms

To consider a depressive episode there should be at least atleast 5 out of 9 symptoms must be present:

- Depressed mood
- Diminished interest or pleasure in everyday activities.
- Loss of appetite.
- Significant weight loss or gain.
- Sleep disturbances.
- Agitation or retardation.
- Poor concentration.
- Feelings of worthlessness and guilt.
- Recurrent thoughts of death.

Dysthymia

Dysthymia means depressed or irritable mood. Present for at least 6-12 weeks.

There should be 2 out of 6 of the following symptoms:

- Poor appetite.
- Insomnia.
- Low energy.
- Low self-esteem.
- Poor concentration.
- Feelings of hopelessness.

Co-morbid Disorders

There are increased rates of co-morbid disorders in depressed children and adolescents than adults.

There is often a overlap of depression and other psychiatric diagnoses such as conduct disorder, anxiety states, learning problems, hyperactivity, anorexia nervosa, substance abuse and school refusal.

Table 35.2 shows the common symptoms of depression.

Table 35.2: Common symptoms of depression

- Irritability
- Sad apthatetic or depressed mood
- Fatigue or loss of energy
- Loss of interest in school, friends, activities
- Impaired appetite or food intake—over eating to comfort oneself
- Weight gain or loss
- Low self esteem
- Bodily preoccupations are common- may worry about his looks, height or acne
- Sense of futility or hopelessness may be present
- Psychomotor retardation or agitation
- Diminished ability to think or concentrate
- Poor academic performance
- Sleep disturbances: insomnia and hypersomnia
- Preoccupation with death or suicide

Table 35.3 shows the identification of mild moderate and severe depression.

Table 35.3: Indentification of mild moderate and severe depression

Mild depression
- Acute identifiable situation
- Transient in nature
- No high-risk behavior
- Minor impairment in functioning
- Low suicidal risk

Treatment
- Supportive counseling

Moderate and severe depression *(Refer to psychiatry)*
- Prolonged mood
- Diminished interest or pleasure
- Weight changes
- Insomnia or hypersomnia
- Fatigue or energy loss
- Psychomotor agitation or retardation
- Worthlessness
- Thinking /concentration reduced
- May have Recurrent thoughts of death

DIAGNOSIS

Interviews in semi-structured format for parents and adolescents.

- Questions and relate to mood symptoms are asked in a way that allows the interviewer to explore significant areas related to those symptoms.
- Information is obtained from teachers and peers.
- Behavioral manifestations of psychiatric symptoms and the temporal course of an illness,
- Subjective symptoms and some vegetative symptoms, such as sleep disturbance.

Self Report Measures

- Useful for detecting and monitoring symptoms in the clinical setting.
- Adolescents depression inventory.
- Beck Depression Inventory (BDI)
- Weinberg Screening Affective Scale (WSAS).

Academic Manifestations

- Often perform poorly in school
- Psychological testing can be useful to determine the influence of mood on cognition.

- Although verbal intelligence is not generally impaired, academic achievement can be adversely impacted by affective illness.
- Recent studies longer duration depressive illness, the greater the negative impact is on academic and social functioning.

Triggering or Provoking Events

Undesirable life events occur in excess in the 12 months before the onset of disorder. e.g. parental loss/death of grandparent., change of residence/ moving out of joint family, change of school.

The best course is to identify depression and refer to mental health professionals for management. If a clinicians decides to treat mild depression they must refresh themselves with the latest drugs their side effects and drug interaction before giving a prescription. Care should be taken to give a very small supply under parental supervision to avoid overdosage by intent or accident

SUGGESTED READING

1. Bhave SY, Nagpal J, Anxiety and Depressive Disorders in College youth; Pediatr Clin N Am PCNA 2005: 52-97-134
2. BirmaherB, Ryan ND, Williamson DE et al. Childhood and adolescent depression: a review of the past 10 years. PartI. Am. Acad Child Adolescent Psychiatry 1996; 35:1427-39.
3. Blackman M, MB, FRCPC, You Asked about .... Adolescent Depression. The Canadian Journal of CME May 1995 Internet Mental Health (http://www.mentalhealth.com/p.html)
4. Caroly S., Pataki, M.D. Mood disorders and suicide in children and adolescents. Kaplan and Sadock's Comprehensive Textbook of Psychiatry 7th (edn). In: Sadock BJ, Sadock VA, (Eds). Philadelphia: Lippincott Williams and Wilkins, 2000: 2740-57
5. Diagnostic and statistical manual of mental disorders, 4th ed.: DSM-IV. Washington, DC: American Psychiatric Association, 1994.
6. Hezell Philip, Depression, Recent Advances in Paediatrics 21, (edn) In: David TJ, (Ed). Royal Society of Medicine Press Ltd. London, 2004; 217: 217-29.
7. John T, Cherian A, Depressive Disorders in the Child and Adolescent Population; Indian Pediatrics 2001; 38: 1211-16.
8. Kroll L, Harrington R, Jayson D, Fraser J, Gowers S. Pilot study of continuation cognitive-behavioral therapy for major depression in adolescent psychiatric patients. J Am Acad Child Adolesc Psychiatry 1996;35:1156-61.
9. Shochet IM, Dadds MR, Holland D, Whitefield K, Harnett PH, Osgarby SM. The efficacy of a universal school based programme to prevent adolescent depression. J Clin Child Psychol 2001;30:303-15.
10. Singhal Sushila, Rao UNB. Psychological concerns. Adolescent concern through own eyes; Kanishka Publishers, Distributors, Delhi © Urivi Vikram Charitable Trust 2004; 157, 139-59.
11. www.clinicaltrials.gov/ct/show/00006286NCT. Questions and Answers about the NIMH Treatment for Adolescents with Depression Study (TADS) Updated: 08/18/2004.

36 Suicide Prevention

Jitendra Nagpal, Swati Y Bhave

INTRODUCTION

Suicide is a major public health problem and needs to be addressed scientifically like any other medical condition. Suicidal behavior is the end result of a complex interaction of psychiatric, social and familial factors.

According to WHO estimates for the year 2020 and based on the current trends, approximately 1.53 million people will die from suicide and 10-20 times more people will attempt suicide worldwide. This represents an average one death every 20 seconds and one attempt every one to two seconds. According to 1999 data from the Center for Disease Control and Prevention, suicide kills more people than homicide. Suicide is the eleventh leading cause of death in adults, the sixth leading cause of death among all those 5-14 years old and the third leading cause of death between 15 to 24 years. Despite increase in the suicide rate among adolescents in past many years our understanding about such adolescent who commits or contemplates suicide is very limited.

Suicide evokes mixed reactions: varying from anger, distress, ridicule, anxiety, tension, ear and sadness. Often, one wonders: Why did it happen?; "Could this have been prevented?"; "Can young lives be saved?" "Was there an alternative solution to the problem?"

Suicidal behavior is defined as an action through which an individual hurts himself whatever the degree of lethal intention and of recognition of genuine reason for this action (Botega et al, 2005). Suicidal behavior may include starting with thoughts of self-destruction, extending to threats, suicidal gestures, suicide attempts, and suicide. Most people who commit suicide have a psychiatric disorder at the time of death. Suicidal ideation is a preoccupation with intrusive thoughts of ending one's own life (Cole et al, 1992) while suicide is the completed act of taking ones life (National Mental Health Association, 2002).

COMMONLY USED TERMS

Suicide: Act of killing oneself intentionally, performed by the person with the full knowledge or expectation of the fatal outcome.

Suicidal attempt: A life-threatening act with a conscious intent to end one's life, requiring medical intervention after the act.

Suicidal ideation: A wish or thought, often setting up the process leading to he ending of one's own life.

Suicidal risk : A characteristic, the presence or absence of which leads to the increase or decrease of the tendency to commit suicide.

Suicidal counters: Set of factors operating within the individual, family or society, likely to prevent suicide.

MISCONCEPTIONS ABOUT TEENAGE SUICIDE

There are many myths and misconceptions. One is the idea that suicide is something teenagers might do on a bad day or in response to some sort of stress. Although an upsetting episode is often the immediate precipitant to suicide, the vast majority of adolescents who commit suicide have relatively longstanding, diagnosable psychiatric disorders, especially depression and substance abuse. Another misconception is that asking kids about suicide will put the idea in their head or lead to an increased risk that they will attempt or commit suicide. But it is not so. Therefore, if parents or teachers are worried that a child may be suicidal, the best thing to do is to ask.

Yet another misconception is that teenage suicide prevention should start in adolescence. Some of the most effective measures for long-term prevention begin in early childhood, or even at the prenatal level with depression screening for pregnant mothers.

PREVALENCE

The occurrence of suicidal behaviors can be divided into behaviors that are successful in ending life (completed suicide) and those that for one reason or another fail at ending life (suicide attempts or parasuicides). Suicide are always underreported and under diagnosed as the cause of death or disability mainly because of the social and legal consequences of the act.

Rates of parasuicides or attempted suicide are significantly higher in adolescents than suicide. Earlier studies reported the ratio of attempt versus success in suicide to be 4:1 to 10:1. While newer studies have seen the ratio of 312:1in a sample of 15 to 18-year-old. The rate of completed suicide increases from early to late adolescents. Boys have killed themselves more than girls with the ratio of 3:1.

Girls are more prone to suicidal thoughts and make attempts more often than do boys (Baker, 1983). According to (Disley, 1994) women are more likely than men to be admitted to a hospital for a suicide attempt, and women in the 15-24 age group are more likely to attempt suicide than are women in other age groups.

RISK FACTORS FOR SUICIDAL IDEATION IN ADOLESCENTS

Adolescents who commit suicide have a long history of difficulties and stressful life experiences. Personality traits are relatively important in predicting who may be likely to develop suicidal ideation. There are lot of factors that may put one to develop suicidal ideation includes family relationships, maternal depression, peer relations, emotional well-being (stress, anger, aggression, impulsivity, and depression), drug use, academic performance, loneliness and hopelessness. Suicidal ideation and attempts are increasing day-by-day among students.

COMMON FACTORS LEADING TO SUICIDAL IDEATION AMONG ADOLESCENTS

Academic Performance

Academic performance has a direct relationship with suicidal behavior among adolescents. Gispert et al (1985) found that academic performance of suicidal adolescents is often poor. Gispert et al (1987) also reported that those who make repeated attempts are less successful in school. Garfinkel and Golombek (1983) observed greater absenteeism among suicidal youngsters. Parental expectation to succeed in competitive exams is also a common factor of suicidal ideation among adolescents. Parents often say that you have to take high marks than neighbor's and children in relationships, which put young children under great pressure and hence suicidal ideation.

There are some significant predictors of suicidal ideation and include job loss, financial loss, child abuse, sex abuse, sexual problems, sexual promiscuity, religious faith and practices, economic hardship, living out of home, legal difficulties, physical complaints (headaches, body pain, etc.), unemployment, sexual orientation (homosexuality, lesbian, etc.), running away from home, excessive, or repetitive coverage of the suicide by media, marital conflicts, hormonal disturbances in the brain, medical illness like epilepsy, schizophrenia, high blood cholesterol levels, HIV/AIDS, and other self-destructive behaviors.

Depression

Depression is one of the important predictor of suicidal ideation and suicidal attempts among adolescents.

Common symptoms of adolescent depression are irritability, hopelessness, anhedonia, changes in sleep and appetite, academic decline, reduced energy, reduced social interactions, somatic symptoms, and suicidal ideation. Many factors may predispose adolescent girls to depression. These include the increase in hormones associated with puberty, changes in body shape and emerging sexual identity, family stressors such as divorce and peer pressure. Boergers et al, (1998) in a study of 120 adolescents found that high levels of depression and anger expression predicted self-reported wish to die. In a similar study of 374 high school students, social support and depression were significantly related to suicidal ideation levels one year later (Mazza and Reynolds, 1998). Family history of depression is also a significant risk factor (Brent et al, 1998) particularly maternal depression (Garber et al, 1998). According to Prigerson and Slimack, (1999) girls are at great risk if they are depressed. (Metha et al, (1998) reported that males progressed from depression to substance use and then to suicide risk, while females progressed directly from depression to suicide risk. Social changes that might be related to the rise in adolescent suicide include family instability, natural disasters, terrorism, etc. also causes depression which contributes to the adolescent's sense of frustration, helplessness, and hopelessness, which, in turn, make adolescents incapable tope with and they turn to escapist measures like drugs, withdrawal, and ultimately suicide.

Stress

Studies have also shown that a naturally stressful demand on youth can be overwhelming to some adolescents and predispose them to thoughts of suicide (Teen suicide, 1998). Researchers (Griffiths et al, 1986; Turner et al, 2002) in their study concluded that the high incidence of adolescent suicide is assumed to be indicative of societal stress in the lives of young people. Academic pressure, work-related problems, interpersonal difficulties, death of loved ones, illnesses, and loss of relationships has been found to be significant stressors on young people (Kurtz and Derevensky, 1993; Mullis et al, 1993; Butler et al, 1994).

Relationships

Relationships in the family and with peers play an important role in suicidal behavior among adolescents. Friendship plays an important role during adolescence. Adolescents particularly girls are more likely have suicidal ideation if they had few close friends or no friends. Romance and dating violence is also a common phenomenon among adolescents. Unsuccessful in love, loss of loved, infatuation, one-sided love, betrayal and other love-hate relationships are important predictors of suicidal ideation and attempted suicide among adolescents.

When emotional needs of children whether from parents or peers, are not met, such children are likely to develop suicidal tendencies. Family relations are also important predictors of suicidal ideation among adolescents. Researchers (Davidson and that suicidal behavior has been observed in children from families where one of the parents is absent due to death, divorce, or separation. Researchers also found that social isolation progressive dissolution of meaningful relationships, loneliness, and alienation (Young, 1985) are associated with suicide. Family economic pressure, parental rejection, parental hostile behavior, discrimination and physical abuse are other significant predictors of suicidal ideation among adolescents.

Personality Factors

1. AHA-syndrome (Anger, hostility and aggression) is the common problem of adolescents in almost every society. Adolescents with hostile behavior pattern and angry temperament are likely to engage in risky behaviors and have suicidal ideation. Studies have shown that adolescents who were depressed were at greater risk if they also manifested high levels of anger and aggression (Stein et al. 1998). In another study, adolescent males were found to be at greater risk for suicide if they were aggressive (Prigerson and Slimack, 1999).
2. Impulsivity is acting on the spur of the movement and don't considering the outcomes of their action. Today's young generation have lower impulse control and engage in many risky behaviors such as smoking, substance abuse, sexual activity, gambling, hyperactivity, etc. resulting in developing suicidal thoughts. Conner et al (2004) found that Impulsivity and irritability were associated strongly with suicidal ideation after accounting for alcohol dependence and other aggression-related constructs including psychopath.

Identity Formation

The identity crisis is significant for adolescents. Adolescence is the period in which the individual must establish a sense of identity, overcoming role diffusion and identity confusion (Erikson, 1950). The search for identity involves establishing a meaningful self-concept in which past, present, and future are brought together to form a unified whole. The adolescent who fails in this task will be susceptible to indulging in a self-destructive activity, including suicide (Baumeister, 1986).

Adolescents with low self-esteem are more prone to have suicidal ideation then with high self-esteem. Adolescents with poor self-esteem doubt themselves and feel helpless in coping with problems. There is growing body dissatisfaction and negative evaluation of themselves among toady's youth and hence increased likelihood of suicidal ideation. Adolescents, particularly girls, who are overweight, are at increased risk for considering suicide and suicide attempts. Wenz (1976) in his study reported that attempters have low self-esteem. De Man, Leduc and Labreche-Gauthier (1993) found that adolescents with low self-esteem or a less internal locus of control have higher suicidal ideation and are more likely to commit suicide.

Drug Abuse

Drug abuse is also an important factor in developing suicidal ideation among adolescents. Young people under depression are likely to progress towards substance use and then to suicidal risk. Family history of substance abuse has also been found to contribute to the risk profile for adolescent suicide (Kosky and Eshkevari, 1998). Alcohol and other drug use are often cited as correlates of adolescent suicidal behavior (Tousignant et al, 1988). For instance, Simon (1991) found linear relationships between suicidal behavior and alcohol and drug abuse, and Corbeil (1984) reported that more than 40% of suicidal adolescents used drugs and approximately 18% consumed alcohol.

PROTECTIVE FACTORS

- Effective clinical care for mental, physical and substance abuse disorders
- Family and community support; and promoting skills in problem solving, conflict resolution and nonviolent handling of disputes.

Addressing the overall health of children has demonstrated success. Providing effective, targeted and community-based mental health services for children and adolescents who are identified to be at risk for suicide is the primary suicide prevention tactic. Research shows that early intervention strategies that target risk factors for depression, substance abuse and aggressive behaviors and building resiliency may have promise in preventing youth suicide.

Successful prevention efforts seek to minimize risk factors and maximize protective factors.

Warning Signs

1. Feelings of worthlessness, helplessness and guilt
2. Loss of interest in activities
3. Diminished ability to concentrate
4. Poor impulse control
5. Anger/aggression
6. Sleeping too much
7. Change in appetite
8. Talking about suicide
9. Feelings of hopelessness
10. Social isolation
11. Boredom
12. Emotional turmoil
13. Sensation seeking behaviors
14. Increased alcohol and drug use
15. Loss of interest in physical appearance
16. Irritability
17. Weight loss or weight gain
18. Fatigue
19. The collection and discussion about the methods of suicide
20. Poor school record.

PREVENTION OF SUICIDE

While the problem is enormous and the loss to the society phenomenal, the obvious question drawing the attention of the public, professionals and societies are "can suicide be prevented?"; "Can lives be saved?"; "Are there effective approaches?" The answer is a definite yes. Each and every member of the society can take effective action, which would lead to saving a life, preventing an act or breaking the suicidal process.

SCHOOL BASED SUICIDAL PREVENTION PROGRAMS

School based suicide prevention programs include both curricula components to teach students about these warning signs and what to do, as well as non-curricula components such as peer groups, hot lines, intervention services and parent training. These programs may include

1. Awareness of suicide risk factors.
2. Identification of students at high risk of suicide and suicide attempts.
3. Enhancing the coping abilities of students.
4. Providing knowledge about the behavioral characteristics ("warning signs") of adolescence at risk for suicide.
5. Providing information to students, teachers and parents on the availability of mental health resources.
6. Training peer counselors.
7. Providing more parental student as well as parental counseling for a healthy relationships and skills for solving problems.
8. Helping the student set up a step by step plan to achieve his/her goals.
9. Get the student involved in positive activities in school or in the community.
10. Providing anger management and stress management techniques to students.
11. Encouraging close relationships between teacher-student and student-student relationships.

INTERVENTION ON THE PART OF PARENTS

1. Recognize the warning sign for suicide among their adolescents.
2. Fostering social skills and competency among adolescents.
3. Listen carefully the needs of risky adolescents.
4. Teach problem solving skills.
5. Do not ignore suicide threats.
6. Take professional including screening, emotional counseling, telephone counseling and other services for risky children.

7. Develop reasons for living among youths.
8. Avoid unnecessary academic pressure.
9. Talk about sensitive issues with youths especially girls who are more depressed during pubertal changes.
10. Restrict access of guns, drugs and other common means of suicide.
11. Reinforce positive behaviors and reward for them and new behaviors.
12. Get involved, available, interested and supportive.
13. Do not discourage and give as much praise as possible.

SUGGESTED READING

1. Ameen S. What parents and teachers should know about suicide in adolescents and young adults. Online 1998.
2. American Psychiatric Association (1998). Teen suicide. Retrieved November 18, 2002 from http://www.psycho.org/public_info/teenag-1.cfm.
3. Allison S, Pearce C, Martin G, Miller K, Long R. Parental influence, pessimism and adolescent suicidality. Arch. of Suicide research. 1995;1: 229-42.
4. Aoki WT, Turk AA. Adolescent suicide a review of risk factors and implications for practice. J. of Psychology and Christianity 1997; 16:273-79.
5. Baumeister R. Identity: Cultural change and the struggle for self. New York: Oxford University Press 1986.
6. Berman AL, Jobes DA. Suicide prevention in adolescents (age 12-18 years) Suicide and life threatening behavior 1991;25: 143-154.
7. Boergers J, Spirito A, Donaldson D. Reasons for adolescent suicide attempts: Associations with psychological functioning. Journal of the American Academy of Child and Adolescent Psychiatry, 1998;37, 1287-1293.
8. Botega NJ, Barros MBA, Oliveira HBO, Dalgalarrondo, P, and Marín-León, L. Suicidal behavior in the community: Prevelance and factors associated with suicidal ideation. Rev Bras. Psiquiatr, 2005;27(1), 45-53.
9. Centers for Disease Control and Prevention. Programs for prevention of suicide among adolescents youth adults. Morb Mortal Wkly Rep CDC Surveill Summ 1994;43, 1-7.
10. Conner KR, Meldrum S, Wieczorek WF, Duberstein PR, Welte JW. The Association of Irritability and Impulsivity with Suicidal Ideation among 15 to 20-year-old-Males. Suicide and life-threatening behavior, 2004;34(4), 363-72
11. Corbeil S. Suicide and adolescence. In: Morisette P (Ed.), Le suicide, demystification, intervention, prevention. Quebec: Garotex 1984; 272-306.
12. Curran DK. Adolescent suicidal behavior. Issues in Mental Health Nursing 1986;8, 275-477.
13. Davidson F, Choquet, M. Adolescent suicide, an epidemiological study. Paris: Les Editions ESF. 1981.
14. De Man AF, Leduc CP, Labreche-Gauthier L. A French-Canadian scale for suicide ideation for use with adolescents. Canadian Journal of Behavioural Science 1993; 25, 126-134.
15. Disley B. Suicide prevention initiatives: Youth suicide - The world and New Zealand wide picture. Community Mental Health in New Zealand, 1994;8(4), 5-11.
16. Erikson E. Childhood and society. New York: Norton 1950.
17. Gary SM, Otto MW Managing approaches to suicide prevention: Application to patients with bipolar disorder J Clin Psychiatr 2001;62: 56-64.
18. Garfinkel BD, Golombek GH. Suicidal behavior in adolescence. In: Garfinkel BD, Golombek GH (Eds.), The adolescent and mood disturbance. New York: International Universities Press 1983;189-217.
19. Gispert M, Wheeler K, Marsh L, Davis MS. Suicidal adolescents: Factors in evaluation. Adolescence 1985;20, 753-762.
20. Gispert M, Davis MS, Marsh L, Wheeler K. Predictive factors in repeated suicide attempts by adolescents. Hospital and Community Psychiatry, 1987;38, 390-3.
21. Mazza JJ, Reynolds WM. A longitudinal investigation of depression, hopelessness, social support, and major and minor life events and their relation to suicidal ideation in adolescents. Suicide and Life-threatening Behavior, 1998;28, 358-74.
22. Mann JJ. A current perspective of suicide and attempted suicide. Ann Int Med 2002;136 (4), 302-11.
23. McKenry D, Tishler C, Kelly C. The role of drugs in adolescent suicide attempts Suicide and Life Threatening behaviour. 1983;13:166-75.

24. Nicholas LM, Goldesn RN. Managing the suicidal patient. J of Psychiatr 2001;3:1-8.
25. NDTV, com, Sanjay Pinto, suicide rate alarming in south India: 6th April 2004.
26. Prigerson, HG, Slimack MJ. Gender differences in clinical correlates of suicidality among young adults. Journal of Nervous and Mental Disease 1999;187:23-31.
27. Preventing suicide: How to start a survivor group. Mental and behavioural disorder. Dept. of Mental health WHO Geneva 2000.
28. Simon R. Survey of suicidal behavior and ideations of 3rd, 4th, and 5th grade high school students of Region 02. Chicoutimi, PQ: Centre de Prevention du Suicide 02;1991.
29. Spirito A. Family therapy techniques with adolescent suicide attempters. 1997a Crisis 18: 106-9.
30. Spirito A. Individual therapy techniques with adolescent suicide attempters. Crisis 1997b;18: 62-4.
31. Saini Sunil. Suicide ideation in AJPP Oct.Dec, issue 2006 (under publication).
32. Saini Sunil. Suicide ideation in AJPP Oct-Dec issue 2006.
32. Stein D, Apter A., Ratzoni G, Har-Even D, Avidan G. Association between multiple suicide attempts and negative affects in adolescents. Journal of the American Academy of Child and Adolescent Psychiatry, 1998;37:488-94.
33. Tan M. An analysis of suicide attempts in 1980-1988. Thesis. Palmerston North: Massey University, New Zealand. AFVT' 1991;70-93.
34. Townsend S. Adolescent health: Youth depression and suicide. New Zealand Practice Nurse, September, 1993;4-5.
35. Tishler CL, McHenry PC. Parental negative self and adolescent suicide attempts. J Am Acad of Child Psychiatr 1982;21:404-8.
36. VanWicklin JE, Adolescent depression: A systemic overview. J of Psychology and Christianity, 1990;9:5-14.
37. Wenz F. Self-evaluation and suicide potential. Psychological Reports 1976;39,289-90.
38. Young TJ. Adolescent suicide: The clinical manifestation of alienation. High School Journal, 1985;69,55-60.

37 Substance Abuse

Jitendra Nagpal, Swati Y Bhave

INTRODUCTION

Substance abuse has a high incidence in adolescent age group, as it forms part of high risk behavior and experimentation prevalent in this developmental stage.

Many adolescents are given to believe that everybody takes drug in some from or the other. To begin with some of their schoolmates and friends prompt and persuade them to start smoking or taking and alcohol which act as *gateway drugs* and they are further driven to take other dangerous substances.

Adolescents who have are not satisfied with the situation at home or school are made to believe that taking to drugs will help them to cope up Teenagers from broken homes, academic failures, mental health problems like depression or psychiatric disorders are more at risk of drug use.

Many also start drug use as they have fear of loosing the peer group or being ostracized by friends they very much like. Taking drugs makes some of them feel is an adult behavior and they will have a tendency to refuse any kind of advise as authoritative and would like to rebel and this encourage them to indulge more in substance abuse. Many of them are not aware of the addiction potential and think that taking drugs once will not make any difference. Many of them are not aware of the long-term side effects and those that are aware lack the skills that empower them to negotiate situations and say NO. Here lies the importance of having life skill education.

Substance abuse is emerging as a major problem. A majority of drug users are below 20 years. Forty percent of them started taking drugs when they were between 15 to 20 years of age (UNODC, 2002). Social factors such as illiteracy, economic hardship, unemployment, rural residence, and family disharmony increase the vulnerability of adolescents to drug abuse.

Various substances can be used for changing the way our body works. According to WHO, a *drug is any substance which, when taken into the body, alters its function physically and/or psychologically, excluding food and water. Drugs can be legal and illegal, medical and non-medical.*

DRUG ABUSE AND ARSH

It has been well documented that drug abuse is associated with increased high-risk sexual behavior. Unprotected sex under effect of drugs increase the risk of sexually transmitted diseases and accidental or unwanted pregnancy. Teenagers who have such problems are likely to go for drugs for solace and the vicious cycle goes on.

When a teenager comes to a clinician for any problems related to sexual and reproductive health it is important for the clinician to very skillfully and in a non threatening manner elicit the history of drug abuse and refer to mental health professionals.

The most compelling reasons that adolescents give for experimenting with drugs and continuing with substance abuse are:

- To feel grown up;
- To take risks and to rebel against authority;
- To fit into and belong to a group;
- To relax and feel good; and
- To satisfy curiosity.

SUBSTANCE ABUSE

Substance abuse is 'the use of illicit drugs or the abuse of prescription or over-the-counter drugs for purposes other than those for which they are indicated or in a manner or in quantities other than directed'.

Generally, when most people talk about substance abuse, they are referring to the use of illegal drugs.

Alcohol, prescription and over-the-counter medications, inhalants and solvents, and even coffee and cigarettes, can be used to harmful excess. Theoretically, almost any substance can be abused.

THE STAGES OF ADOLESCENT SUBSTANCE USE

- Curiosity or pre-abuse: Opportunity for prevention;
- Experimentation: Tried it for fun and peer acceptance; no associated behavioral changes;
- Actively seeking drugs: More drugs needed (increased tolerance); to escape reality; to escape from problems at home and school;
- Preoccupation with drugs: Experiences loss of control over drug use; faces legal and relationship problems;
- Dependence: Drugs are used all day, every day.

WHO IS AT RISK FOR DEVELOPING SUBSTANCE ABUSE?

Teenagers are at a particular risk of developing substance abuse problems particularly if the following personal, behavioral and environmental factors mentioned below apply to them: Various factor leading to substance above are summarised in Table 37.1.

SUBSTANCE DEPENDENCE

Substance abuse leads to substance dependence with the development of increased tolerance and withdrawal symptoms.

Substance dependence is defined as 'compulsively seeking to use a substance, regardless of the potentially negative social, psychological, and physical consequences'.

Tolerance is defined as the need for increased amounts of the substance to achieve the desired levels of intoxication as before.

Withdrawal symptoms occur when the user who is dependent on a substance stops using it. Withdrawal symptoms range from mild tremors to convulsions, severe agitation, and sometimes even death. Withdrawal symptoms vary depending upon the substance abused, the duration of substance abuse, and the quantity of the substance abused.

Regular and excessive abuse of drugs leads to physical and psychological dependence. Some drugs produce only physical dependence while others produce both physical and psychological dependence.

A list of frequently abused drugs and their adverse effects are given in Table 37.2.

PSYCHOLOGICAL DEPENDENCE

When psychological dependence develops, the substance abuser becomes mentally 'hooked' to the drug. He/she constantly thinks only about the drug and has a continuous uncontrollable craving for it. This state is characterized by mental and emotional preoccupation with the drug.

PHYSICAL DEPENDENCE

Physical dependence denotes a state when the body of the abuser requires the continuous presence of the drug within it. With prolonged use the body becomes so used to its functioning

Table 37.1: Various factors leading to substance abuse

Personal factors	*Behavioral factors*	*Environmental factors*	*Physiological factors*
Beliefs and perceptions about the benefits of substance use Lack of knowledge of consequences of substance use Low self-efficacy Personality factors, e.g. depression, low self-esteem Poor psychological well-being Academic under achievement (statistically low achievement = higher risk.	Teenagers engage in heavy and frequent use of substances as compared with adults Teenagers often use more than one substance Teenagers tend to engage in high-risk behavior more than adults Teenagers may lack well-developed self-control and may behave more impulsively than adults Curiosity leads to experimentation Lack of various life skills, including critical thinking, ability to cope with stress	Attitudes and values of parents and peers regarding substances Substance use by parents, sibling, and peers Influence of advertising and media Easy accessibility of substances or drugs Pro-social and cultural norms towards substance use Factors such as low socio-economic status are statistically related to the tendency to use substances	Developing brains and growing bodies are more sensitive to substances that can be abused

Table 37.2: Frequently abused substances and their adverse effects

Drug name/class	*Commercial and/or street names*	*Effects of intoxication*	*Adverse health consequences*
Marijuana Cannabinoid	Dope, pot, joint, grass, reefer, weed	Euphoria, slowed thinking and reaction time, confusion, impaired balance and coordination	Cough, frequent respiratory infections, impaired memory and learning, increased heart rate and anxiety, panic attacks
Cocaine Stimulant	Blow, candy, coke, crack, rock, snow	Increased heart rate, blood pressure, temperature, and metabolism, feelings of exhilaration and energy, increased mental alertness	Rapid or irregular heart beat, reduced appetite, weight loss, heart failure, nervousness, insomnia, chest pain, respiratory failure, nausea, abdominal pain, strokes, seizures, headaches, malnutrition, panic attacks
Amphetamines Stimulant	Biphetamine, Dexedrine, black beauties, crosses, hearts, speed, truck drivers, uppers	Increased heart rate, blood pressure, metabolism, feelings of exhilaration, energy, increased mental alertness, rapid breathing	Rapid or irregular heart beat, reduced appetite, weight loss, heart failure, nervousness, insomnia, tremor, loss of coordination, irritability, anxiousness, restlessness, delirium, panic, paranoia, impulsive behavior, aggressiveness, psychosis
Barbiturates Depressant	Amytal, Nembutal, Seconal, Phenobarbital, barbs, reds, yellow jackets	Reduced anxiety, feeling of well-being, lowered inhibitions, slowed pulse and breathing, lowered blood pressure, poor concentration, sedation, drowsiness	Fatigue, confusion, impaired coordination, impaired memory and judgement, depression, unusual excitement, fever, irritability, slurred speech, dizziness, life-threatening withdrawal symptoms, respiratory depression and arrest, death

Contd...

Contd...

Drug name/class	*Commercial and/or street names*	*Effects of intoxication*	*Adverse health consequences*
Benzodiazepines Depressant	Ativan, Librium, Valium, Xanax, downers, sleeping pills	Reduced anxiety, feeling of well-being, lowered inhibitions, slowed pulse and breathing, lowered blood pressure, poor concentration, sedation, drowsiness	Fatigue, confusion, impaired coordination, impaired memory and judgement, sedation, drowsiness, dizziness, respiratory depression and arrest, death
Heroin Narcotic (Opioid).	Diacetyl-morphine, brown sugar, dope, junk, smack, white horse	Pain relief, euphoria, drowsiness, unsteady gait	Nausea, constipation, confusion, sedation, respiratory depression and arrest, tolerance, unconsciousness, coma, death
LSD Hallucinogen	Lysergic acid diethylamide, acid	Altered states of perception and feeling, nausea, increased body temperature, heart rate, blood pressure, loss of appetite, sleeplessness, numbness, weakness, tremors, persistent mental disorders	Persisting perception disorder (flashbacks)
PCP Dissociative anesthetics	Phencyclidine, angel dust	Increased heart rate and blood pressure, impaired motor functioning, possible decrease in blood pressure and heart rate, panic, aggression, violence	Memory loss, numbness, nausea and vomiting, loss of appetite, depression
Inhalants	Solvents (paint thinners, gasoline, glues), gases (butane, propane, aerosol propellants, nitrous oxide), nitrites (isoamyl, isobutyl, cyclohexyl), laughing gas, poppers, snappers, whippets		Unconsciousness, cramps, weight loss, muscle weakness, depression, memory impairment, damage to cardiovascular and nervous systems, sudden death
Anabolic steroids	Anadrol, Oxandrin, Durabolin	No intoxication effects	Hypertension, blood clotting, changes in cholesterol, liver cysts and cancer, kidney cancer, hostility and aggression, acne; in adolescents, premature stopping of growth; in males, prostate cancer, reduced sperm production, shrunken testicles, breast enlargement; in females, menstrual irregularities, development of beard and other masculine characteristics

under the influence of the drug that it is able to function normally only when the drug is present. After the user becomes physically dependent on drugs, he/she develops withdrawal symptoms if the intake of the drug is stopped abruptly. The withdrawal symptoms (i.e. when the abuser stops using the substance) may include mild tremors, convulsions, severe agitation, and fits. The withdrawal symptoms and their intensity depend on the type of drug abused and the amount and duration of drug intake.

Table 37.3 list sign and symptoms of drug abuse parents should know. Table 37.4 lists the physical signs and symptoms that should alert a clinician for drug abuse.

Table 37.3: Signs and symptoms of dependence which parents should know

- Losing interest in previously enjoyed activities like sports, homework, or hobbies
- Deterioration in work or school attendance and academic grades non-completion of home work,
- Indulging in any acts that gives money, e.g. frequently borrowing money or stealing items from home or school
- Driving under the influence or sexually risky behavior
- Mood changes temper outbursts, irresponsible behavior, personality change, hostility, defiance, acute anxiety, depression, blaming, lying, making excuses, emotional detachment
- Deterioration of physical appearance and grooming.
- Change of friends, new friends likely to be known users
- Secrecy in respect of possessions and actions such as repeated trips to toilet, locking room and personal things, suspicious behavior like insisting on going out of the house at particular hours, tremendous resistance to give an account of his/her movements, etc. Withdrawal from family environment and non-participation in family work.
- Needing to use more of the substance of choice to achieve the same effects
- Pressuring others to use and talking about the substance constantly
- Looking exhausted, depressed, feeling hopeless, or suicidal
- Presence of needles, syringes and strange packets at home.

These withdrawal symptoms make it difficult for the user to give up drugs. The user is caught in a vicious circle of his/her own making. He/she wants to avoid the experience of suffering

Table 37.4: Physical signs and symptoms

- Running nose, congestion, coughing, pale face, circles under eyes
- Reddening and puffiness of eyes, unclear vision
- Messy appearance, lack of cleanliness
- Loss of appetite, significant weight loss or gain
- Slurring of speech
- Drowsiness or sleeplessness, lethargy and passivity
- C/o Nausea, vomiting, body pain, profuse sweating
- Fresh or old injection marks on veins
- Blood stains on clothes or body
- Impaired memory and lack of concentration

unbearable withdrawal symptoms, and hence continues taking the substance. The addict is thus forced to continue with substance abuse even when he/she realizes that the substance is dangerous.

Many adolescents are given to believe that everybody takes drug in some form or the other. To begin with some of their schoolmates and friends prompt and persuade them to start smoking or taking alcohol which is easily available, accessible and affordable for teenagers. Alcohol and tobacco also known as *gateway drugs* are the stepping stones into the arena of other dangerous substances.

The following table lists some of the other frequently abused substances, the colloquial names, their effects and adverse health consequences. (http://www.drugabuse.gov Drug Pages/DrugsofAbuse.html, National Institute on Drug Abuse).

Advise effects of tabacco and smoking are given in Table 37.5.

SMOKING AND TOBACCO USE

Out of the 1.1 billion smokers worldwide, 16.6% live in India. Everyday about 80, 000 to 100, 000 young people initiate smoking, out of which around 5500 are from India.

A Global Youth Tobacco Survey (GYTS) was conducted by WHO and CDC, Atlanta in 2002-2004 in India. The results showed that tobacco use among school going youth (13-15 years) was 17.5%, 30% in boys and 16% in girls. Smokeless tobacco (pan masala, gutka, zarda, etc) was used

Table 37.5: Adverse effects of smoking and tobacco use

Respiratory	Decreased rate of lung development Decreased pulmonary function Decreased exercise tolerance. Increased incidence of respiratory infections. Worsening of existing asthma and chronic cough. Chronic obstructive pulmonary disease
Cardiovascular risk	Increased serum LDL and triglycerides Decrease in HDL Predisposition to coronary artery disease
Pregnancy and newborn	Abortion, ectopic pregnancy, fetal malformation. Low-birth-weight babies Increased risk of STDs
Malignancy	Oral cavity, pharynx, larynx, esophagus and lungs
Reproductive health	Impotence Combined with contraceptive pills can increase risk of myocardial infarction
Smokeless tobacco	Gingivitis, periodontal disease, leukoplakia, oral precancerous lesions
Enviornmental Tobacco	Increased prevalence of lower respiratory tract infection
Smoke (ETS)	Middle ear infection Hyper-reactive airway disease. Increase the risk of coronary artery disease in later life

by 14.6% while 8.3% were smokers. Survey showed highest prevalence of 58.9%, in Bihar with some children starting as early as 8 years. In the capital city of New Delhi it was 4.5% and 4 in 10 of them reported freely purchasing tobacco products in a store.

Various Factors that Lead Adolescents to Smoking

Adolescents smoke because of curiosity; and peer pressure. The other risk factors are impact of media and advertising. Smoking by parents and role models also influence adolescents to smoke. Other risk factors are poverty, illiteracy; poor hope for future; easy availability of tobacco. Personality factors like rebelliousness, alienation and co-morbidities like depression and conduct disorders, poor value system, lack of life skills with poor knowledge of smoking risks also lead to smoking.

Preventive Programs

It is very important to make adolescent aware of the hazards of smoking as Nicotine is highly addictive and dependence is common after one smokes as few as 100 cigarettes. A 90% of the adolescent smokers become adult smokers.

At the first opportunity the clinician should elicit history of tobacco use. Studies have shown brief physician delivered intervention even as short as 3 minutes for smoking cessation in a primary care setting can significantly increase patient's smoking cessation rates.

Anticipatory guidance should be provided to prepare adolescents for the social pressures that they would face from peers and other environmental sources.

Smoking parents should be warned of the effects of passive smoking and being a negative role model.

Various school based programs have shown to be very effective at prevention, e.g. KS Reddy et al Hridaya program.

Legislation 'The Cigarettes and Other Tobacco Products Act 2003' came into force on 1st May 2004 in India: prohibition of selling tobacco products to persons less than 18 years, total ban on advertisements of any tobacco product and sponsorship of any sport or cultural event by tobacco companies and making smoking in public places punishable.

ALCOHOL

Teenagers begin consumption of alcohol generally for relaxation or to feel grown up or simple under peer pressure. Some teenagers from affluent families may be encouraged to start drinking when they are grown up as a social norm and custom. Very often there is a well stocked bar in the house itself.

Harmful drinking of alcohol can mean many things: excess consumption with inappropriate behaviors or drinking under dangerous circumstances like driving, under situation of pregnancy, binge drinking, daily heavy consumption, etc.

A person is called alcoholic if she/he has alcohol dependence.

Alcohol dependence consists of craving, impaired control, physical dependence or withdrawal symptoms and increasing tolerance *This is a chronic progressive disease.*

Social drinking soon crosses into alcohol dependency without the person getting aware that she or he is going into a phase of daily consumption of significant amount of alcohol.

MIXING DRINKS

Drinks can be mixed with water soda, fruit juice, etc. there is dilution and a greater volume that is consumed over a longer time slowing the immediate effects of alcohol by slower absorption. The alcohole content of various beverage is given in Table 37.6.

Drinks can be mixed by sequential drinking or mixing together different varieties like rum, vodka whisky beer, etc .Whether you drink huge quantity of the same drink or drink sequentially, what matters ultimately is the total amount of ethyl alcohol that goes into the body.

What is more dangerous is mixing alcohol with other substances abuse drugs and medications like barbiturates and anxiolytics, painkillers, etc. Most teenage morbidity and mortality is due to mixing alcohol with substance abuse and then leading to death by intoxication or road accidents.

TEEN AGE GIRLS

need be specially cautioned about alcohol use as it has been seen that due to the lesser body weight and water ratio women tend to get more intoxicated for the same amount of alcohol as compared to a man. Drinking during pregnancy can lead to fetal alcohol syndrome.

SCREENING FOR DRINKING PROBLEM

Clinicians can use the CAGE test developed by Dr John Ewing for a quick screening for drinking problems.

Do you feel that you should **Cut** down on your drinking?

Do you feel **Annoyed** when other people comment about your drinking habits?

Do you ever feel bad or **Guilty** about your drinking?

Do you ever need a drink (**Eye** opener) first thing in the morning to steady your nerves or to get rid of a hangover?

A "yes" to any one of these question suggests possible alcohol-related problems.

More than one "yes" answer means it is highly likely that the person is abusing alcohol.

Table 37.6: Alcohol content of various alcoholic beverage

Arrack—50-60%
Vodka 35-60%
Brandy whisky (scotch) rum —40-55%
Gin 40-50%
Wine port sherry champagne, etc 10-22%
Toddy 5-10%
Beer 4-8%
Breezer 3-5%

Various measures

T standard bottle of beer is 285 ml
Single measure or peg of alcohol is 30 ml
One glass of wine is 120 ml
One measure of aperitif is 180 ml
1 unit of alcohol is approximately 10 gm of alcohol
12 ounce of beer is equal to one peg of whisky

Source: Alcohol use and abuse what you should know alcohol series -4 WHO Regional office for southeast Asia 2006

TREATMENT METHODS FOR TEENAGERS DEPENDING UPON THEIR STAGE OF DRUG AND ALCOHOL USE

1. **Experimental/recreational use:**
   Education helps adolescents and parents learn about alcohol and drugs and their detrimental effects. This along with counseling, i.e. talking with the adolescent about his life and drug use.
2. **Regular use:**
   Individual, group and family therapy—done by mental health professional.
   Abstinence contract—written agreement not to use drugs, to have regular urine drug screens and abide by home rules (privileges and consequences) as developed by the parents and the adolescents.
3. **Preoccupation with use:**
   12-Step program—attending regular meetings of alcoholics anonymous or narcotics anonymous and completing the steps.
4. **Chemical dependency:**
   Hospital program—acute and intermediate level of care
   Residential program—long-term intermediate level of 24 hours care and therapeutic program.

SUMMARY

There is no denying the fact that treatment methods for substance abuse are costly and relapse rates are high.

Prevention programs which are aimed at delaying the onset of substance abuse and focus on knowledge, attitude and skill and are initiated in early adolescence before the experimentation starts are more helpful.

It is not enough to have knowledge about the hazards of drug abuse, but to keep away from drugs adolescents to have skills to deal with friends who pressurize for drinks or smoke.

Glamorization of alcohol, cigarette and other substances in media, films, etc. also is a great influencing factor.

Hence it is important for them to learn certain refusal skills. Saying "No" in different situations in part of life skill education program.

Family support is essential to help teenagers who are indulging in alcohol, tobacco or other drugs. If their friends are doing so they must also persuade them to confide and take support of the family.

SUGGESTED READING

1. Adolescence Education. Knowledge Base, Part II, NCERT, New Delhi, 1999 (a Package of Basic Materials)
2. Addiction Recovery Agency. Frequently asked questions about alcohol.
3. Arora M, Reddy KS. GYTS, Delhi. Indian Pediatr 2005; 42: 850-51.
4. Desai NG, Nawamongkolwattana B, Ranaweera S, Shrestha DM, Sobhan MA. Prevention of harm from alcohol use: get high on life without alcohol.New Delhi: World Health Organization, Regional Office for South-East Asia.Document SEA/Ment/122, 2003.
5. Doyon S. The many faces of ecstasy. Curr Opinion Pediatr: 2001;13: 170-76.
6. Galagali P smoking in adolescents in Bhaves textbook of Adoelscent Medicine 1st edition Swati Y Bhave Jyapee Publishers New Delhi 2006;920-28.
7. Greydanus DE, Patel DR. Substance abuse in Course Manual for Adolescent Health Part –1. IAP-ITPAH. In: Greydanus DE, Patel DR, Prat H, Bhave S. (Eds). 2002;480-88.
8. Greydanus DE, Yadav Sangeeta. Substance Abuse disorders in Bhaves Text book of adolescent medicine 1st ed. Jaypee Brothers New Delhi. Chapter 23.1 800-06
9. Greydanus DE (Ed). Caring for your Adolescent. Second Edition, American Academy of Pediatrics and Bantam Books (NY), 2003.
10. Greydanus DE, Patel DR. Sports doping in the adolescent athlete. Asian Journal of Paediatric Practice 2000;4(1): 9-14.
11. Greydanus DE, Substance Abuse in Adolescents: Basic chemistry lessons gone awry. International Pediatrics 2002;17(1): 3-4.
12. Heyman RB. Reducing tobacco use among youth. Pediatr Cli of Nor Am 2002; 49: 377-388.

13. Klein DJ, Kodjo CM. Prevention and risk of adolescent substance use: the role of adolescents, families and communities. Pediatr Cli of Nor Am 2002; 49: 257-68.
14. Hogan MJ: Diagnosis and treatment of teen drug use. Med Clin No Amer 2000;84 (4): 927-66.
15. (http://www.addictionrecovery.org.uk/ACAD-BAS-FAQPage.html, accessed 15 June 2006).
16. http://www.MonitoringTheFuture.org
17. Jenkins RR: "Substance abuse" In: RE Behrman, RM Kliegman and HB Jenson (Ed). Nelson Textbook of Pediatrics, 17th Edition, Philadelphia: WB Saunders Co., 2004;105:653-62.
18. Johnston LD, O'Malley PM Bachman JG. The Monitoring the Future Study: National Survey Results on Adolescent Drug Use. Overview of Key Findings. University of Michigan Institute for Social Research, 1999.
19. National Institute on Drug Abuse: www.nida.gov/NIDAHome.html
20. National Clearinghouse on Alcohol and Drug Information:www.health.org
21. National Institute on Alcohol Abuse and Alcoholism: www.niaaa.nih.gov
22. Obot IS, Saxena S. (Eds). Substance use among young people in urban environments. Geneva: World Health Organization, 2005.
23. Patel DR, Greydanus DE. Substance abuse: A pediatric concern. Indian J Pediatr, 1999.
24. Reddy KS, et al. Tobacco and alcohol use outcomes of a school based intervention in New Delhi. American Journal of Health Behavior 2002; 26: 173-81.
25. Reddy KS, Arora M. Tobacco use among children in India: a burgeoning epidemic. Editorial. Indian Pediatr 2005; 42: 757-61.
26. Schydlower M (Ed). Substance Abuse: A Guide for Health Professionals. American Academy of Pediatrics. Elk Grove Village, IL, 2000
27. Singh G, et al. Use among 10-12 year old school students in Patna district, Bihar, India. Indian Pediatr 2005; 42: 805-10.
28. World Health Organization. Regional Office for South-East Asia. Facts on alcohol use and abuse. New Delhi, 2003.
29. WHO Regional Office for South East Asia. Alcohol use and abuse—what you should know alchohol series—2006;4.

38 Psychiatric Problems Related to ARSH

PC Shastri, Jay P Shastri

DEVELOPMENT OF SEXUALITY IN ADOLESCENT

Adolescence can be viewed as comprising of three phases, each of which has a specific relationship to sexual development and behaviour.

1. *The early phase (12 to 14 years)*: This phase is marked by changes associated with puberty. The changes are related attractiveness, size and maturation rate and the relationship of these issues to self-esteem and body image.
2. *The middle phase (14 to 16 years)*: This phase is marked by closeness with the peer group, increase use of abstract ability mainly to distinguish them from the parents. General theme of sexual issues during this phase includes dating competence, sexual orientation, and exploratory sexual behaviour. Other issues that can complicate the sexual development in this phase include separation from family and continuous comparison of oneself to the peer group.
3. *The late Phase (16 to 19 years)*: This phase is associated with setting pattern and plans for work and establishing patterns of more intimate interpersonal relationship. This phase is characterized by increasing wishes and ability for emotional and sexual intimacy and fewer needs of familial base.

MASTURBATION

Is a normal physiological process but if indulged in too often at the cost of normal daily activities or if it is associated with extreme guilt and depression it will fall into the abnormal category.

Masturbation is the manual excitation of the sexual organs, usually to the point of orgasm. It can refer to excitation either by oneself or by another. It is part of a larger set of activities known as autoeroticism which also includes the use of sex toys and non-genital stimulation.

Masturbation and sexual intercourse are the two most common sexual practices, but they are not mutually exclusive (for example, many people find the sight of their partner masturbating highly erotic). Some people are able to achieve orgasm only through masturbation and not sexual intercourse.

Masturbation is the most common source of orgasm in boys. By age of 14 years, 80% have masturbated, and by age 18 years, 90 to 98% have masturbated. At the same time, more than 50% of boys experience guilt in relation to this activity. According to few reports available, masturbation occurs less frequently in girls than in boys.

Though masturbation can be regarded as an normal sexual activity there are certain deviant behaviors that might indicate the shift.

Culturally the significance of semen ("Dhat" in native hindi) is extremely large in Indian society. The syndrome called " Dhat Syndrome" is highly prevalent in Indian culture where semen is given more importance than blood and the loss of semen through masturbation or otherwise provokes extreme high anxiety states. This is more seen in adolescent population. The management requires insight oriented psychotherapy with use of psychotropic medications in case of co-morbid psychiatric illness like depression and anxiety are present.

SEXUAL DYSFUNCTIONS

A sexual dysfunction is characterized by a disturbance in the processes that characterize the sexual response cycle or by pain associated with sexual intercourse.

The sexual response cycle can be divided into following four phases.

a. **Desire:** This phase is characterized by fantasies about sexual activity and the desire to have sexual intercourse. This phase marks the mental preparedness for the upcoming sexual activity which leads to the next phase of excitement.
b. **Excitement**: This phase consists of a subjective sense of sexual pleasure and accompanying physiological changes. The foreplays that partners in the sexual intercourse undertake forms the major portion of subjective experiences during this phase. In males there is erection of penis following increased in the blood supply to that region. While in females this phase is marked by vasocongestion in pelvis, vaginal lubrication and expansion and swelling of external genitals.
c. **Orgasm:** This phase is marked by peaking of sexual pleasure, with release of sexual tension and rhythmic contraction of the perineal muscles and reproductive organs. In males there is a strong need to ejaculate, which is followed by the act of ejaculation. In females the outer one-third of vaginal wall contracts.
d. **Resolution**: This phase consists of a sense of muscular relaxation and general satisfaction. During this phase males are physiologically refractory to further erection and orgasm for a variable period of time. In contrast, females may be able to respond to additional stimulation almost immediately.

Sexual dysfunction may occur during one or more of these phases and it is also possible to have more than one sexual dysfunction in an individual.

- There is no described norm as to frequency, setting, activities and types of sexual intercourse. The decision is made clinically taking into consideration factors like, age, experience, culture, etc.
- Sexual dysfunction can be life long when it is present from the onset of sexual activity or acquired when it appears after a long duration of normal sexual activity.
- When it appears across all the situations and with all the partners it is called generalized, If difficulties are experienced in specific situation, type of stimulation and partner it is called situational sexual dysfunction.
- Etiologically psychological factors, presence of general medical conditions and/or presence of substance use can be related to presence of sexual dysfunction.

Depending on the various stages of sexual cycles and the etiological factors the disorders are divided into:

1. **Sexual Desire Disorders**
   i. Hypoactive sexual desire disorder
   ii. Sexual aversion disorder
2. **Sexual Arousal Disorder**
   i. Female sexual arousal disorder
   ii. Male erectile disorder
3. **Orgasmic Disorder**
   i. Female orgasmic disorder
   ii. Male orgasmic disorder
4. **Premature Ejaculation**
5. **Sexual Pain Disorder**
   i. Dyspareunia
   ii. Vaginismus
6. **Sexual disorder due to general medical condition**
7. **Substance-induced sexual disorder**

SEXUAL DESIRE DISORDERS

Hypoactive Sexual Desire Disorder

It is characterized by deficiency or absence of sexual fantasies and desire for sexual activity. The individual does not normally initiate sexual activity and generally does not participate actively when it is initiated from partner. Sexual desire disorder is frequently associated with sexual arousal and orgasmic difficulties.

Sexual Aversion Disorder

The essential feature of sexual aversion disorder is the aversion to and active avoidance of genital sexual contact with a sexual partner. The individual reports anxiety, fear, or disgust when confronted by a sexual opportunity with a partner.

Management:

Hypoactive sexual desire disorder has been the most difficult to treat of all sexual dysfunctions. The most effective treatment involves combination of therapy to deal with maladaptive beliefs, behavioral treatment and couple therapy.

In case of sexual aversion disorder the main goal of management is to reduce the patient's fear and avoidance of sex. This goal can be accomplished by systemic desensitization.

The use of tricyclic antidepressant along with sex therapy has also shown positive results.

SEXUAL AROUSAL DISORDER

Female Sexual Arousal Disorder

This disorder is marked by presence of a persistent or recurrent inability to attain, or maintain until completion of the sexual activity, an adequate lubrication-swelling response to sexual excitement. The individual may have little or no sense of sexual arousal. The disorder may result in painful intercourse, sexual avoidance and disturbed relationship.

Male Erectile Disorder

The essential feature of male erectile disorder is a persistent or recurrent inability to attain, or maintain until completion of the sexual activity, an adequate erection. There are different patterns of erectile dysfunction.

Some adolescent may report the inability to obtain any erection from the outset of the sexual experience, while others will complain about losing the erection during penetration or anytime during thrusting before ejaculation.

Losing of masturbatory erection is extremely uncommon.

It is frequently associated with sexual anxiety, fear of failure, concerns about sexual performance, and decreased subjective sense of sexual excitement and pleasure.

Management

Sexual arousal disorders are better handled in presence of partner. The psychotherapeutic approach like behavioral assignments to reduce performance anxiety, sensate focus exercises, systematic desensitization, group therapy and couple therapy has been used with considerable amount of success.

Somatic treatments like vasoactive injections and tropical application of medications that results in relaxation of arterial smooth muscle have met with limited success.

Drugs like sildenafil citrate has been effective in both the sexes in adult population as seen in many randomized controlled trails. *However, its use in adolescent population has not been well documented.*

ORGASMIC DISORDER

Female Orgasmic Disorder

This disorder is characterized by presence of persistent or recurrent delay in, or absence of, orgasm following a normal sexual excitement phase. The diagnosis of female orgasmic disorder should be based on the clinician's judgment that the female's orgasmic capacity is less than would be reasonable for her age, sexual experience, and adequacy of sexual stimulation that she receives.

According to controlled studies, orgasmic capacity is not correlated with vaginal size or pelvic muscle strength. Since orgasmic capacity in females increases with sexual experience, female orgasmic disorder may be more prevalent in younger women.

Once the female learns how to reach orgasm it is uncommon for her to lose that capacity.

Male Orgasmic Disorder

The essential of male orgasmic disorder is a persistent or recurrent delay in, or absence of, orgasm following a normal sexual excitement phase. As with females the clinical diagnosis of male orgasmic disorder should take into consideration his age, and adequacy, focus and intensity of stimulation. Many such males describe the act of coitus as mere formality after having a normal arousal pattern to start with. In male orgasm can occur in the absence of emission of semen.

Management

Orgasmic disorders are best treated through a program of directed masturbation. Use of exercises to strengthen pubococcygeal muscles in case of females has shown better results when coupled with masturbatory program. Use of sensate focus technique in both the sexes has been found useful.

Here too sildenafil has been shown to be effective in both the genders in adult population.

Premature Ejaculation

This disorder is characterized by persistent or recurrent onset of orgasm and ejaculation with minimal sexual stimulation before, on, or shortly after penetration and before the person wishes it.

The majority of individuals with such disorder can delay orgasm during self-masturbation for a considerably longer time than during the coitus.

Partner's estimates of the duration of time from the beginning of sexual activity until ejaculation as well as judgment of whether premature ejaculation is a problem can be quite varied.

Typically, premature ejaculation is seen in adolescents or young men and is present from their first attempts at intercourse.

Some young males hesitate to begin dating new partners out of fear of embarrassment from the disorder. This can further contribute to social isolation.

Management

The management includes raining of an individual to high levels of excitement without ejaculating and reducing anxiety associated with sexual arousal.

Other successful interventions are "Start and Stop Technique" and "Squeeze Technique". Somatic treatments like papaverine injections and use of medicines have shown results with related difficulties.

SEXUAL PAIN DISORDERS

Dyspareunia

The cardinal feature of this disorder is the pain associated with sexual intercourse. Although it is most commonly experienced during coitus, is may also occur before or after intercourse. The disorder can occur in both males and females.

In females, the pain might be described as superficial during the foreplay, while it is described as deep during the act of intercourse. The intensity of pain can range from mild discomfort to sharp pain. It rarely presents as a chief complain in medical settings. The repeated experience of pain during the sexual act can lead to avoidance of sexual experience, disruption of existing sexual relationships or limiting the development of new sexual relationships.

Vaginismus

The core symptom of vaginismus is the recurrent or persistent involuntary contraction of perineal muscles surrounding the outer third of vagina when vaginal penetration with penis, finger, tampon, or speculum is attempted.

In some females, even the anticipation of vaginal insertion may result in muscle spasm. The contractions may range from mild, inducing some tightness and discomfort, to severe, preventing penetration.

Other sexual responses may not be impaired until penetration is attempted or anticipated. The disorder is more often found younger than older females, in females with negative attitude towards sex and in females who have a history of being sexually abused or traumatized.

Management

Systemic desensitization is found to be successful in the treatment of sexual pain disorder especially vaginismus. Therapy oriented to individual and couple's psychosexual issues generally helps in treating such disorders.

SEXUAL DISORDER DUE TO GENERAL MEDICAL CONDITION

The essential feature of this type of sexual dysfunction is presence of general medical condition whose direct physiological effect can cause it. The history, physical examination and laboratory findings should reflect the same.

Although there are no set rules which guides us regarding the relationship between the sexual dysfunction and medical conditions, there are certain considerations that might help clinician to establish the connect between the two.

One consideration is the presence of a temporal association between the onset, exacerbation, or remission of the general medical condition and that of sexual dysfunction.

A second consideration is the presence of features that are atypical of the primary sexual dysfunction like age of onset and course of the dysfunction.

The variety of general medical conditions that can cause sexual dysfunctions are neurological disorders (neuropathy, temporal lobe lesion, multiple sclerosis), endocrine disorders (juvenile onset diabetes mellitus, hypothyroidism, pituitary dysfunction), vascular conditions and genitourinary conditions.

For physically ill children, the type of problems with sexual issues experienced during the early phase of adolescence is governed largely by the impact their illness or its treatment has on their pubertal development.

These effects might include influences on the timing of puberty and associated secondary sexual characteristics, body size, or the development of dysmorphic physical features. In boy illnesses that make them shorter and thinner have a powerful negative impact on their developing image of themselves as sexual and male. For girls, illnesses or treatments that cause weight gain or facial changes are particularly troubling.

SUBSTANCE INDUCED SEXUAL DISORDER

When the sexual dysfunction is judged to be fully explained by the direct physiological effects of the substance (drug of abuse, a medication or toxin exposure) it is called Substance-Induced Sexual Dysfunction.

Substance–Induced Sexual Dysfunctions usually have their onset during Substance Intoxication. The following classes of substances are known to produce sexual dysfunction: alcohol, amphetamine and related substance, cocaine, opioids, sedatives, hypnotics and anxiolytics and other or unknown substances.

Acute intoxication with or chronic abuse of or dependence on substances of abuse has been reported to decrease sexual interest and cause arousal problems in both sexes.

Side Effects of Prescribed Medications

The decrease in sexual interest, arousal disorders and orgasmic disorders can also be cause by prescribed medications including antihypertensive, histamine H_2 receptor antagonists, antidepressant (especially SSRI's), neuroleptics, anxiolytics, anabolic steroids and antiepileptic.

The onset of sexual dysfunction with prescribed medications must have with the initiation of the drug and would subside within few days once the drug is stopped or withdrawn.

PEDOPHILIA

- Among the long list of sexual perversions, pedophilia needs special mention here as the victim is always an adolescent but the victimizer can also be adolescent in certain cases. The pedophilia involves sexual activity with a prepubescent child generally age 13 years or younger.
- The individual with pedophilia must be age 16 years or older and at least 5 years older than the child.
- The female victims are usually between the ages of 8 and 10 years and male victims are usually slightly older.
- Pedophilia involving female victims is reported more often than pedophilia involving male victims.
- Most pedophiles have low self-esteem and begin the behavior in adolescence.
- The frequency of pedophilic behavior often fluctuates with psychosocial stress.
- The course is usually chronic, especially in those attracted to males.
- Management mainly includes skill training and cognitive restructuring to change the individual's maladaptive beliefs and aversive therapy.
- Role of medications like SSRI's are mainly based on case reports.

SUGGESTED READING

1. Althof SE, Turner LA, Levine SB, et al. Sexual, psychological, and marital impact of self injection of papaverine and phenotolamine: a long-term prospective study. J. Sex Marital Ther 1991;17:101-12.
2. American Psychiatric Association. Diagnostic Statistical Manual of Mental Disorders, 4th Edition, Text Revision. Washington, DC, American Psychiatric Association, 2000.
3. Araji S, Finkelhor D. Explanations of pedophilia: review of empherical research. Bulletin of American Association of Psychiatry and the Law 1985;13 17-37.
4. Baum N, Spieler B. Medical Management of premature ejaculation. Medical Aspects of Human Sexuality 2001;1:15-25.
5. Berman JR, Berman LA, Lin H. et al. Effect of Sildenafil on subjective and physiologic parameters of the female sexual response in women with sexual arousal Disorder: J Sex Marital Ther 2001; 27:411-20.
6. Cocores JA, Millers NS, Pottash AC, et al. Sexual Dysfunctions in abusers of cocaine and alcohol. Am J Drug Alcohol Abuse 1988;14: 169-173.
7. Fein RL. Intracavernous medication for treatment of premature ejaculation. Urology; 1990;35: 301-3.
8. Finger WW. Antidepressants and sexual dysfunction: managing common treatment pitfalls. Medical Aspects of Human Sexuality 2001; 1:12-8.
9. Graziottin A. Clinical approaches to dyspareunia. J Sex Marital Ther 2001;27: 489-501.
10. Greil W, Horvath A, Sassim N, et al. Disinhibition of libido: an adverse effect of SSRI? J Affect Disord 2001;62:225-228.
11. Leiblum SR, Rosen RC. Couples therapy for erectile disorders: conceptual and clinical considerations. J Sex Marital Ther 1991;17: 147-59.
12. LoPiccolo J, Stock WE. Treatment of sexual dysfunction. J Consult Clin Psychol 1986; 54:158-67.
13. Metz ME, Pryor JL. Premature ejaculation: a psychophysiological approach for assessment and management. J Sex Marital Ther 2000;26:293-320.
14. Montejo-Gozalez AL, Llorca G, Izquierdo JA, et al. SSRI-induced sexual dysfunction: Fluoxetine, paroxetine, sertraline, and fluvoxamine in a prospective, multicenter, and descriptive clinical stuy of 344 patients. J Sex Marital Ther 1997;23: 176-94.
15. Salerian AJ, Vittone BJ, Geyer SP, et al. Sildenafil for psychotropic induced sexual dysfunction in 31 women and 61 men. J Sex Marital Ther 2000;26: 133-40.
16. Seidman SN, Roose SP, Menza MA, et al. Treatment of erectile dysfunction in men with depressive symptoms: results of a placebo controlled trial with sidenafil citrate. Am. J Psychiatry 2002;158:1623-30.
17. Weiss JN, Ravalli R, Badlani GH. Intracavernous pharmacotherapy in psychogenic impotence. Urology 1997;37:441-43.
18. Yates A. Childhood sexuality. In: Lewis M, (Ed). Child and Adolescent Psychiatry: A Comprehensive Textbook. Baltimore: Williams and Wilkins 1991;195-214.
19. Zucker KJ, Green R. Psychosexual disorders in children and adolescents. J Child Psychol Psychiatry 1992;33:107-51.

39 Sexual Aggression

Sunil Saini, Swati Y Bhave

INTRODUCTION

Sexual aggression is a major social problem around the world. Sexual aggression and victimization against women and children are increasing day by day. Newspaper and media coverage are full of story of attempted rapes and rapes at college and university, girl child molestation at school by teachers and older students, and other many such cases in rural areas. Most of the cases are unreported to police. Protective factors against sexual aggression are summarised in Table 39.1.

Researchers have found sexually aggressive youth to be poorly socialized and to have inadequate peer relationships (Ford and Linney, 1995). A large-scale survey in the United States suggests that approximately 27% of females and 16% of males have experienced some form of sexual abuse as children (Finkelhor et al. 1990).

In a survey of over 2, 800 college women conducted by the Centers for Disease Control and Prevention, 71% of women who reported rape were victimized before the age of 18, mainly in the teen years, and an additional 22% were of college age [19-24 years] (Brener et al 1999).

SEXUAL AGGRESSION

Sexual aggression is generally a man's attempts, whether successful or not, to coerce, threaten, or force a woman to engage in sexual acts against her will. Studies have shown that most sexual aggression is committed by acquaintances (e.g. 84%, Koss, 1988). Sexual aggression is perpetrated by a large number of people with varying motivations (Hall and Hirschman, 1991) and in different circumstances. It may involve a variety of different behaviors designed to achieve the goal of sexual intercourse with an unwilling woman. These behaviors may include physical aggression, psychological aggression, taking advantage of intoxication, sexual misperception, acid throwing, incest, child molestation, attemp-

Table 39.1: Protective factors

• Healthy parent child relationships	• Healthy marital relationships
• Recreational activities	• Social skills
• Conflict management skills	• Empowerment
• Well-integrated sense of identity	• Social support system Self-confidence
• Self-esteem	• Safe dates
• Sense of morality	• School counselor
• Strong judiciary system	
• Community development programs like workshops accepting professional help at the right time	

Table 39.2: Various factors that may have influence on sexual aggression

• Parent child relationships	• Domestic violence
• Harsh discipline	• Family history of sexual abuse
• Child maltreatment	• Anger
• Hostility	• Aggression
• Impulsivity	• Sensual sensation seeking
• Dominance	• Emotional constriction
• Peer pressure	• Social competence
• Attitude towards sex	• Personality traits
• Cognitive factors	• Loneliness
• Rejection	• Neglect
• Parental separation	• Gender discrimination
• Poor academic achievement	• School problems
• Juvenile Delinquency	• Criminal history
• Environmental factors	

ted rape, rape, verbal coercion, and other sexually aggressive behaviors.

Similarly Ouimette (1997) found that college men who reported rape or attempted rape were significantly more likely to meet diagnosis for alcohol abuse or dependence (53%) compared with men from the same population who reported only nonviolent sexual intercourse (25%). Various factors that can influence sexual aggression are summarised in Table 39.2.

SEXUAL AGGRESSION OF WOMEN AGAINST MEN

General views and researches are mainly concerned with men's sexual aggression on women. It is generally cited that men are responsible for sexual assault on women. In Germany, the penal code was changed in 1997 to remove the restriction of sexual victimization to female victims of extramarital sexual assault and allow both women and men to be acknowledged as victims of sexual violence, both within and outside marital relationships (Krahe et al. 2003).

Women's use of sexual aggression is generally neglected due to widespread preoccupation of men's physical aggression toward women (Eagly and Steffen, 1986; Hyde, 1984). However, if other forms of aggressive behavior are considered, such as verbal aggression, indirect aggression (e.g. spreading rumors), or relational aggression (e.g. exclusion), it becomes clear that girls and women engage in these forms of behavior to a substantial degree (Bjorkvist, et al. 1994; Crick and Grotpeter, 1995).

Cultural difference is likely to play an important role in women's sexual aggression toward men. As Frieze (2000) noted, cultural norms are likely to play an important part in explaining gender differences or similarities with regard to aggressive behavior. Sarrel and Masters (1982) presented 11 cases that documented that men might be made to show sexual responses (i.e., erections, ejaculations) against their will. Indeed, such sexual reactions can be triggered not only by sexual stimulation but also by intense feelings of fear or anger.

In one of the first prevalence studies of female on-male sexual aggression, Struckman-Johnson (1988) found that 2% of the 355 female college students in her sample reported that they had "forced sex on a dating partner" at least once in their lifetime. Poppen and Segal (1988) reported an overall percentage of lifetime prevalence (including both verbal coercion and physical assault) of 14%. In a survey of 171 female college students, Shea (1998) obtained a lifetime prevalence rate of 19% for verbal coercion. Hogben et al. (1996) found an overall lifetime prevalence rate of 24% for women having made a man engage in sexual activity against his will. Similarly In a sample of 212 female participants studied by Anderson and Aymami (1993), 28.5% reported the use of verbal coercion, 14.7% had coerced a man into sexual activity by getting him intoxicated, and 7.1% had threatened or used physical force.

DOMESTIC VIOLENCE

Domestic violence is a crime created by men against women and can involve behaviors such as threatening, psychological abuse, physical abuse, verbal abuse, financial abuse and sexual assault. Youth exposure to domestic violence has been linked to an array of mental health and behavioral problems in adolescents and adults including anxiety and depression, posttraumatic stress, anger and aggressive behavior, and sexual aggression (Blumenthal et al. 1998; Fantuzzo and Mohr, 1999; McGruder-Johnson et al. 2000; Spaccarelli et al. 1997).

Another study (Becker, 1986) has shown that juvenile sexual aggression has been associated with a history of sexual or physical abuse during childhood, exposure to family violence, and alcohol use during adolescence Young male victims of sexual abuse often demonstrate acting-out behaviors, sexualization, and identification with the offender (Watkins and Bentovim, 1992).

The newly introduced domestic violence bill is biased towards women and can promote its misuse. There should be equality given to both genders for domestic violence. Majority of domestic violence that occurs, is of the man hitting his wife and children. However, there are increasing numbers of Indian husband today that are emotionally abused by wife threatening to withhold sexual intimacy, threatening to leave home and children at the smallest disagreement, threats of self-injury or suicide, shouting and screaming and creating scenes when the husband does not agree to her unreasonable demands. There are many women who scratch, beat, bite, hit and throw things at men in fits of temper tantrums . Many men are silent sufferers because they do not like the public image of a harassed husband.

DATING VIOLENCE

Romantic relationships are the important aspects of adolescents. High school students spend between five and eight hours per week thinking about actual or potential romantic partners (Richards et al. 1998). The other sex is a frequent source of strong emotions. The majority of these emotions are positive but a substantiation proportion is negative. Increased prevalence of teen pregnancies, abortions, early sexual maturity, early sexual relationships, multiple sex partners, and sexually transmitted diseases including HIV/AIDS are clearly linked with romantic involvement of adolescents and lead to substantive damage to reproductive health.

More than 25% of adolescents are victims of dating violence or aggression (Wolfe and Feiring, 2000). Between 9 and 46% of high school students are involved in dating violence (Watson et al 2001). 89% of teenagers between the ages of 13 to 18 say they have been in dating relationships and nearly 80% who have been physically abused on dating continue to date their abusers The high dating violence victimization rates for adolescents suggest that this topic is a serious social issue (Chase et al. 2002).

Dating violence is a pattern of violent behavior that someone uses against a girlfriend/boyfriend. Dating violence can take many forms like physical aggression, psychological aggression and sexual coercion. There are many reported cases in newspapers, magazines and in other media. Dating violence including slapping, kicking, tearing hair, pushing and pulling, hitting, acid throwing, forced kissing, touching, petting, attempted rape, rape, date rape, group rape, drug abuse, aggression and even murder. Young girls are most vulnerable to this.

Teenage girls who have sex with more than one partner in a short period of time are more likely to engage in other risky behaviors, such as fighting, binge drinking, smoking cigarettes, using cocaine or sniffing glue, according to a new study by two Universities of Maryland researchers.

Adolescents who experience dating violence, report isolation, sad/hopeless or depressed feelings, suicidal behavior, emotional outbursts, eating disorders, poor self-esteem. Adolescents indulging in substance use, (Foo and Margolin, 1995) multiple sex partners, and unprotected sex are more likely to report being a victim of dating violence (Silverman et al. 2001; Ackard et al. 2003). It has also been linked to poor academic performance (Bergman, 1992), and later marital violence (Henton et al 1983).

DRINKING AND AGGRESSION

Alcohol is commonly viewed as increasing sexual arousal and contributing to consensual and nonconsensual activity (Abbey et al 1999). Studies have shown that alcohol consumption is frequently considered and invoked as a contributor to sexual aggression (Abbey et al. 1994; Lightfoot and Barbaree, 1993; Seto and Barbaree, 1995).

Tyler et al (1998) considered the role of perpetrator alcohol use as a predictor of three different sexually aggressive strategies among college men: physical force, verbal coercion, and victim intoxication. Perpetrator's use alcohol or drug as a strategy to obtain sex. Cognitive and motor impairment are associated with high level of intoxication. Fischer (1996) found that college men who reported excessive alcohol use were more likely to report lying or making false promises to obtain sex, most of these lying took place at parties.

In 2001, the Youth Risk Behavior Survey determined that 25.6% of high school students had consumed alcohol or drugs before their last sexual intercourse (Grunbaum, 2002). Gudjonsson and Sigurdsson (2000) found that alcohol was much more likely to be used at the time of the offense among men convicted of rape and other violent crimes (75% and 90%, respectively) than among convicted child molesters (13%), who tended to victimize someone they knew well.

Similarly, female college students reported that incidents involving rape or attempted rape were more likely to involve alcohol use on the part of the perpetrator (56%) than were sexual coercion incidents (30%, Abbey et al. 1996). Norries et al. (1999) found that that men who consumed alcohol judged the female victim to be less upset and less disgusted with the perpetrator than sober men.

DRINKING AND DRIVING

Alcohol consumption is one of the most prevalent health risk factors among adolescents. One of the most serious effects of alcohol consumption among adolescents is drunken driving, road rage, road accidents leading to injuries and death. Since alcohol impairs judgment, reduces intellectual functioning, and affects cognitions and emotions, it may release pent-up anger and frustrations, thus inducing violence.

Young people are at an increased risk of motor vehicle injuries when alcohol is involved, owing to their inexperience in drinking coupled with their inexperience in driving and (Mayhew et al. 1986,) and risky driving style Williams and Preusser, 1997).). Alcohol has been found to be a factor in more than one-third of motor vehicle deaths among adolescent drivers. Nighttime crash risk is particularly elevated for teenage drivers, more so if even a little alcohol has been consumed (Keall and Frith, 2004). High teenage driver risk is due to a combination of their inexperience and risky driving style.

Younger adolescents are found to be more involved in behaviors such as horn honking, tailgating, fast overtaking, night drinking driving, etc.

Conditions associated with chronic alcohol abuse, such as depression (Miczek, et al. 1993), sleep withdrawal (Pernanen, 1976), and paranoia (Potter-Efron and Potter-Efron, 1991) might also increase rage and violence, suggesting that alcohol abusers were likely to display violence not only while intoxicated, but also in the absence of alcohol consumption or intoxication.

SEXUAL BULLYING IN SCHOOL AND COLLEGE

Sexual bullying is a common practice in school and college campus in today's urbanization. Child molestation in school by teachers is an emerging issue nowadays. Recently one such a case of happened in a senior secondary school in India. The director of a school education board was found to be abusing 5th and 6th class girls over a prolonged duration One of the victims confided in her parents .A local media person encouraged them to disclose the matter to public and police. In another casein the same school it was found that young girls used to entertain visual images and movie on cell phones of school car driver. The case in under jurisdiction and school is under government administration.

Sexual aggression in college/university campus has been a topic of discussion since a long time. It is generally seen that dating aggression is commonly accepted among adolescents, which further leads to sexual aggression. There have been many cases of girl rape at campus in New Delhi and other parts of India. Recently court gave a death penalty to a famous case, in which a law student was raped and murdered at home. Researchers have found many factors influencing sexual aggression among college/university student. For example, Koss and Gaines (1993) identified athletic involvement, particularly in revenue producing sports, as a predictor of sexual aggression. The association between athletics and sexuality is not a recent phenomenon: the use of athletics and sexuality as outlets for aggression has been widespread for years (Naison, 1972). Sigelman et al. (1984) noted an association between sexual and physical aggression in college men. Similarly other findings have shown that sexual aggression is motivated by aggression rather than by sexuality (Bianchi, 1976; Briere and Malamuth, 1983; Brownmiller, 1975).

PORNOGRAPHY

Pornography industry is growing very rapidly in different forms. Nowadays, pornography material is easily accessible to young boys and girls, even at their home on Internet and CDs. Violent pornography refers to sexually explicit material portraying sexual aggression, typically enacted by men against women (Marshall and Barrett, 1990). Violent pornography is more likely to aroused sexual aggression.

Pornography has a negative impact on intimate relationships, which leads to negative interaction between the partners. Zillmann and Bryant (1988) in their study found that both male and female participants were less satisfied with their sexual partners' appearance, affection, and sexual performance after repeated exposure to pornographic films.

Court (1976) found a positive association between availability of pornography and sex crime rate in a study using data from seven countries, and Jaffee and Strauss (1987) found a positive association between sex magazine readership and rates of reported rape across the American states. Carter and colleagues found that, as adults, their sample of 26 child molesters used more pornography than their sample of 38 rapists, and were more likely to incorporate pornography in their sexual offending, for example, viewing photographs before having contact with the victims (Carter et al. 1987).

Pornography usually arouse physiological arousal, excitation transfer theory predicts that this arousal could be attributed to anger if participant is subsequently provoked. As suggested by M. Allen et al. (1995), excitation transfer theory predicts that: (a) previously angered subjects will manifest higher levels of aggression after pornography exposure (b) as the level of provocation (i.e., anger) prior to exposure to pornography increases, the greater the manifestation of aggression after the exposure.

Feminist theory have suggested that pornography is responsible for three kinds of harm. First, pornography may cause direct harm to women. Cole (1989) has claimed that the majority of women involved in the sex trade are there because of their experience of sexual abuse as children.

Second, pornography is seen as promoting violence directed against women, through its effects on attitudes and beliefs (Dworkin and MacKinnon, 1988).

Finally, pornography is seen as causing social harm. Therefore, from feminist theories we can predict that: (1) the higher the consumption of pornography, the higher the rate of sexual violence against women, at both the aggregate and individual level; (2) pornography negatively alters both male and female perceptions of women; and (3) sexual arousal toward aggression against women occurs in tandem with attitudes supportive of violence against women (Baron and Straus, 1984).

Social learning theory suggests that violent pornography can increase subsequent aggressive behavior because it portrays this behavior as rewarding. As stated by M. Allen et al. (1995), we can also predict that: (a) sexually aggressive behavior will increase after exposure to violent pornography; (b) the degree of increase in sexual aggression after exposure to violent pornography will be directly related to the level of identification experienced by the viewer; and (c) aggressive behavior will not increase after exposure to nonviolent pornography.

SUMMARY

It is concluded that sexual aggression especially among school, college and university students is becoming a common practice nowadays, which is a major danger for the whole society. Research has shown that physical aggression, masculinity, attitude towards women, acceptance of interpersonal violence, parental negligence, domestic violence marital conflicts, parental alcoholism, dating relationships, pornography, etc. are the major predictors of sexual aggression. More and more preventive efforts are required to modify attitude towards other sex, dating violence, resolving marital conflict, pornography, etc., to help prevent the development of aggression among adolescents. Therefore, it is suggested here that more and more research is required on adolescent aggression, its development, and prevention.

SUGGESTED READING

1. Abbey, A, McAuslan, P, Ross, LT, and Zawacki, T. Alcohol expectancies regarding sex, aggression, and sexual vulnerability: reliability and validity assessment. Psychology of Addictive Behaviors 1999; 13, 174-82.
2. Abbey, A, Ross, LT, and McDuffie, D. Alcohol's role in sexual assault. In: R R Watson (Ed.), Drug and alcohol abuse reviews: Addictive behaviors in women (pp. 97–123). Totowa, NJ: Humana Press. 1994; 5: 97-123.
3. Ackard, DM, Neumark-Sztainer, D, and Hannan, P. Dating violence among a nationally representative sample of adolescent girls and boys: Associations with behavioral and mental health. Journal of Gender Specific Medicine 2003; 6: 39-48.
4. Allen, M, D'Alessio, D, and Brezgel, K A meta-analysis summarizing the effects of pornography.II: Aggression after exposure. Human Communications Research 1995a; 22, 258-283.
5. Baron, L, Straus, MA. Sexual stratification, pornography, and rape in the United States. In: N. M. Malamuth and E. Donnerstein (Eds.), Pornography and sexual aggression. Orlando, FL: Academic Press 1984; 185-209.
6. Bergman, L. Dating violence among high school students. Social Work 1992; 37:21-27.
7. Bianchi, EC. The super-bowl culture of male violence. In: D. F Sabo and R. Runfola (Eds.), Jock Sports and male identity. Englewood Cliffc, NJ: Prentice-Hall 1976.
8. Bjorkqvist, K, Osterman, K, and Lagerspetz, K. Sex differences in covert aggression among adults. Aggressive Behavior 1994; 20:27-33.
9. Blumenthal, DR, Neemann J, and Murphy, C M. Lifetime exposure to interparental physical and verbal aggression and symptom expression in college students. Violence Vict. 2998;13(2):175-96.
10. Briere J, and Malamuth, N, Self-reported likelihood of sexually aggressive behavior: Attitedinal vs sexual explanations. Journal of Research in Personality, 1983; 17:315-23.
11. Brownmiller, S. Against our will: Men, women and rape. New York: Simon and Schuster. 1975.

12. Carter, DL, Prentky, RA, Knight, RA, Vanderveer, P L, and Boucher, R J. Use of pornography in the criminal and developmental histories of sexual offenders. Journal of Interpersonal Violence 1987; 2:196-211.
13. Cole SG. Pornography and the sex crises. Toronto: Amanita Enterprises, 1989.
14. Court JH. Pornography and sex-crimes: A re-evaluation in the light of recent trends around the world. International Journal of Criminology and Penology 1976; 5:129-157.
15. Crick NR, Grotpeter JK. Relational aggression, gender, and social-psychological adjustment. Child Development, 1995; 66:710-22.
16. Dworkin A, MacKinnon C A. Pornography and civil rights: A new day for women's equality. Minneapolis, MN: Organizing Against Pornography 1988.
17. Eagly AH, Steffen, FJ. Gender and aggressive behavior: A meta-analytic review of the social psychological literature. Psychological Bulletin, 1986; 100:309-30.
18. Fantuzzo, JW, Mohr, WK. Prevalence and effects of child exposure to domestic violence. Future Child. Win 1999; 9(3):21-32.
19. Finkelhor D, Hotaling G, Lewis, I A, and Smith, C. Sexual abuse in a national sample of adult men and women: Prevalence, characteristics, and risk factors. Child Abuse and Neglect, 1990;14:19-28.
20. Foo L, Margolin G. A multivariate investigation of dating violence. Journal of Family Violence 1995; 10:351-77.
21. Ford ME, Linney, JA. Comparative analysis of juvenile sexual offenders, violent nonsexual offenders, and status offenders. Journal of Interpersonal Violence 1995; 10:56-70.
22. Frieze IH. Violence in close relationships—Development of a research area: Comment on Archer (2000). Psychological Bulletin, 2000;126, 681–84.
23. Grunbaum JA, Kann L, Kinchen, S. Youth Risk Behavior Surveillance—United States, 2001. MMWR CDC Surveill Summ, 2002; 51, 1–64
24. Gudjonsson GH, Sigurdsson, JF. Differences and similarities between violent offenders and sex offenders. Child Abuse and Neglect 2000; 24, 363–72.
25. Hall GCN, Hirschman, R. Toward a theory of sexual aggression: A quadripartite model. Journal of Consulting and Clinical Psychology, 1991;59, 662–69.
26. Henton J, Cate R, Koval J, Lloyd S, Christopher, S. Romance and violence in dating relationships. Journal of Family Issues, 1983; 4:467-82.
27. Hogben M, Byrne D, Hamburger ME. Coercive heterosexual sexuality in dating relationships of college students: Implications of differential male–female experiences. In: ES Byers and LF O'Sullivan (Eds.), Sexual coercion. New York: Haworth 1996; 69-78.
28. Hyde JS. How large are gender differences in aggression? A developmental meta-analysis. Developmental Psychology, 1984; 20:722-36.
29. Jaffee D, Straus MA. Sexual climate and reported rape: A state-level analysis. Archives of Sexual Behavior 1987; 16:107-23.
30. Keall MD, Frith, WJ. Drink-driving behavior during the main drinking times in New Zealand and its implications for enforcement countermeasures. In Proceedings of the Seventeenth International Conference on Alcohol, Drugs and Traffic Safety, 2004.
31. Koss MP, Gaines JA. The prediction of sexual aggression by alcohol use, athletic participation, and fraternity affiliation. Journal of Interpersonal Violence, 1993; 8:94-108.
32. Koss MP, Hidden rape. In: A. W. Burgess (Ed.). Rape and sexual assault (pp. 3–25). New York: Garland 1988; 3-25.
33. Krahe B, Waizenhofer, E., and Moller, I. Women's Sexual Aggression Against Men: Prevalence and Predictors. Sex Roles 2003; 49:5/6.
34. Lightfoot LO, Barbaree HE. The relationship between substance use and abuse and sexual offending in adolescents. In: H. E. Barbaree, W. L. Marshall, and S. M. Hudson (Eds.). The juvenile sex offender. New York: Guilford 1993; 203-24.
35. Marshall, WL, and Barrett, S. Criminal neglect: Why sex offenders go free. Toronto: Doubleday. 1990.
36. McGruder-Johnson AK, Davidson, ES, Gleaves DH, Stock W, Finch JF. Interpersonal violence and posttraumatic symptomatology: The effects of ethnicity, gender, and exposure to violent events. J. Interpers. Violence 2000; 15(2):205-21.
37. Miczek KA, Weerts EM, DeBold JF. Alcohol, aggression and violence: Biobehavioral determinants. In: S. E. Martin (Ed.). Alcohol and interpersonal violence: Fostering multidisciplinary perspectives (NIAAA Research Monograph. Rockville, MD: National Institute on Alcohol Abuse and Alcoholism 1993; 24: 83-119.

38. Naison, M, Sports, women, and the ideology of domination. In: D. F. Sabo and R. Runfola (Eds.). Jock Sports and male identity, Engiewood Cliffs, NJ: Prentice-Hall, 1972.
39. Norris J, George WH, Davis KC, Martell J, Leonesio R J. Alcohol and hypermasculinity as determinants of men's empathic responses to violent pornography. Journal of Interpersonal Violence 1999; 14:683-700.
40. Ouimette PC, Psychopathology and sexual aggression in nonincarcerated men. Violence and Victims 1997; 12:389-95.
41. Pernanen K. Alcohol and crimes of violence. In: B. Kissin and H. Begleiter (Eds.). The biology of alcoholism. New York: Plenum Press, 1976.
42. Poppen PJ, Segal NJ. The influence of sex and sex role orientation on sexual coercion. Sex Roles, 1988; 19:689-701.
43. Potter-Efron PS, Potter-Efron RT. Anger as a J. Yu et al. / Journal of Criminal Justice 32 (2004) 421-30, 429 treatment concern with alcoholics and affected family members. Alcoholism Treatment Quarterly 1991; 8:31-46.
44. Richards MH, Crowe PA, Larson R, Swarr R. Developmental partterns and gender differnces in the experience of peer companionship during adolsnence. Child Development, 1998; 69:154-63.
45. Sarrel PM, Masters WH. Sexual molestation of men by women. Archives of Sexual Behavior 1982; 11: 117-31.
46. Seto MC, Barbaree HE. The role of alcohol in sexual aggression. Clinical Psychology Review 1995; 15: 545-66.
47. Shea MC. When the tables are turned: Verbal sexual coercion among college women. In: PB. Anderson and C. Struckman-Johnson (Eds.), Sexually aggressive women. New York: Guilford Press, 1998; 96-104.
48. Sigelrnan CK, Berry CJ, Wiles KA. Violence in college students' dating, relationships. Journal of Applied Social Psychology, 1984; 14:530-48.
49. Silverman JG, Raj A, Mucci, LA, Hathaway JE. Dating violence against adolescent girls and associated substance use, unhealthy weight control, sexual risk behavior, pregnancy, and suicidality. Journal of the American Medical Association, 2001; 286:372-79.
50. Spaccarelli S, Bowden B, Coatsworth J D, Kim S. Psychosocial correlates of male sexual aggression in a chronic delinquent sample. Crim. Just. Behav 1997; 24(1):71-95.
51. Struckman-Johnson C. Forced sex on dates: It happens to men, too. Journal of Sex Research 1988; 24:234-41.
52. Taylor SP, Leonard KE. Alcohol and human physical aggression. In: RG Green, EI Donnerstein (Eds.), Aggression: theoretical and empirical reviews. San Diego, CA: Academic Press, 1983.
53. Watkins B, Bentovim A. The sexual abuse of male children and adolescents: A review of current research. Journal of Child Psychology and Psychiatry, 1992; 33:197-248.
54. Watson JM, Cascardi M, Avery-Leaf S, O'Leary KD. High school students' responses to dating aggression. Violence and Victims 2001; 16:339-48.
55. Williams AF, Preusser DF. Night driving restrictions for youthful drivers: a literature review and commentary. Journal of Public Health Policy 1997; 18:334-45.
57. Wolfe DA, Feiring C. Dating violence through the lens of adolscent romantic relationships. Child Maltreatment 2000; 5:360-63.
58. Zillmann D, Bryant J. Pornography's impact on sexual satisfaction. Journal of Applied Social Psychology, 1988; 18:438-53.

40 Eating Disorders

Sangeeta Yadav

INTRODUCTION

Eating disorders are primarily characterized by severe disturbances in eating behavior and are typically applied to the syndromes of anorexia nervosa and bulimia nervosa. Eating disorders (EDs) are generally believed to be increasing in frequency especially among young women and are now established as the third most prevalent chronic health condition in the west among adolescent females, after asthma and obesity.[1-3] Eating disorders most commonly first present during adolescence. EDs are primarily considered psychiatric disorders, but they have significant medical and organ system complications and thus require the medical and psychiatric teams to work together for successful management.

EPIDEMIOLOGY

The incidence of eating disorders has increased 2 to 5 fold since the mid 1960s.[4] Prevalence rates among women are around 1%.[5] The prevalence rates of anomalous eating behavior was 2.8 percent in a study conducted by the author on 300 girls 12-15 years in schools of Delhi.[6]

Anorexia nervosa is typically seen between the ages of 14 to 18 years and is ten times more common in females.[7] It is seen more commonly in sisters and mothers of those with anorexia nervosa.[8]

Around 90-95% of anorexia nervosa patients are females, 80 percent of bulimia nervosa patients are females and perhaps 60 percent of binge eating disorder are females. Recent evidence suggests that all social economic classes and ethnic groups are affected, and not just the socioeconomically advantaged people as was previously thought.[9]

Bulimia nervosa has its onset during mid to late adolescence and is 20 times more common in females. It is rare to see bulimia nervosa before 14 years of age.[1] It has also been observed that there is higher incidence of major depressive disorders in first degree relatives of patients with bulimia nervosa.[10]

Weight and body image concerns develop early in children and are well established by puberty. Several studies have associated problem eating behavior in infancy and childhood with higher incidence of abnormal eating behavior in adolescence[11-13] thus describing eating disorders as a continuum of developmental psychopathology. In a study by Maloney et al in the age group of 7-13 years, 55% girls wanted to be thinner and 40% girls reported some weight loss activities.[14] Several studies[14, 15] have explicitly identified that pubertal concerns are the most frequent precipitant of eating disorder. The onset of puberty has been recognized as a critical period for the development of disordered eating in girls. Among adolescent females more than two-thirds were dissatisfied with their weight and more than one third expressed the desire to loose weight. In our study 30% school going girls expressed concern about being overweight despite having normal weight for age.[16]

ANOREXIA NERVOSA (AN)

AN represents a complicated web of events that begins on a societal level, extends through the family to the individual and eventually becomes expressed through the hypothalamic-pituitary-adrenal axis in life threatening consequences. Anorexia, usually is not associated with the course of illness until late. The term anorexia is somewhat misleading because patients experience real hunger and obsession for food but deny their initial urges.

AN is a syndrome that includes[17]

1. A marked fear of fatness, a disturbed perception of body size (body image), and an obsessional desire to lose increasing amounts of weight.
2. Self starvation with significant weight loss, usually less than 75% below normal weight for height and age.
3. Amenorrhea
4. Physical signs of starvation, physical hyperactivity and sleep disturbances
5. Other mental changes, including bizarre behaviors and attitudes about food, sometimes accompanied by self induced vomiting and binge eating and a stubborn denial of illness
6. No known physical or other psychiatric illness that accounts for the weight loss and other symptoms and signs.

ETIOLOGY

AN is a complex syndrome with multicentric etiology.[1] Despite many studies, there is no proven causal link between body image and weight concerns and development of disordered eating in adolescents.[18] Nevertheless a plethora of cross sectional and longitudinal studies in adult women, suggests a path in which body image and weight concerns, mediated by low self concept and self esteem, may lead to dysfunctional eating attitudes and, eventually, to unhealthy eating behavior.

Many studies over the past and in recent years have supported the role of mass media influences in the onset of eating disorders.[19, 20] As the incidence of eating disorders has increased, society's ideal body type has become progressively slimmer. In a male dominated society, women frequently define themselves in terms of how attractive they appear to men. Women's magazines are filled with shapely, computer enhanced images of models whose average weight is 23% less than the average women.[21] Television and radio also contributes to the problem by glorifying thinness in its portrayal of young women. In a recent study conducted in Spain, frequent reading of girls magazine or listening to radio programs were considered as important risk factor in the development of eating disorders.[19]

Family studies indicate that the patient may be the identified problem in already troubled families.[10] Alternatively, one parent may also be suffering from an eating disorder. Similarly, sexual abuse is also frequently identified in patients with disordered eating and at rates higher than those in the population.[22]

BULIMIA NERVOSA

Bulimia nervosa and binge eating disorder, occur less commonly in adolescents.[5]

Bulimia is episodic binge eating, often accompanied by purging. Although only 1 to 5% of adolescent girls meet the DSM-IV criteria for bulimia, as many as 10 to 50% reportedly engage in occasional self-induced vomiting or binge eating.[1, 23] Bulimia nervosa is a syndrome seen mostly in older adolescent and young adults.

EPIDEMIOLOGICAL FEATURES

Using fixed DSM-IV criteria, an estimated 1 to 5% of adolescent and college women and up to 0.4% of young men suffer from bulimia nervosa.[24, 25]

However, many more college men (41-60%) and women (26-79%) demonstrate occasional bulimic behaviors (e.g. binging and purging to achieve desired weight for wrestlers, group binging among college women).[26] In addition, 13% of adolescents report engaging in some sort of purging behavior at some time.[23]

ETIOLOGY

Bulimia is a relatively newly described disorder, and so its definition is still being revised and refined. As such, far less is understood about its etiology than about anorexia nervosa. Adolescents with bulimia have a high prevalence of depression (35%) and of affective disorders in first-degree relatives (50% or more).[10] Again, society is thought to play a key role: weight control is synonymous with self-control and attractiveness. Adolescent girls in particular are unhappy with their weight.[27]

PSYCHOLOGICAL PROFILE

Psychologically, the bulimic patient differs from the anorectic patient. In the former, there is an increased history of childhood maladjustment and family psychiatric disorders. Bulimics describe their mothers as being more emotionally distant and seem to experience greater rejection and blamed as youngsters.[28] Bulimic women are also more prone to have been obese, are more extroverted, and are more likely to abuse alcohol, steal, be sexually active, or attempt suicide than patients with anorexia nervosa.[29] The association between bulimia and a history of childhood sexual abuse remains controversial.[30] Bulimia therefore appears to be more of a disorder in regulation of affect and impulse control.

CLINICAL PRESENTATION

Young patients with EDs are more likely to present with nausea, abdominal pain, or dysphagia. They are also likely to present with comorbid psychiatric symptoms especially obsession or depression. They may also present with physiologic disturbances. They are less likely to report disturbances in body image or concerns about weight.

Growth development and puberty is impaired. Amenorrhoea is a constant feature of the syndrome. *In a recent study, it was found to be the most likely reason for consulting the gynecologist and therefore it should alert them to the possibility of an underlying eating disorder.*[31]

ANOREXIA NERVOSA

The syndrome of AN often begins when a young teenage girl sees herself as being overweight and begins dieting. Dieting is endemic among female adolescents and is a substantial risk factor.[32] In fact, dieting may account for much of the gender difference in prevalence of eating disorders as women are far more likely to diet than men.

The main factor which separates the casual or even the recurrent dieter from the anorectic is the profound distortion in self image, a preoccupation with thinness and an extreme change in eating habits. Patients with AN continue to diet well past the normal end point, and they actually perceive themselves to be fat even when they are severely underweight. In addition, obsessive athletic activity allows them to keep their weights under control. Patients with restrictive AN severely curtail their caloric intake whereas those with binge eating/purging form regularly engage in self induced vomiting or misuse of laxatives, diuretics or enemas.[8] The latter begin to resemble bulimics, being older and less isolated socially but having greater family and behavioral instability.

The signs and symptoms of malnutrition and involvement of other organ systems predominate (Table 40.1). They are often motivated by issues of eating behaviors like avoidance of junk food, low fat diet and physical fitness.

The patients with AN exhibit a spectrum of disease and progress at different rates, therefore the clinician should not necessarily wait for all the official criteria listed above, to appear before suspecting the diagnosis and deciding to intervene. The nutritional impact of disordered

Table 40.1: Physical symptoms and signs in anorexia nervosa

Presenting physical symptoms
- Weight loss
- Amenorrhea, no cyclic symptoms or menstruation (Anovulatory).
- Hyperactivity (mental and motor).
- Aberrant behavior, irritability, isolation or withdrawal, sleep disturbances
- Hyperacusis or optic hyperesthesia

Physical signs
- Cachexia, emaciation, debilitation or dehydration, or impending shock.
- Infectious processes (pneumonia or sepsis).
- Immunologic problem (late) anergy negative skin tests
- Skin changes (dryness, yellowish palms and soles, desquamation, edema)
- Scalp and pubic hair loss or lanugo hair or increased pigmented body hair
- Hypothermia (rectal temperature below 96.6°F).
- Bradypnea (respiratory compensation for alkalosis).
- Bradycardia, (decreased basal metabolic rate) pulse below 60 bpm usual
- Hypotension often below 80/50 mm Hg
- Signs of estrogen deficiency (skin dryness, osteoporosis; small uterus and cervix; vaginal mucosa is pink, dry and gross and microscopic evidence of deficient estrogen.
- Signs of decreased androgen (no acne, no oily skin).

Table 40.2: Laboratory findings in anorexia nervosa

- Normal results on most laboratory tests early in process
- Elevated BUN levels, secondary to dehydration
- Hypercarotenemia
- Elevated serum cholesterol level (early; may decrease later.
- Decreased transferrin (a late and ominous sign).
- Depressed magnesium and calcium levels (calcium may be elevated).
- Possible depression of plasma zinc, and urinary copper levels.
- Endocrine
- Low luteinizing hormone (LH); low or pseudo-normal follicle-stimulating hormone(FSH); deficiency of gonadotropin-releasing hormone (GnRH); normal prolactin; low testosterone in men and low estradiol in women
- Elevated circulating cortisol (normal production; does not suppress with dexamethasone.
- Low normal fasting glucose (increased insulin binding by red blood cells and growth hormone deficiency reported.
- Low normal thyroxine (T): reduced triiodothyronine (T3); elevated reverse T3; normal TSH Possible elevation of parathyroid homrone (PTH) secondary to hypomagnesemia with hypercalcemia
- Elevated growth hormone levels

  Hematologic
- Very low erythrocyte sedimentation rate, Anemia Leukopenia with lymphopenia

eating on younger patients may also be unusual or misleading. Many will not have lost sufficient weight to qualify for a diagnosis of AN according to DSM-IV. Any weight loss is concerning in children and adolescents who should be expected to be growing and gaining weight.

The diagnosis of AN is made based on a constellation of historical findings, in combination with a careful physical examinations. Various laboratory tests which assist in diagnosis are shown in Table 40.2. However, in most cases, an extensive workup is not required.

BULIMIA NERVOSA

The typical patients of bulimia are females, in late teens or early twenties, slightly overweight, and with a history of unsuccessful dieting. They try to control weight through self-induced vomiting or the use of cathartics. Unlike the anorectic patient, who almost by definition is asexual and isolated, these patients are usually extroverted and have heterosexual relationships. However, they rapidly becomes preoccupied with planning for binges, which are usually solitary and involve junk food. They may have other impulsive behaviors as well, such as drug use or shoplifting. They may binge recurrently or binge and purge using syrup of ipecac, laxatives, or diuretics. After binging, they feel out of control and ashamed and yet they are unable to tell others of their behavior. Overall, their personality is more labile than an anorectic's and they are is more likely to attempt suicide.

Unless a patient confesses to such behavior or a specific question is asked and answered truthfully, bulimia is unlikely to be discovered until it has become a chronic problem.[33] A number of clinical clues and diagnostic criteria exist for the diagnosis of bulimia nervosa as shown in Tables 40.3 and 40.4.[5]

Table 40.3: Diagnostic criteria: bulimia

1. Recurrent episodes of binge eating
2. A feeling of lack of control over eating behavior
3. Regularly engaging in either self-induced vomiting, use of laxatives or diuretics, strict dieting or fasting, or vigorous exercise to prevent weight gain.
4. At least two binging episodes a week for at least 3 months.
5. Persistent over concern with body shape and weight

Table 40.4: Clinical clues to the diagnosis of bulimia

History	Abdominal bloating or pain, muscle aches or stiffness weakness
Skin	Calluses on knuckles from self-induced vomiting, edema of feet or hands
Oral	Dental caries erosion of enamel, parotid hypertrophy
Renal	Hematuria, pyuria, or proteinuria
Electrolytes	Metabolic alkalosis, decreased Na, Cl, K
Electrocardiogram	Wandering atrial pacemaker, prolonged QTc
Chest X-ray	Mediastinal emphysema

DIFFERENTIAL DIAGNOSIS

The list of differential diagnosis is given in Table 40.5.[34] The differential diagnosis is not usually difficult in typical patients because teenagers who suffer from AN secondary to depression or a chronic disease have a normal self image and are quite concerned about their weight loss.

TREATMENT

TREATMENT OF ANOREXIA NERVOSA

requires a multidisciplinary approach, with contribution from a physician, psychiatrist, pediatrician, nutritionist, gynecologist, and skilled nursing. The primary care physician should consult the adolescent specialist while treating a patient of AN.

- The first goal in management is vital sign stabilization and weight rehabilitation to > 75% of ideal body weight. The weight gain should be approximately 1 kg/month. Long term goal is to normalize weight and nutrition in anorectic patients and resumption of normal menses.

Table 40.5: Differential diagnosis: anorexia nervosa

Organic disease	
Endocrine	
Hypothyroidism	
Hyperthyroidism	
Diabetes	
Addison's disease	
Central nervous system:	
Tumor	
Intracranial infarcts	
Increase intracranial tension	
Gastrointestinal	
Inflammatory bowel disease	
Gastroesophageal reflux	
Genitourinary	Pregnancy
Neoplastic	Any malignancy
Psychiatric disease	
Depression	
Anxiety disorder	
Schizophrenia	
Mood disorder	
Substance abuse	
Posttraumatic stress disorder	

- Patient with AN can usually be managed on outpatient basis but sometimes they need to be hospitalized depending on the clinical status and associated complications. The indications for hospitalization are given in Table 40.6.[5]
- If the patient is managed on an out patient basis, then frequent visits are required to establish a good rapport with adolescent and also relate to the usual challenges of a teenager.
- Treatment modalities range from individual to group and family therapy, and from behaviour modification techniques to pharmaco-

Table 40.6: Indications for hospitalization

1. Severe malnutrition (weight < 75% ideal body weight.
2. Dehydration
3. Electrolyte disturbances
4. Physiologic instability
5. Severe bradycardia
6. Hypotension
7. Hypothermia
8. Orthostatic changes
9. Acute food refusal
10. Acute medical complication of malnutrition (e.g. pancreatitis, syncope, cardiac failure.
11. Acute psychiatric emergencies (e.g. suicidal ideation, acute psychosis.
    Failure of outpatient treatment

therapy. Renutrition, psychotherapy and family therapy remain the cornerstones of treatment of AN.

According to recent studies family therapy has emerged as the treatment of choice in managing early onset AN.[34] Individual supportive therapy tended to be more effective in older patients.

- It has been found that lasting symptomatic improvement and remission require the addition of psychological treatments in the form of cognitive and interpersonal psychotherapy.[35]
- Regarding pharmac xotherapy, controlled and uncontrolled studies testing antipsychotic, antidepressant, weight promoting and prokinetic drugs have demonstrated that the core symptoms of AN are refractory to currently available psychotropic medication. For relapse prevention, however, antidepressant medi-cation may be useful.[36]
- For problem of amenorrhea and osteopenia due to estrogen deficiency states in AN, oestrogen replacement therapy has not shown to be an effective treatment and so *gynecologist should avoid simply prescribing estrogen replacement therapy without referring the patient for comprehensive treatment of the eating disorder*.

TREATMENT OF BULIMIA PATIENTS

- Counseling or therapy is unlikely to fall within the purview of the average practicing physician. Referral to an expert in psychotherapy with young women with eating disorders probably is indicated.[37] Such patients maybe difficult to keep in therapy because of their low frustration tolerance. Nevertheless, the clinician can play an important role in the medical follow-up of the patient, especially in monitoring the patient's weight and electrolyte status, and in providing family support.
- Because of the known association between bulimia and depression, psychiatrists have been more aggressive with using antidepressants. Many controlled studies find improvements (reduction in binging, improvement in mood, less preoccupation with weight) with use of tricyclic antidepressant.[38] Fluoxetine (Prozac) has also been demonstrated to be effective.
- However, studies also show that psychotherapy is most important and that drugs alone are not effective.[39]

PROGNOSIS

Over 100 studies have been published in the literature to date on the course and outcome of eating disorders. These have generally shown that approximately 50% of patients do well over time, approximately 30% do reasonably well but continue to have symptoms and approximately 20% do poorly.[17]

Also it is seen that adolescents do, in fact, have a somewhat better prognosis than adults. Good prognostic factors among adolescents are a lower co-morbidity, a shorter duration of illness, less familial psychotherapy and a higher minimal weight.

The mortality in AN is about 5% with suicide being the most common cause of death. Other causes are severe fluid electrolyte disturbances and cardiac arrhythmias.

In general, BN approximately 50% of patients report no binging or purging behavior 2 to 10 years after cognitive behavioral therapy, 20% remain persistently symptomatic, and 30% seem to have remissions and relapses.[40] Certainly bulimic patients who have an affective disorder or features of anorexia nervosa fare more poorly.

CONCLUSIONS

Eating disorders in young adults are serious health problems with substantial morbidity and mortality. The etiology of disordered eating is multifactorial and complex, current systems of classification are sub optimal, and our under standing of both remain to be refined. There is often a significant delay in diagnosis, making it crucial that clinicians maintain a high index of suspicion, screen aggressively, and respond immediately when signs and symptoms of disordered eating are present.

It requires an interdisciplinary treatment team. Earlier treatment seems to improve response. There is growing evidence that family therapy is the best form of psychotherapy and the literature appears to confirm that adolescents do somewhat better than adults.

REFERENCES

1. Fisher M, Golden NH, Katzman DK, et al. Eating disorders in adolecents: A background paper. J Adolesc Health 1995;16:420-37.
2. Lucas AR, Beard CM, O'Fallon WM, Kurland LT. 50-year trends in the incidence of anorexia nervosa in Rochester, Miunnesota: A population -based study. Am J Psychiatr 1991;148:917-22.
3. Society for Adolescent Medicine. Eating disorders in adolescent. J Adolesc Health 1995;16:476-80.
4. Crisp AN, Palmer RL, Kalucy RS. How common is anorexia nervosa? A prevalence study. Br J Psychiatry 1986;148:268-74.
5. Practice guidelines for the treatment of patients with the eating disorders. Revised edition. American J of psychiatry 2000;137 (supplement): 1.
6. Aggarwal N, Yadav S. To assess eating behaviour among school adolescents girls. Thesis for Doctor of Medicine, A. University of Delhi 2005.
7. Comerci GD, Greydanus DE. Eating disorders: Anorexia nervosa and bulimia. Chapter 31, pp 683. In Hofmann AD, Greydanus DE (Eds). Adolescent Medicine Appleton and Lange, Stamford, CT, USA 1997; 31:683 3/e.
8. American Psychiatric Association. Eating Disorder Diagnostic and Statistical Manual of Mental Disorders. American Psychiatric Association, Washington DC 2000, 4/e.
9. Powers PS, Santana CA. Eating disorders: A guide for the primary care physician. Prim Care 2002;29(1):81-98.
10. Swift WJ, Andrews D, Barklage NE. The relationship between affective disorder and eating disorders: a review of the literature. Am J Psychiatry 1986;143:290.
11. Dahl M, Rydell AM, Sundelin C. Children with early refusal to eat: Follow-up during primary school. Acta Paediatr 1994 83:54-58.
12. Marchi M, Cohen P. Early childhood eating behaviors and adolescent eating disorders. J Am Acad Child Adolesc Psychiatry 1990;29:112-17.
13. Maloney MJ, McGuire J, Daniels SR, Specker B. Dieting behavior and eating attitudes in children. Pediatrics 1989;84:482-89.
14. Killen JD, Hayward C, Litt I, et al. Is puberty a risk factor for eating disorders? Am J Dis Child 1992 146:323-25.
15. Moore DC: Body image and eating behavior. Am J Dis Child 1988 1421114-18.
16. Gupta A, Yadav S. Health profile of students in mid and late adolescence in schools of Delhi. Thesis 2002.
17. Fisher M. The course and outcome of eating disorders in adults and in adolescents: A review. Adolescent Medicine 2003;14:149-58.
18. Ricciardelli LA, McCabe MP. Children's functioning and life events in the outcome of adolescent anorexia nervosa. Br J Psychiatr 1997; 171:545-9.
19. Mertinez MA, Gual P, Lahortiga F, et al. Parental factors, mass media influences and the onset of eating disorders in a prospective population based cohort. Pediatrics 2003;111(2):315-20.
20. Mcknight. Risk factors for the onset of eating disorders in adolescent girls: Results of the Mcknight longitudinal risk factor study. Am J Psychiatry 2003 Feb; 160(2):205-07.
21. Kilbourne J. Killing us softly; gender roles in advertising. Adolescent Medicine: State of the Art Reviews 1993;144:635.
22. Wonderlich S, Crosby R, Mitchell J, et al: Pathways mediating sexual abuse and eating disturbance in children. Int J Eat Disord 2001;29:270-279.
23. Whitaker AH. An epidemiologic study of anorectic and bulimic symptoms in adolescent girls: Implications for pediatricians. Pediatr Ann 1992;21:752.
24. Kreipe RE. Eating disorders among children and adolescents. Pediatr Rev 1995;16:370.
25. Schotte DE, Stunkard AJ. Bulimia vs, bulimic behaviors on a college campus, JAMA 1987; 258: 1213.
26. Marchi M, Cohen P, Early childhood eating behaviors and adolescent eating disorder. J Am Acad Child Adolesc Psychiatry 1990;29:112.
27. Moses N, Baniliry MM, Lifshitz E. Fear of obesity among adolescent girls, Pediatrics 1989;83:393.
28. Humphery LL. Relationships within subtypes of anorexics, bulimics, and normal families. J Am Acad C Adolescen Psychiatry 1998;27:544.

29. Garfinkel PE, Garmer DM, Goldbloom DS, Eating disorders: implications for the 1990s. Can J Psychiatry 1987;32:624.
30. Pope HG, Hudson JL, Is childhood sexual abuse a risk factor for bulimia nervosa? Am J Psychiatry 1992;149:455.
31. Golden NH. Eating disorders in adolescence and their sequelae. Best Pract Res Clin Obstet Gynaecol. 2003;17(1):57-73.
32. Story M, Rosenwinkel K, Himes JH, et al. Demographic and risk factors associated with chronic dieting in adolescent. Am J Dis Child 1991;145:994.
33. Bursten MS, Gabel LL, Brose JA et al. Detecting and treating bulimia nervosa: how involved are family physicians? J Am Board Fam Pract 1996; 9:241.
34. Levine RL. Eating disorders in adolescents: a comprehensive update. International Pediatrics 1995;10:327.
35. Rosen DS. Eating disorders in children and young adolescents: Etiology, classification, clinical features and treatment. Adolesc Med 2003; 14(1):49-59.
36. Casper RC. How useful are pharmacological treatments in eating disorders? Psychopharmacol Bull. 2002;36(2):88-104.
37. Fairburn CG. Short-term psychological treatment for bulimia nervosa. In: Brownell KD, Fairburn CG, (Eds). Eating disorders and obesity a comprehensive handbook. New York: Guilford Press: 1995;344.
38. Walsh FT. Pharmacotherapy of eating disorders. In: Brownell KD, Fairburn CG, (Eds) Eating disorders and obesity a comprehensive handbook, New York: Guilford Press. 1995;313.
39. Agras WS, Rossiter EM, Arnow B, et al. Pharmacologic and cognitive-behavioral treatment for bulimia nervosa: a controlled comparison. Am J Psychiatry 1992;49:82.
40. Hus LKG. Outcome of bulimia nervosa. In: Brownell KD, Fairburn CG (Eds). Eating disorders and obesity: comprehensive handbook. New York: Guilford Press 1995;238.

41 Gynecological Malignancies in Young Women

Murad E Lala

INTRODUCTION

Genital tract tumors in the adolescent and young women are fortunately rare. The adolescent, while still retaining some propensity for the preponderate tumors of childhood, shows a pattern which more closely resembles that seen in the women of reproductive age. Though most of the genital neoplasms in this age group are benign the possibility of malignancy must be kept in mind. Genital tumors in young women pose a special challenge since the need for organ and function preservation needs to be balanced against the need for complete tumor excision.

TYPES OF TUMORS

VULVAL TUMORS

Vulval viral warts affect older girls or adolescents. They are the typical condylomata acuminata and may be few in numbers or present in very large masses. They are commonest on the vulva but not confined to it, being present in the vagina or on the cervix on occasions. Treatment may be by chemical destruction (podophyllin), cryocauterization or excision.

TUMORS OF THE VAGINA

The mesodermal mixed tumor of the vagina and cervix (often referred to as the botryoid sarcoma or as the rhabdomyosarcoma) is a highly malignant tumor of the young child. Equally important is clear-cell adenocarcinoma of the vagina related to the administration of diethylstilbestrol (DES) to the mother during pregnancy.

Benign tumors of the cervix and vagina during adolescence are extremely rare and any apparently innocent tumor encountered during this time must be regarded with deep suspicion until it is proved beyond doubt that it is not malignant.

The important clinical feature of the mesodermal mixed tumors of the vagina is bleeding. Whatever its characteristics, bleeding per vaginum is potentially a very serious symptom. Whenever there is vaginal bleeding in a young adolescent, immediate investigation is essential to exclude malignancy.

Treatment

In recent years the management of the mesodermal mixed tumor of the vagina or cervix in children and adolescents has undergone a marked change. In former times only early and radical surgery was likely to offer any hope of cure, the necessary surgery often being an anterior or posterior exenteration.

Now-a-days combination chemotherapy (vincristine, actinomycin D and cyclophosphamide) with radiotherapy is given. The response to this treatment will determine the extent of surgery.

If the tumor becomes resectable, as the majority do, the surgery is nowadays limited to an extended hysterectomy and vaginectomy.

CANCER OF THE CERVIX

Cervical, ovarian and breast cancers are the main cause of cancer related morbidity and mortality amongst women globally. Cervical cancer is the most common form of cancer in women in virtually all developing countries.

The high-risk factors for cervical cancer are:

- Onset of coitus at an early age
- Multiple sexual partners
- Partner who has multiple sexual partners
- History of STD
- Cigarette smoking/tobacco chewing
- History of HPV infection
- History of prior CIN/VIN.

HPV AND CANCER CERVIX

HPV 16 and 18 are the first and second most common types of HPV seen in cervical cancer and together cause about 71% of all cervical cancers. Prevalence of HPV is greatest in women aged less than 25 years and the virus can be acquired by mere skin-to-skin contact also. Thus condoms are useful but not fully effective.

Cervical Cancer Screening Recommendations

Effective screening for cervical cancer by taking regular PAP smears has led to early detection and better outcomes in developed countries. The recommendations for young women as laid down by the American College of Obstetricians and Gynecologists are as follows:

First screen: Screening of cervical cytology (cervical cells) should begin by approximately 3 years after first sexual intercourse or by age 21, whichever comes first (Previously, ACOG called for screening by the onset of sexual activity or by age 18, whichever occurred first).

Women under age 30 have a higher likelihood than older women of acquiring high-risk types of HPV that cause premalignant cervical disease, which should be ruled out before extending the testing intervals.

Colposcopy should be carried out in all cases of abnormal cytology as well as suspicious cervix on examination. Combining colposcopy with PAP smear reduces the false negative and false positive results. Colposcopy locates the exact site for biopsy and helps in selecting patients for conservative management in cases of cervical intraepithelial neoplasia (cryocauterization, large loop excision of transformation zone, laser ablation).

Treatment

Early cervical cancers can be treated with Wertheims's hysterectomy. In young women the ovaries can be preserved to prevent early menopause. The ovaries can be transposed high in the abdomen to remain out of the radiation portals in case adjuvant radiotherapy is required. In cases of advanced cervical cancer, concurrent radiotherapy and chemotherapy is given. Radiation can be in the form of teletherapy with brachytherapy boost.

UTERINE TUMORS

Carcinoma of the endometrium is uncommon in young women. However with the rising incidence of polycystic ovarian syndrome (PCOS) in young girls, a rise in the occurrence of uterine cancers is expected as unopposed estrogenic action in PCOS may lead to hyperplasia of endometrium if neglected.

Risk Factors for Endometrial Cancer

- Early menarche, late menopause
- Infertility and sub-fertility (pregnancy has a protective effect)
- PCOS
- Tamoxifen
- Corpus cancer syndrome (obesity, diabetes, hypertension)
- Breast ovarian cancer syndrome (mutation of BRCA-1 gene).

Young women presenting with persistent irregular bleeding per vaginum with thickened endometrium on sonography will require diagnostic curettage with hysteroscopy to rule out endometrial carcinoma.

Treatment

MRI scans help us to accurately predict the extent of tumor invasion in the endometrium and thus to plan treatment.

The standard treatment for early endometrial cancer is surgery.

However, in young women seeking children, there may be a role of conservative treatment in Grade 1 lesions with progestins and close follow-up.

Once child bearing is complete, these women should go in for a hysterectomy.

OVARIAN TUMORS

Ovarian tumors tend to be asymptomatic till they attain a large size. A strong clinical suspicion and attention to vague symptoms will help pick up these tumors at an early stage. Ultrasound abdomen and pelvis has contributed significantly towards this.

The pathology of ovarian neoplasms of this period of life is most interesting. Germ cell tumors and sex-cord stromal tumors predominate over the epithelial and other growths. The germ cell tumor category of the WHO histological classification comprises the dysgerminoma, endodermal sinus tumor, embryonal carcinoma, teratoma and mixed forms; closely related is the gonadoblastoma which however, appears in a separate WHO category.

The sex-cord stromal types include the granulosa cell tumor, thecoma, fibroma, Sertoli- Leydig cell tumors, notably the teratoma and the dysgerminoma, have an unusual preponderance in the young. As adolescence is reached, however, the pattern of tumors more closely relates to that found in the adult. For example, epithelial tumors in the 15 to 17 year-old age group comprised 28% of tumors, as compared with 16% at the age of 10 to 14 years and 0.5% below nine years.

BENIGN TERATOMA

Also known as dermoid cyst, it is usually unilateral but may be bilateral or more than one cyst may occur on the same side. The tumors are small (~10 cm) with a translucent lining through which hair and the fatty contents of the cyst are visible. At one point on the surface the thickened area of the remaining normal ovarian tissue can be discerned fading off into the cyst wall around the central thicker area. The cut surface contains a glairy fatty fluid, and at one point there is usually a papilla where hair and sebaceous material can be distinguished and sometimes tooth and cartilaginous structure as well. These are the commonest ovarian growths in childhood and are benign. Malignant change has been reported rarely (1-2%) in adults but is unknown in adolescence. Keeping this in mind, ovarian cystectomy is recommended. Meticulous hemostasis and appropriate reconstruction of the substance of the ovary may have an important bearing on successful future fertility.

DYSGERMINOMA

Usually unilateral but occasionally bilateral, most tumors are of moderate size (~15 cm), firm or solid, rubbery smooth or lobulated. These tumors are of malignant nature; recurrence in the residual ovary may occur even years later. The treatment is oophorectomy and as the tumor is remarkably radiosensitive, a tumor dose of 3000 rad is curative in almost all cases. The five-year survival for Stage I is around 95%.Stage III disease also carries an excellent prognosis (80%) unless there are intraperitoneal metastases. In such cases chemotherapy with VAC (vincristine, actinomycin D, cyclophosphamide) or VBP (vinblastine, bleomycin, cisplatin) is the treatment of choice.

GONADOBLASTOMA

The gonadoblastoma may be so small as to be microscopic or up to 10 cm in size. It is rounded, smooth or bossed in appearance and gray or grayish-pink on its cut surface. One-third of the tumors are bilateral. Gonadoblastomatous and dysgerminomatous areas are seen in the same tumor in 50 % of cases. Nearly 90 % of cases are seen in gonadal dysgenesis especially XY females or XO/XY mosaics and ambiguous genitalia are common. The gonads should be removed as early as possible because of the risk of malignancy.

GRANULOSA/THECA TUMOR

The granulosa cell tumor is usually unilateral, only 5% or so being present on both sides. It is encapsulated with a smooth or lobular surface. All granulosa cell tumors should be considered actually or potentially malignant, but the degree of malignancy is low.

The thecoma is usually bilateral. It may be very tiny, is usually some 5 to 8 cm or so in diameter, but can rarely be extremely large. The histological appearance of a thecoma is often very similar to that of a fibroma. The diagnosis may rest on the finding of large pale cells usually with abundant lipid, and without this fat content one is not prepared to make the diagnosis. Mixed granulosa/theca cell tumors are uncommon.

Both thecomas and granulosa cell tumors frequently produce oestrogen and 70% present with precocious or irregular menstruation in adolescence. Thus estrogen may be a useful tumor marker.

Treatment

Treamtent of granulosa cell tumors is salpingo-oophorectomy. Subsequent adjunctive chemotherapy with VAC or VBP will depend on the degree of spread and the stage of the disease. The five and ten years survival of Stage I disease is 95%, although Stages II and III are 55 and 25%, respectively. Fortunately, 85% of cases are Stage I. The prognosis is also associated with rupture of the tumor, which decreases the survival.

The thecoma is also managed by salpingo-oophorectomy but adjuvant therapy is unnecessary if the histological examination reveals a pure thecoma and a low (< 3 mitoses/hpf) mitosis count, as the vast majority are benign.

ENDODERMAL SINUS TUMOR

This is one of the most malignant tumors of the ovary and occurs almost exlusively in children and teenagers. It is usually confined to one ovary, although rupture and ascites are common. The tumor produces α-fetoprotein (AFP), and this is a good tumor marker. Treatment is by surgical removal of the ovary and subsequent chemotherapy with VAC or more successfully recently, VBC. As in all cases when chemotherapy is necessary, the effect on subsequent fertility must be explained to the parents and, if relevant, the patient. There are numerous reports of pregnancy following VAC and appropriate counseling must be given.

The current standard for the treatment of all germ cell tumors, even in advanced stages, in women who wish to maintain fertility is a unilateral salpingo-oophorectomy and staging procedure consisting of an omentectomy, cytologic washings, peritoneal biopsies, and pelvic and para-aortic lymph node sampling.

The contralateral ovary is not biopsied unless grossly involved with tumor in an attempt to preserve future fertility by reducing the potential for adhesions. As these tumors are rarely bilateral, the patient is left with one ovary, one tube, and an intact uterus for future childbearing.

The ideal treatment for low malignant potential tumors is unilateral salpingo-oophorectomy, with cystectomy reserved for those with a recurrent low malignant potential tumor, with a previous history of contralateral/unilateral salpingo-oophorectomy and a strong desire to preserve future fertility.

A laparoscopic approach is becoming more and more popular. The concerns for laparoscopy are tumor rupture and spillage, resulting in upstaging the patient and trocar implants.

PRESERVING FERTILITY AFTER CANCER

In the past, the primary goal of cancer therapy—survival—tended to overshadow survivorship considerations. However, with recent advances in oncology, survival rates are increasing, and therefore, issues affecting long-term cancer survivors become more important and more widely recognized.

As an increasing number of young people survive cancer, *addressing the psychosocial issues and concerns of adolescents and young adults assumes greater importance. With the cure rate for many pediatric malignancies now between 70 and 90%, infertility becomes an increasingly important issue.*

Phases

Strategies for preserving fertility in girls and adolescent women occur in two distinct phases.

The first phase includes oophorectomy (usually unilateral) and cryopreservation of ovarian cortex slices or individual oocytes; ultrasound-guided needle aspiration of oocytes, with or without *in vitro* maturation (IVM), followed by cryopreservation; and ovarian autografting to a distant site.

The second phase occurs if the woman chooses to pursue pregnancy, and includes IVM of the oocytes, followed by *in vitro* fertilization (IVF) and transfer of any created embryos to the woman's uterus (or to a surrogate's uterus if the cancer patient's uterus has been surgically removed or the endometrium destroyed by radiotherapy).

Damage Induced by Radiation to the Pelvis or Chemotherapy for any Malignancy

It is progressive and irreversible in the ovary, resulting in *amenorrhea and infertility*. Although younger women (~age 35 years) tend to have resumption of normal menses, they still remain at risk for infertility and premature menopause.

Direct effects on the uterus after abdominal radiation in young girls being treated for childhood cancers have included irreversible changes in uterine musculature and blood flow.

Significantly decreased uterine volume (up to 40% of normal adult size), which is unresponsive to hormone therapy, has been observed in girls who received abdominal radiation.

Spontaneous abortions occur at a rate of 38% compared with 12% in the general population, preterm labor 62% compared with 9%, and low-birth-weight infants 62% compared with 6%.

However, there is no increased risk of subsequent teratogenicity as long as radiation is not administered during a pregnancy.

Older age, higher doses, and longer duration all increase the toxic effects of chemotherapy on the ovary. Although there is ovarian damage from chemotherapy, there seems to be no risk of toxicity to future offspring of women treated with these agents before pregnancy.

Most chemotherapeutic drugs are excreted in the urine within a few days.

Significant toxicity has been attributed specifically to alkylating agents, which act on undeveloped oocytes and possibly pregranulosa cells of primordial follicles and do not require cell proliferation for their cytotoxic action.

CONCLUSIONS

As the demand for fertility-sparing options grows among young women with cancer, the medical community has responded to these demands with more conservative surgical and medical therapies. Patients need to be made aware of their options. Reproductive endocrinologists continue their efforts to perfect cryopreserving technologies to retain ovarian function. Conservative treatment is an option in highly motivated young women desiring future fertility with certain cancers of the reproductive tract. Informed decision making is essential. Patients must be aware of the standard therapies, risks and benefits of conservative treatment, and need for careful follow-up.

SUGGESTED READING

1. Andersen BL, Green DM. Fertility and Sexuality After Cancer Treatment. In: Lenhard RE Jr, Osteen RT, Gansler T (Eds). Clinical Oncology. Atlanta, GA: American Cancer Society, 2001:853-71.
2. Beth Simon, Stephanie Joi Lee, Ann Hart Partridge, Carolyn D Runowicz. Preserving Fertility after Cancer. CA Cancer J Clin 2005;55;211-28.
3. Coeland LJ, Gershenson DM, Saul PB, Sneige. N, Stringer CA, Edwards CL. Sarcoma botryoids of the female genital tract. Obstetrics and Gynaecology, 1985;66:262.
4. Critchley HO, Bath LE, Wallace HB. Radiation damage to the uterus—review of the effects of treatment of childhood cancer. Hum Fertil 2002;5:61-6.
5. Herbst AL, Anderson D. Clinical correlations and management of vaginal and cervical clear cell carcinoma. In developmental effects of diethylstilboestrol (DES) in Pregnancy Herbst AL, Bern HA), (Eds) Thieme-Stratton Inc., NY, 1981.
6. Maurer HM, Moon T, Donaldson M, et al. The intergroup rhabdomyosarcoma study: A preliminary report. Cancer, 1977;40:2015.
7. Meirow D. Ovarian injury and modern options to preserve fertility in female cancer patients treated with high dose radio-chemotherapy for hemato-oncological neoplasias and other cancers. Leuk Lymphoma 1999;33:65-76.
8. Meistrich ML, Byrne J. Genetic disease in off-spring of long-term survivors of childhood and adolescent cancer treated with potentially muta-genic therapies. Am J Hum Genet 2002;70:1069-71.
9. Morice P, Carmatte S, Hassan JE, et al. Clinical outcomes and fertility after conservative treat-ment of ovarian borderline tumors. Fertil Steril 2001;75:92-6.
10. Sanders JE, Hawley J, Levy W, et al. Pregnancies following high-dose cyclophosphamide with or without high-dose busulfan or total body irradiation and bone marrow transplant. Blood 1996;87:3045-52.
11. Schilder J, Thompson A. outcome of reproductive age women with Stage IA or IC invasive epithelial ovarian cancer treated with fertility sparing therapy. Gynecol Oncol 2002; 87:1-7.
12. Schwartz PE. Combination chemotherapy in the management of ovarian germ cell malignancies. Obstetrics and Gynaecology 1984;64:564.
13. Tscherne G. Female genital tract malignancies during puberty. Uterine and cervical malig-nancies. Ann NY Acad Sci 1997;816:331-7.
14. Young RH, Dickensin GR, Scully RE. Juvenile granulosa cell tumor of the ovary. American Journal of Surgical Pathology 1984;8:575.
15. Zaloudek C, Norris HJ. Granulosa cell tumors in young children. American Journal of Surgical Pathology, 1982;6:513.

42 Lifestyle Disease Prevention by Early Intervation

Swati Y Bhave

INTRODUCTION

There are many diseases that are caused by a unhealthy lifestyle that tracks through childhood into adolescence and into adult onset diseases

These are obesity, Type 2 diabetes mellitus (T2 DM) Hypertension, coronary heart disease (CHD) and stress related disorders

Lifestyle' risk factors developed during childhood/adolescence (unhealthy food habits, alcohol, smoking, poor physical activity, drugs etc) also track through into adult life.

By adopting a healthy lifestyle from child hood especially adolescence it is possible to prevent these diseases.

Clinicians dealing with adolescents are in a excellent position to sensitize their patients about a healthy lifestyle specially when they come with problems related to high risk behaviors like substance abuse, junk food and lack of exercise

Asian and also Indians are at a high risk for insulin resistance (syndrome X).

Metabolic syndrome is associated with increased risk of obesity, insulin resistance, Type 2 diabetes mellitus and cardiovascular disease.

As per the new 2005 International Diabetes Federation definition the criteria for the diagnosis of the metabolic syndrome are:

1. Central obesity (waist circumference > 90 cm for males/> 80 cm for females)
2. Any two of the following four factors:
   a. Raised serum triglycerides 150 mg /dl,
   b. Reduced serum HDL cholesterol < 45 mg/dl,
   c. Raised blood pressure BP systolic > 130, and diastolic > 85 mm Hg), and
   d. Raised fasting blood sugar level > 100 mg/dl).

ADDITIONAL FEATURES ASSOCIATED WITH METABOLIC SYNDROME

1. Insulin resistance (fasting insulin, HOMA IR).
2. Dyslipidemia (in addition to above, increased small dense LDL).
3. Hypercoagulability of blood (increased plasminogen activator inhibitor).
4. Vascular dysregulation (beyond elevated blood pressure) endothelial dysfunction-micro-albuminuria.
5. Inflammatory state-raised high sensitive C-reactive protein, TNC-alpha and IL 6.
6. Polycystic ovarian disease (PCOS).
7. Acan-thosis nigricans.

OBESITY

There is increasing evidence of overweight and obesity in our country specially in the affluent children and adolescents. Many studies show high prevalence. In a Chennai study of school children over weight/obesity was seen in 4.5 %

in LSE group, 15% in MSE group and as high as 22% in the HSE group. In an urban Delhi obesity and overweight was seen in 45% of females and 25% males.

A Delhi study in young adults showed that an increase of BMI of 1 SD from 2 to 12 years of age, increased the odds ratio for disease (IGT/DM) by 1.36. Further, continuing cohort studies in Pune suggest that accelerated growth in childhood specially in low birth weight is associated with early puberty and greater risk of obesity.

It is important to understand that we need to watch carefully if any child or adolescent starts crossing his centiles of growth and be especially alert to the 'healthy' weight gain during adolescence.

TYPE 2 DIABETES (T2 DM)

Type 2 DM has an insidious onset and patients may have hyperglycemia for a number of years before diagnosis. It constitutes high risk for cardiovascular and cerebrovascular mortality and morbidity. Obesity particularly of the central type appears to be a direct correlate of type 2 DM. Obese children are insulin resistant and have up to 40% lower glucose utilization than non-obese children. Acanthosis nigricans is an early marker of insulin resistance and can prove as a simple screening tool for syndrome X.

Polycystic ovarian syndrome (PCOS) is a constituent of metabolic syndrome and often exhibits in adolescent girls with irregular periods, hirsutism, obesity and infertility.

Early puberty has also been correlated with insulin resistance. Puberty is also the peak age of presentation of childhood type 2 DM.

HYPERTENSION AND OTHER CVS RISK FACTORS (HYPERLIPIDEMIA, HYPERCOAGULABILITY)

The high incidence of mortality and morbidity due to myocardial infarctions and stroke in young adults shows that these problems start insidiously in childhood/adolescence and are asymptomatic for long periods.

Indian cohort studies have suggested that high risk factors for CVS diseases are associated with both fetal origins and later lifestyles.

WHAT CLINICIANS DEALING WITH ADOLESCENTS CAN DO TO PREVENT DISEASES CAUSED BY METABOLIC SYNDROME?

Help increase awareness by advocacy programs in schools and community for adolescents, parents and community regarding these diseases

- Use the visit of the adolescents to check height and weight and chart his/her BMI and advise him/her accordingly. Compare with past records if available.
- Check the blood pressure and keep a annual record.
- Take a good family history for cardiovascular disease and diabetes and if positive and/or the adolescent is obese, check for lipid profile and do in glucose tolerance test.
- In obese girls look for acanthosis nigricans and signs of PCOS and treat accordingly.
- If any features of metabolic X syndrome are detected, subject to additional tests to rule out associated features.

ADVISE

- To cut down sedentary activities like TV, computer, video games, etc.
- Healthy diet giving the food pyramid eating plenty of fresh fruits vegetables whole grains. avoiding junk food heavy greasy fried food.
- Refrain from smoking, alcohol consumption and substance abuse.
- Physical activity for at least one hour daily.

ARSH DISEASES ASSOCIATED WITH LIFESTYLE

If one wants to keep away from the risk of sexually transmitted diseases including HIV and unwanted pregnancy then one has to adopt a lifestyle that of responsible sexual behaviors. This translates into delaying the initiation of the first sexual encounter as long as possible, always practicing safe sex, sticking to one sexual partner, not indulging in alcohol and substance abuse before after and during sex. If one adapts a lifestyle of high-risk sexual behaviors which means sex with strangers, multiple sexual partners, not practicing safe sex, not using contraception, having sex while under influence of drugs and alcohol then one is going to have the negative consequences some time or the other

At every encounter with the adolescents clinicians must open up this topic and sensitize them about the hazards to of risky sexual behavior.

STRESS AND DISEASE

Adolescent life has conflicting demands from parents, teachers, and friends that gives a lot of stress. Stress is a challenge to the body homeostasis and this causes a biological and biochemical reaction that begins in the brain and causes an autonomic nervous system effect, causing hormone release and adversely affecting the immune system- the "Neuro-Endocrine Immuno axis".

Stress can be physical, psychological, and psychosocial.

Stresses can manifest as Eustress, i.e. the positive stress which motivates our everyday actions. Inability to cope up with stress means Distress. The key to good health, is learning how to turn bad stress (distress) into good stress (eustress)

The body response to stress is called the general adaptation syndrome. Chronic stress can cause chronic health problems, as wellness cannot be maintained when a large percentage of body energy is channeled into coping with stress.

Stress affects the whole body: causing gastrointestinal disturbances (dyspepsia, peptic ulcer, irritable bowel syndrome) neuromuscular disorders (chronic back pain, vague aches and muscle pains, migraine), sleep disorders, inability to concentrate on performing well academically and other extracurricular activities, cardiovascular disease (hypertension, coronary disease) allergic disorders, and recurrent infections due to depressed immunity.

Teenagers can manifest stress with a variety of psychosomatic symptoms (pertaining to any systems) and these may mislead the diagnosis to somatic illness hence, a pediatrician dealing with the adolescents must go deep into the proper history.

Teenagers stress can come from various factors: biological, family, peer factors, societal, etc. Most teenagers turn to tranquilizers to manage stress and so it is important to teach them how to manage stress without drugs which should become a lifestyle that will prevent stress related diseases. If stress is not properly managed it can result in depression, suicidal behavior, drug or alcohol abuse, eating disorders. It has been found that day-to-day stress are more difficult for adolescents than major life events.

Adolescents generally cope with stress by listening to music and watching television. They must also be helped to find a meaning in stressful experience. Table 42.1 lists how to empower adolescents to deal with stress.

Table 42.1: Empower adolescent to deal with stress

- They should develop coping skills
- They should seek adult support and help when needed
- They should maintain perspective in various situations
- Work on values and purposes in life
- They should learn various stress reduction techniques

The best way to deal stress is to get into the relaxation response which means one brings down the heart rate with breathing exercises and relaxation techniques and mentally decide that the situation is not stressful. Table 42.2 lists various stress reduction techniques.

RELIGION AND SPIRITUALITY

These are known to give mental peace and keep a person on the right track in life. However, adolescents are used being extremely involved and intense about the activities they undertake

Table 42.2: Stress reduction techniques

- Learn time management
- Exercise regularly
- Have a healthy nutritious diet
  Avoid excess caffeine intake that can cause anxiety and agitation
- Don't use illegal drugs, alcohol and tobacco.
- Learn relaxation exercises (abdominal breathing and muscle relaxation techniques)
- Learn life skill approach
- Learn practical coping skills
- Learn positive self-talk, decrease negativity in attitude.
- Learn to find activities that are stress busters for you, e.g. music, painting, reading, etc
- Build a network of friends, who help you cope in a positive way

and care has to be taken that they do not become religious fanatics or indulge in religious bigotary.

Care also has to taken that they do not come under the influence of unscrupulous people that can pose as religious leaders to exploit the innocent

YOGA MEDITATION, PRANAYAMA AND ART OF LIVING

These are known to reduce stress and induce positive thinking in life and adolescents should be encouraged to learn and practice these arts.

SUMMARY

A lot of diseases have their origin in childhood that track through adolescence into adulthood.

Fortunately many of them are preventable by a healthy lifestyle that includes healthy eating habits, exercise, effective stress management and avoidance of alcohol and substance abuse.

Clinicians dealing with adolescents should help them to understand the importance of healthy lifestyle for prevention of disease and clinically monitor them to detect early signs. Stress management should form a important part of daily life.

SUGGESTED READING

1. Asterita MF. The physiology of stress. New York. Human Sciences Press 1985;4-5.
2. Bansal CP, Bhave Swati Y. Stress in adolescents in Bhave's Textbook of Adolescent Medicine 1st (ed.), New Delhi, Jaypee Brothers Medical Publishers 2006;24.5 844-54.
3. http://www.aacap.org/publications/factsfam/66.htm, Helping Teenagers with Stress.
4. International Diabetes Federation. The IDF consensus worldwide definition of the metabolic syndrome. Brussels: IDF, 2005. http://www.idf.org/webdata/docs/IDF-Metasyndrome-definition.pdf(May 2005).
5. Johnson Jacquleine learn to take control of your reactions, cope with what you cant change http://www.billingsgazette.com/tempo/991218_temp01.html
6. Pandit AN Bhave S Bavadekar Fetal origin of adult onset disease in Bhave's Text book of adolescent medicine 1st (ed.) New Delhi, Jaypee Brothers Medical Publishers 2006; 3.6: 104-09
7. Ramachandran A, Snehalatha C, Kapur A, Vijay V, Mohan V, Das AK, et al. High prevalence of diabetes and impaired glucose tolerance in India: National urban diabetes survey. Diabetologia, 2001; 9: 1094-111.
8. Ramachandran A, Snehalatha C, Vinitha R, Thayyil M, Sathish Kumar CK, Sheeba L, et al. Prevalence of overweight in urban Indian adolescent school children. Diabetes Res Clin Pract 2002;57:185-90.
9. Reddy KS. Cardiovascular diseases in developing countries: Dimensions, determinants dynamics and directions for public health action. Pub Hlth Nut 2002; 5:231-37.
10. WHO/NMH/NPH/ Life course perspectives on coronary heart disease, stroke, and diabetes. WHO, Geneva, 0.1.4:2001.
11. Yajnik CS. The insulin resistance epidemic in India: Fetal origins, Later lifestyle, or both ? Nutr Rev 2001; 59: 1-9.
12. Yajnik CS, Fall CHD, Koyaji KJ, Hirve SS, Rao S, Barker DJP, et al. Neonatal anthropometry: The thin-fat Indian baby. The Pune Maternal Nutrition Study. Int J Obes 2003;27:173-80.

43 Premarital Counseling

Sheela V Mane

INTRODUCTION

Premarital counseling tackles concerns relating to the impending marriage, clears up misconceptions about sex, talks about issues like interpersonal relationships and family planning and in short, prepares a person for marriage. Parents may, at times, be unaware of certain conflicts and concerns that their children have with regard to marriage. It has been established that those youngsters, who have been exposed to premarital counseling have better chances of coping successfully with their marriage, than those who have not.

WHAT IS THE PURPOSE OF MARRIAGE?

The definition of "Marriage" states that marriage is the pledging of two people to have a meaningful partnership to form a family and to make a home. Marriage is a social and legal commitment to share their lives and family responsibilities.

People get married for love, companionship, social and emotional security, support and parenthood, not merely to satisfy the sexual needs.

WHAT IS THE APPROPRIATE AGE TO GET MARRIED?

The Indian law states that a woman can get married when she is 18 years or above and a man when he is 21 years or above.

But this is not the only criteria, both need to be self-supporting, financially stable and able to share responsibilities of home and children. So a woman can get married at 20-28 years and a man at 24-30 years.

DIFFERENCE IN THEIR AGE?

A woman should be about 2 to 5 years younger to the man because the mental maturity of women is much earlier than that of the men and the fertility age of women is much less than that of the men.

OTHER PREREQUISITES FOR MARRIAGE

A person with sound physical and mental health, maturity of mind, financial stability, ability for emotional involvement, ability to share marital responsibilities on finding a judiciously selected life-partner.

MARRIAGE—LOVE OR ARRANGED

Love does not shower like sudden rain but grows slowly like a sapling nurtured in the soil. True love is kind, patient, hopeful, with endurance, not rude, never selfish and keeps no store of wrongs. It grows in stages of acquaintance, companionship, friendship, liking the person, understanding the qualities of the person, and ultimately marriage. Two people having similar lifestyles, believing in secularism and not strictly following religious rituals may not find difficulties in adjustment after the marriage. But if their attitudes are traditional or conservative they should not go for inter-caste or inter-religious marriage.

FACTORS FOR A SUCCESSFUL MARRIAGE

LOVE

Those individuals who come from loving homes will make their marriage happy. People who receive love from their parents during childhood can share love with their spouse during their adulthood.

SIMILARITY

Similarly in social class, lifestyle attitudes, values, interests, thoughts and equal intelligence is always better.

ABILITY

The abilities that a couple must possess are those of adjustment, flexibility, adaptability, emotional stability, problem solving and believe in caring and sharing.

PERIOD OF COURTSHIP

Frequently meeting at each other's home to understand each other's personality, socio-cultural background, values and dear ones, ways of communication, thoughts and beliefs, ideas and behavior can go a long way in building a rapport between two people who want to spend the rest of their lives together.

Meeting in a coffee shop or a restaurant which may be more appealing, may miss some of the opportunities to know the other person better.

PHYSICAL HEALTH

The foundation of a happy marriage is a healthy lifestyle.

Diseases like diabetes, high blood pressure, insomnia, TB, epilepsy, STD, HIV, skin problems, sexual problems, hereditary diseases must be considered.

A complete physical examination including genital examination should be done. Menstrual history of the female should be noted.

The following investigations may be carried out:

- A simple semen examination of the groom-to-be and a simple sonography examination of the uterus and ovaries of the bride-to-be may be recommended as screening tests to assess the reproductive ability of a couple.
- Two HIV tests with the gap of three months are also recommended. Very rarely people are aware that pre-test counseling is very necessary before every HIV testing and it is a responsible and a sensitive task.
- It is also necessary to test for one more fatal disease that is transmitted sexually—hepatitis B. A carrier of hepatitis B appears healthy outwardly but could transmit the deadly disease to the partner through sexual contact.
- VDRL test or TPHA test for syphilis can be asked for.
- Though everybody must know his or her blood group, due to availability of anti-D injection the problem of Rh incompatability is no more considered significant.
- Test for thalassemia and hemophilla may be included.

MENTAL HEALTH

The symptoms of sound mental health are:

- Desire to survive.
- Experiences happiness, tranquility and contentment.
- Ability to face day-to-day problems.
- Shoulders family and social responsibilities.
- Independent and bold.
- Has friends.
- Normal mental functions.

Diseases like schizophrenia, mania, depression and personality disorders could be suspected during a conversation.

Suspicious signs are sad, lethargic, unclean, suicidal thoughts, disturbed thinking, emotions, laughs/cries without reason, suspicious, tense, looks frightened, unreliable, violent, sleeplessness.

A WOMAN MUST HAVE THE QUALITIES OF A GOOD MOTHER

These are: intelligence, dedication, confidence, perseverance, discipline, hard work, planning, punctuality, devotion, affection and ambition.

THE FIVE "T"S FOR A HAPPY MARRIAGE

Trust, Time, Togetherness, Talk, Touch.

DOES EVERY PERSON NEED TO GET MARRIED?

Not necessarily, marriage is not for everyone. People with personality problems should never marry. Some may not find a person with whom they can be happy. There is nothing wrong with choosing to be single under these circumstances.

HUMAN SEXUALITY

MAN

A man is pleasure-loving, rational, proud, authoritative, aggressive, egoist, tends to hide emotions, likes to be dominant, has higher sexual desire, gives priority to education and intelligence, likes to see pornography, deeply interested in penetrative sex, seeks variety in sex and has possibility of premarital or extramarital sex.

Man is biologically weaker than woman. Masturbation is a common sexual behavior in men. Nearly 93% men masturbate. Man is invariably a polygamist (having sex with many females).

WOMAN

A woman is soft, emotional, loves romance, instinctual, talkative, jealous, feelings are hurt easily. Sheds tears easily, fond of love, has tolerance, likes beauty, priority to marriage and motherhood. Not much interested in penetrative sex, fond of fashion and cooking, not interested in extramarital sexual experience.

HEALTHY SEXUAL RELATIONSHIP

A healthy sexual relationship is defined by the WHO as integration of social, intellectual, physical and emotional aspects of human being in ways that enhance personality, communication and love.

COMMON CAUSES OF MARITAL CONFLICTS

Misunderstandings during the marriage

- Dowry,
- Irresponsible parents, troublesome in-laws,
- Suspicious spouse,
- Infertility,
- Extramarital relationship.
- Difference in religion/caste, difference in behaviours,
- Over expectations,
- Mental illness,
- Financial problems,
- Sexual dysfunction,
- Addiction.

COMMUNICATION

- There are several ways to communicate - letter writing, telephone, e-mail, chatting, SMS, etc.
- Do not hurt the sentiments of the person or family members.
- Talk about your future and your family. Maintain dignity.
- This is a period when sexual feelings and intimate physical contact is highest. But it should be avoided as it may lead to a lot of complications and embarrassments.

POINTS TO REMEMBER

- If you do not approve of a person to be your partner, be bold to reject. Similarly, if he rejects you for whatever reason, do not feel offended.
- Never presume that your partner will mirror your ideas, values, likes and dislikes.

- Nobody is perfect. Perfection and idealism are found only in novels and films.
- Never ask about his past love affairs (which would mostly be infatuation).
- Do not have false hopes that you will change him after the marriage. He or she may not change. Try to adjust.
- Happy marriage does not mean marriage without conflicts. Efforts are required to make the marriage work.
- Marriage works only if both are determined to make it a success, come what may.
- "Give to Get" is the mantra for a happy married life.

SEX EDUCATION

It is necessary to explain to the couple especially the women about the external and internal genital organs.

CONTRACEPTION

The couple must be told about suitable contraceptive methods that they can use after marriage for the purpose of family planning.

It is said that "a Wedding is an event but a marriage is an achievement".

There are a great many factors generating the marital relationship and these must be worked out efficiently.

SUGGESTED READING

1. Marriage Guidance for "To Be Married and Newly Married", Dr Vithal Prabhu and Dr Padmini Prasad, Bangalore.
2. Education in Human Sexulaity. A sourcebook for educators by Ms. Dhun Parithaki. Second edition, April 2005. Published by FPA India, Bajaj Bharan, Mumbai.

44 Life Skills Training Programs ARSH

Swati Y Bhave, Jitendra Nagpal

INTRODUCTION

In adolescents there is a direct correlation between high risk taking behavior and ARSH related issues. High risk taking behavior can reduced by teaching adolescents life skills. Hence, teaching of life skills are extremely important if we want to reduce morbidity and mortality related to ARSH like unwanted teen age pregnancy, sexually transmitted diseases and drug abuse *Life skills can be used for promotion of age appropriate responsible sexual behaviors and enhance gender sensitivity.*

EQ, i.e. emotional quotient and SQ, i.e. social Quotient is increasingly being assessed by multinational companies in selection of their employees in addition to their qualifications and work experience and very important aspect of adolescent development.

Life skills give a person psychosocial competence, This will lead to *behavior reinforcement or change* which leads to *positive health behavior* and will ultimately result in **prevention of health problems.**

Psychosocial competence is a person's ability to deal effectively with the demands and challenges of everyday life. It is a person's ability to maintain a state of mental well being and to show this in adaptive and positive behavior while interacting with others. An adolescent with good psychosocial competence will have minimal adjustment problems and is less likely to participate in high risk taking behavior.

DEFINITIONS OF LIFE SKILLS

There are a number of definitions:

World Health Organization (WHO) defines life skills as "the abilities for adaptive and positive behavior that enable individuals to deal effectively with the demands and challenges of everyday life". Table 44.1 shows kinds of life skills.

UNICEF defines "life skills-based education as basically being a behaviors change or behaviors development approach designed to address a balance of three areas: knowledge, attitude and skills. The UNICEF definition is based on research evidence that shifts in risk behaviors are unlikely if knowledge, attitudinal and skills based competency is not addressed.

HOW DOES LIFE SKILL EDUCATION EMPOWER ADOLESCENTS?

Life skills enable individuals to translate knowledge, attitudes and values into actual abilities—i.e., what to do and how to do it. Effective acquisition and application of life skills can influence the way we feel about others, ourselves and equally will influence the way we are perceived by others, ourselves and others.

Table 44.1: Kinds of life skills

Communication and Interpersonal Skills	*Decision-making and Critical Thinking Skills*	*Coping and Self-management Skills*
• Interpersonal communication skills • Verbal/nonverbal communication • Active listening • Expressing feelings; giving feedback (without blaming) and receiving feedback • Negotiation/refusal skills • Negotiation and conflict management • Assertiveness skills • Refusal skills • Empathy building • ability to listen, understand another's needs and circumstances, and express that understanding • Cooperation and teamwork • Expressing respect for others' contributions and different styles • assessing one's own abilities and contributing to the group • Advocacy skills • influencing skills and persuasion • Networking and motivation skills	• Decision-making/ Problem solving skills • Information-gathering skills • Evaluating future consequences of present actions for self and others-determining alternative solutions to problems • Analysis skills regarding the influence of values and of attitudes about self and others on motivation • Critical thinking skills • analyzing peer and media influences • Analyzing attitudes, values, social norms, beliefs, and factors affecting them • Identifying relevant information and sources of information	• Skills for increasing personal confidence and abilities to assume control, take Responsibility, make a difference, or Bring About Change • Building self-esteem/confidence • Creating self-awareness skills, including awareness of rights, influences, values, attitudes, rights, strengths, and weaknesses • Setting goals • Self-evaluation/self-assessment/ self-monitoring skills • Skills for managing feelings • Managing anger • Dealing with grief and anxiety • Coping with loss, abuse, and trauma • Skills for managing stress • Time management • Positive thinking • Relaxation techniques

LIFE SKILLS

- Are abilities that enable individuals to behave in healthy ways, given the desire to do so and given the scope and opportunity to do so. They are not a panacea.
- Are abilities that help promote mental well being and competence in young people as they face the realities of life. The promotion of mental well being contributes to motivation to look after oneself and others, in prevention of mental disorders, and in the prevention of health and behavior problems.
- Contribute to perceptions of self-confidence and self-esteem.
- Can be utilized in many content areas, issues, topics or subjects such as in prevention of drug abuse, sexual violence, teenage pregnancy, HIV/AIDS/STD prevention, suicide prevention, etc.
- In short, life skills empower young people to take positive actions to protect themselves and to promote health and positive social relationships.

EXPECTED OUTCOMES OF LIFE SKILLS DEVELOPMENT

- Enhanced self-esteem
- Self-confidence
- Assertiveness
- Ability to establish relationships
- Ability to plan and set goals
- Acquisition of knowledge related to specific content areas.

THE METHODOLOGY

- The life skill is taught depending on the cultural and social factors, e.g. eye contact may be encouraged in boys for effective communication, but not for girls in some societies. The exact content of life skill education has to be determined in a more local context. Life skills are being taught in such a wide variety of countries and still have relevance across cultures.

- Life skills lessons are designed to allow opportunities for practice of skills in a supportive learning environment.
- Lessons are both active and experiential. In passive learning, the teacher passes on knowledge and the learner is the recipient of information. Active learning, however, engages the teacher and children in a dynamic process of learning by using methods such as brainstorming, group discussion and debates.
- Life skills are taught by interactive teaching—learning process. Methods used are brainstorming, group discussion, debates. Experiential learning is based on actual practice or what is being taught by games and role-plays. Structure is provided through the use of processing questions. They help in student involvement and reflection. Practice of skills in a supportive learning environment.

OPTIMAL STRATEGY FOR LIFE SKILL EDUCATIONS

- Given the wide ranging relevance of life skills, an optimal strategy for the introduction of life skills teaching would be to make it available to all children and adolescents in schools.
- The school is an appropriate place for the introduction of life skills education because schools have access to children and adolescents on a large scale, experienced teachers and infrastructure is in place.
- The place of life skills teaching in the school curriculum can very greatly. When the life skills program is included as a part of the school curriculum, it is referred to as "integrated". Life skills can also be taught within the academic subjects, such as the teaching of communication skills in the context of language classes. Taught in this way life skill education is "infused" into the existing curriculum. Life skill education may also be implemented as an extra-curricular activity. Framework for life skill education for AEP is shown in Figure 44.1.

LIFE SKILLS EDUCATION IN ARSH

- In the United States, a CDC study in 1999 of nearly 6,000 students from 56 schools over a three-year intervention study showed that LST had a significant impact on reducing cigarette, marijuana, and alcohol use. Results of the six-year follow-up indicated that the effects of the programme lasted until the end of the twelfth grade

Fig. 44.1: Framework of life skills for adolescent education program AEP

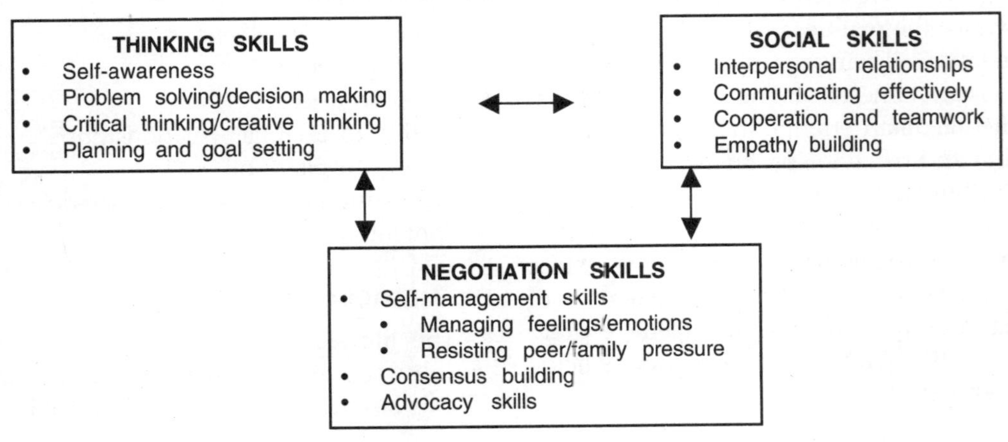

- Kirby and DiClemente in 1994 found that negotiation skills enhance students' ability to delay sex or to use condoms.
- Wilson and colleagues in 1992 found that female student teachers in Zimbabwe who participated in a skills-based AIDS intervention were more knowledgeable about condoms and their correct use, had a higher sense of self-efficacy, perceived fewer barriers, and reported fewer sexual partners four months after the intervention than their colleagues who participated in a lecture.
- A meta-analysis of adolescent psychosocial smoking prevention programs by Hwang et al in 2004) examined 65 adolescent psychosocial smoking prevention programs (1978 to 1997) among students in Grades 6 to 12 in the United States. Adolescent smoking reduction rates were improved by using either cognitive behavior or life skills program modalities and/or a school-community-incorporated program setting.
- Tobler in 1992 in a meta-analysis of 207 school-based drug prevention programmes concluded most successful of the interactive programmes are the comprehensive life skills-based education programmes that incorporate the refusal skills offered in the social influences programs and add skills such as assertiveness, coping, communication skills, etc.
- Perry and Grant in 1991 in Australia, Chile, Norway, and Swaziland collaborated in a pilot study which showed that peer-led education appears to be effective in reducing alcohol use across a variety of settings and cultures.
- 'Expressions' (Nagpal, Bhave and Prasad., 2005) is a school based project on mental health and life skills education. It is a very successful peer educator program to reduce substance abuse, HIV/AIDS, anger and stress management, coping with failures, etc.
- In a panel study of 2222 youth by Magnani et al in 2005, showed good impact of school-based life skills education on reduction of HIV risk.

LIFE SKILL TRAINING IS BEST GIVEN BY PEER EDUCATORS

A true peer is a person who is considered a member of a particular group, both by themselves and by other group members. A near peer is similar but differs in some small way, for example they may be a few years older.

Peer educators may act in different roles, such as facilitators, counselors, sources of information, support workers or tutors. Teenagers are more likely to hear and personalize messages, and thus to change their attitudes and behaviors, if they believe the messenger is similar to them and faces the same concerns and pressures. Peer educators themselves benefit from programs by receiving special training in making decisions, clarifying values, and acting in accordance with those values.

A Cascade Strategy for disseminating the training is used. Peer trainers go on to train others using the same, or a similar, training schedule. Care has to be taken however, to maintain the quality of the training at all levels.

SUMMARY

Life skill education can be used as a preventive strategy to empower adolescents to deal with the various problem situation in life. Life skills can be used for promotion of age appropriate responsible sexual behaviors and enhance gender sensitivity. Life skill approach has been effective in reduction of HIV/AIDS and other ARSH issues.

SUGGESTED READING

1. AEP training modules developed by Expressions for AEP program (MHRD-NACO) supported.
2. Centers for Disease Control and Prevention (CD). (1999). Adolescent and School Health. Available on-line: http://www.cdc.gov/nccdp-hp/dash.
3. Hwang MS, Yeagley KL, Petosa R. A meta-analysis of adolescent psychosocial smoking prevention programs published between 1978 and 1997 in the United States. Health Educ Behav. 2004;31(6):702-19.

4. Kirby D, DiClemente RJ, School-based interventions to prevent unprotected sex and HIV among adolescents. in RJ, DiClemente and JL. Peterson (Eds.), Preventing AIDS: Theories and methods of behavioural intentions, pp. 7-139. New York: Plenum Press, 1994.
5. Magnani R, Macintyre K, Karim AM, Brown L, Hutchinson P, Kaufman C, Rutenburg N, Hallman K, May J, Dallimore A. The impact of life skills education on adolescent sexual risk behaviors in KwaZulu-Natal, South Africa.; J Adolesc Health 2005;36(4):289-304.
6. Nagpal J, Prasad DS. Life skills training programs, Chapter in Bhaves Text Book of Adolescent Medicine 1st ed. New Delhi, Jaypee Brothers 2006;8(4):299-303.
7. Nagpal Jitendra, Bhave Swati Y, Prasad Divya S, Parental Management Training In School Mental Health - The Indian Experience, American Academy of Pediatrics - Section on Adolescent Health Newsletter, Autumn 2005;29(1).
8. Perry CL, Grant M, (1991). A Cross-cultural pilot study on alcohol education and young people. World Health Statistics Quarterly—Rapport. Trimestriel de Statistiques Sanitaires Mondiales. As cited in Hubley, 2000;44, 70-73.
9. Tobler N, Drug Prevention Programmes can Work: Research findings. Journal of Addictive Diseases;1992; 11 (3).
10. Wilson D, Mparadzi A., Lavelle E. An experimental comparison of two AIDS preventions interventions among young Zimbabweans. Journal of Social Psychology 1992;132 (3):415-17.
11. World Health Organization (WHO) - Information Series on School Health, Document 9, Skills for Health—Skills-based health education including life skills: An important component of a Child-Friendly/Health-Promoting School. http://www.who.int/school_youth_health/media/en/

45 Value Education and Spirituality in Adolescent and Young People

Roza Olyai

INTRODUCTION

When it comes to realizing the grave challenges surrounding mankind, a common mistake we all do is to identify the problems in the external phenomena and then put all our energies on addressing these superficial problems. Whereas the truth is that our most basic problems lie in the depths of our thoughts and aptitude. Medical Science is the part and parcel of an evolving human society which is passing through a moral crisis.

New thought patterns and life-styles are casting their most powerful Influence on our adolescent minds because they are in a vulnerable age-group. The so-called 'open-mindedness' of a fastly narrowing world mounted on the winged vehicle of media (especially television and cinema) is revolutionizing the way our adolescent citizens are living their lives. Sex is widely portrayed in this media invasion but its true meaning and true educative measures are missing.

Therefore, the adolescents, enchanted by the ulterior shining of this forbidden Pandora's box, are not aware fully what stings and miseries will follow their curiosity. So what is the remedy? Should be shut down the 'Idiot Box' and warn our children not to go near them? Or we confine them within such narrow walls where no win of change can dare enter? Rousseau said: "If you close the door to keep away errors, even the truth will remain outside". The remedy is in accepting this basic truth that our adolescents need to be educated ... and education that does not lay emphasis just on fact-sharing but in changing the attitudes. Once they are equipped with a sound moral vision, they will be in a better position to discern the good and the evil.

WE NEED MORE THAN A SUPERFICIAL CALL FOR 'MORALITY'

In many societies one hears the call of "Our young people have forgotten their culture and should return to the age old values of the past". No doubt, spirituality and moral education have fallen by the wayside in our materialistic times. Science has sent religion to the sidelines and any talk of spirituality is seen as unscientific and irrelevant. On the other hand, societies and communities that have tried to go back to the 'old religious values of the past' have fought a losing battle, with young people still finding a way to access drugs and alcohol and take part in risky behaviors.

WHAT IS SPIRITUALITY?

The basic assumption of the author is that all religions have been sent to humanity by one

Creator and contain universal spiritual truths that apply to all of God's creation. From this perspective, let us look at what is really meant by spirituality. A brief look at the Holy Books of the world's religions show that all religions teach about the existence of a soul that is immortal:

"The Spirit that is in all beings is immortal in them all: for the death of what cannot die, cease thou to sorrow." 2:30 Bhagavad Gita (Muscaro translation)

All religions teach that the purpose of desire is to direct it towards spiritual behavior or righteousness. That only by 'hungering and thirsting' after right behavior will we become fulfilled. "Blessed are they which do hunger and thirst after righteousness: for they shall be filled." Matthew 5:6

The religions teach that good words and good deeds are recognized by God and rewarded. This is the source of real greatness.

"If any one desireth greatness, all greatness is in God. The good word riseth up to Him and the righteous deed will He exalt." Qur'an, 35:11 (Rodwell translation)

Overall, the religions teach us that real happiness is only attained through spiritual behavior."...human happiness is founded upon spiritual behavior." Baha'i Writings (Abdu'l-Baha)

On the other hand, today's society teaches the youth that our physical bodies are of the utmost importance, that without a job and money you are nothing. Society shows how success can be attained by any means and that happiness can be bought or acquired through material pleasures.

THE SPIRITUAL NATURE OF MANKIND

The basis of such empowerment should be understanding of this fact that every human being is basically a spiritual creature. As Benson wrote: "Spiritual development is likely a well-spring for the best of human life (e.g., generosity, unity, sacrifice, altruism, social justice) as well as for our darkest side (e.g., genocide, terrorism, slavery). Using social science to examine this potent force in society and individual lives of young people has been neglected for too long."

When it comes to improving the reproductive health of adolescents, programmes in India inevitably focus on either information; for example - sex education, or on service delivery; for example – distribution of condoms, family planning clinics or the recent upsurge in research into microbicides for women.

Research has proven time and again that information and service-based programmes are not effective in bringing about a change in behavior. On the other hand, programmes that empower adolescents by examining their internal beliefs and values and equip them with skills will protect them from risk behaviors. The need for understanding the social, cultural, educational and spiritual needs of the 'target population' and making interventions relevant to their experiences has been recommended in many Indian studies.

The Search Institute (1996) uses the term 'Assets' to measure the likelihood of youth taking part in risky behavior and explains that External assets are support from family and others while Internal assets are commitment to education and learning, development of spiritual values to guide choices and developing a positive identity. Yet debate and scientific research about the 'spiritual' nature of the human being is sorely lacking.

The worldwide moral and spiritual crisis is manifesting itself in varied forms such as alcohol and drug abuse, violence, crime, promiscuity, sexually transmitted diseases, prejudice, injustice and a multitude of other social ills. At present, we are trying to resolve each problem separately without realizing that they are all symptoms of an underlying disease, moral crisis. While we try to resolve each social ill separately, the moral crisis continues to rage out of control. It is evident that for a moral crisis, we need a moral solution. The moral solution is to give moral education to children. Arm them with moral fortitude and they will shun all the evil desires. Moral education of children is the responsibility of every member of society. Unless and until moral education is part of a child's education at home, at school and in the society, the current crisis will continue to worsen.

Moral education is basically a process of helping children acquire virtues such as uprightness, truthfulness, trustworthiness, kindliness, respect, courtesy, obedience, courage, cooperation, justice, unity, purity, faithfulness, loyalty, generosity, service to others, perseverance, pursuit of excellence, etc. These virtues are universal. They are acceptable to all traditions, cultures, religions, nations and people. They are a part of the human character that needs to be nurtured and developed. When children acquire virtues as part of their character, they will have the moral force necessary to make moral decisions and act upon them.

RELIGION AT THE CORE OF MORAL REARING

As the famous poem "Pippa Passes" puts in : "God is in His heaven and all is well with the world". For many of us, religion means this much. We go to temples, churches, mosques and gurdwaras and then come back home satisfied that 'all is well with the world'. But God has given us religion as a means for divine education of the children of man and for serving mankind. If religion fails to fulfill this mission, its very purpose is defeated. All great religions of God emphasize this need and lay stress on setting up high moral standards for human beings. Lord Buddha put morality at the core of religion when He said : "Though one were to live a hundred years immoral and with a mind unstilled by meditation, the life of a single day is better if one is moral and practises meditation.". (Dhammapada).

A righteous conduct is loved by God above all things. Therefore, He said in the Bible: "Thou hast loved righteousness, and hated iniquity; therefore God, even thy God, hath anointed thee with the oil of gladness above thy fellows." (Bible: Hebrews). In Hinduism, religion is directly related with the practice of such vows as Ahimsa (non-violence), Satya (truthfulness), Asteya (non-stealing),

Brahmcharya (sexual chastity) and Aparigraha (non-accumulation of excessive wealth). These are the five moral codes mentioned in 'Manu Smriti' along with other virtues such as Tapa (austerity), Swadhyaya (deep study of Holy Texts), Shaucha (cleanliness), Kshama (forgiveness), Daya (kindness), etc. Baha'u'llah, the latest in the Prophetic cycle, specifies : "All men have been created to carry forward an ever-advancing civilization. The Almighty beareth Me witness: To act like the beasts of the field is unworthy of man. Those virtues that befit his dignity are forbearance, mercy, compassion and loving-kindness towards all the peoples and kindreds of the earth." (Gleanings from the Writings of Bahá'u'lláh, p. 214)

THE JUNIOR YOUTH EMPOWERMENT PROGRAM

As we saw, moral empowerment is stressed in all religions of God. However, we seldom find a systematic moral empowerment programme in all the religions. To some extent, the Christians have some integrated activities for children and youth and they hold Sunday schools on these themes. Yet, a more comprehensive outlay is visible in India and the world in the "Junior Youth Empowerment Program (JYEP)" run along Baha'I principles. JYEP focuses on junior youth aged 12 to 15. Over years of testing and development, the JYEP has been found to equip junior youth with a profound understanding of their own potentialities and empower them to engage in acts of service to the community. Four books are currently in use for study by the junior youth groups:

Breezes of Confirmation and Glimmerings of Hope for 12 year olds;

Walking the Straight Path for 13 year olds;

Drawing on the Power of the Word for 14 year olds.

The entire curriculum helps the junior youth discover moral and spiritual realities for themselves, assisted by the Animator or the facilitator of the class who is a trained personnel. Since a participative method is applied, the study of these books also helps develop the junior youth's powers of expression and comprehension. Developing these powers can have beneficial effects on their intellectual abilities in other areas of study. Some 100 Baha'i-inspired schools all over India have either started or are in the process of starting JYEP. One leading high school in Madhya Pradesh launched this program systematically early September in Gwalior city with the help of two trained animators who are now successfully holding the classes on weekly basis and this is amply helping the junior youths in becoming their own change-agents and acquiring the skill for self decision making after careful discernment of the right and wrong.

Some 90 students are benefiting from this endeavour. In addition, various local Baha'I communities of India are running on a regular and systematic basis hundreds of 'Youth Year of Service' projects in which young souls are encouraged to pick up some nearby communities and extend some sort of service such as holding of children's moral classes, devotional meetings, etc. All this is revolutionizing the lives of the adolescents who are involved and harnessing their energies into creative and self-rewarding avenues.

MORAL EDUCATION IN SCHOOLS: SOME CASE STUDIES

AUSTRALIA

About 6,000 primary school children in Australia are attending Moral classes, which are offered in more than 300 state-run schools. More than 90 percent of the children in these classes are from families with different religious background.

NUR UNIVERSITY, ECUADOR

Nur University believes that an indispensable element for the achievement of sustainable development is the exercise of a moral and ethical leadership, a leadership that is based on universal principles, such as justice, and oriented towards the common good. To this effect, the university offers well-stipulated courses. The moral leadership course has six elements: the purpose of leadership, personal and social transformation, service-oriented leadership, the fundamental moral responsibility to investigate and apply truth, belief in the essential nobility of the human being, transcendence and the development of capabilities.

ROLE OF PARENTS AND FAMILIES AS WELL AS COMMUNITIES

As back as in 1997, Newsweek asked some 500 parents about their most important goal as a parent. The most common response, given by 48% of the parents, was making sure their child grows up to be a moral person. Unfortunately, this goal is becoming harder for parents to achieve. Traditionally, parents and their children were embedded in a network of family and community that contributed to the moral upbringing of children. Families, however, are becoming more and more isolated. The difficult task of raising moral children is compounded by other forces in the lives of children and parents (e.g., culture, media, peers, etc.) that promote unethical, immoral, and self-focused behavior.

However, there is no reason to lose hope. Parents still continue to be the role models for their children and just by their exemplary behavior they can contribute to a great deal in moral rearing of their children. Several parenting behaviors have been shown to promote moral conduct. Parents who model pro-social behavior promote children acting in the same way (Kohn, 1990). Several studies support the importance of a nurturant rearing figure who is explicit in his or her pro-social training, using inductive and effective communications (Radke-Yarrow & Zahn-Waxler, 1984). Other results suggest that structural family characteristics are far less important than the quality of family relationships in the development of adolescent moral reasoning (Speicher, 1992).

However, moral education of children is not the sole responsibility of parents alone. In fact, every member of society should feel responsible for this. No one should be indifferent to the great suffering that diseases like HIV/AIDS, alcohol and drug abuse, hatred and prejudice have brought upon humankind. Unless and until moral education is part of a child's education at home, at school and in the society, the current crisis will continue to worsen.

CLINICAL RELEVANCE OF SPIRITUALITY AND MORAL EDUCATION

HIV is probably the most pertinent of the many conditions that can be prevented by moral education. This is well documented by the experience in Uganda in 1989. A Senior consultant, Dr. Davachi, suggested to the government to begin a campaign of abstinence before marriage and faithfulness during marriage, to children before puberty since all other awareness campaigns were aimed at youth and adults. President Museveni agreed and started a massive campaign across the country, teaching abstinence and faithfulness in every school. The results now coming from the World Health Organization indicate that in 1991 the rate of infection in girls, 15 to 19 years of age in some antenatal clinics was 38%. In 1998, the infection rate in girls of the same age group, in the same clinics, fell to 7.3%. This represents an 80% decrease in infection, a figure that has no equal anywhere else in the world. The girls 15 to 19 years of age who had 80% less infection were only 6-10 years old when the campaign began in 1989. Yet the "abstinence and faithfulness" components of HIV prevention remain controversial due to the aforementioned fear of broaching the subject of moral education.

THE DAUNTING TASKS

As said above, the most basic belief that should guide our efforts in fostering moral values among our adolescents will be that all of us are created noble. All have the potential to show forth the spiritual qualities in our character. All have been given talents and gifts that can be used to benefit the world of humanity. These qualities are latent in every child, but they need to be developed. The Baha'i writings state: "Regard man as a mine rich in gems of inestimable value. Education can alone cause it to reveal its treasures and enable mankind to benefit therefrom." These gems of inestimable value are the spiritual qualities of love, kindness, truthfulness, trustworthiness, sincerity and integrity to name but a few.

Every day as we nurture our young children, we must help them discover these gems that are already within them and assist them to polish and develop these "gems" until they can apply them in their lives. Then we will begin to educate spiritual beings who are guided in their actions by betterment of the world. A child is like a young plant, it will grow in whatever way we train it. It just needs tender handling, that we can determine the way it grows firmly. We should never treat it roughly or harshly, or it would never survive. We must not censure or vilify our children. They must not be subjected to blows or verbal abuse or their character will be totally perverted.

We must be firm in the principles we believe in and agree that these spiritual qualities are necessary for the education of our children. If we want our children to solve their problems through the power of words, uttered with respect and clarity; then we must discipline them with words uttered with respect and clarity. If we want our children to be constant and determined, then we must be consistent, patient, and diligent in our task. A child learns what he lives and if we are striving for a more peaceful world where spiritual principles guide our actions and decisions; then we must begin with the young children. So let us strive to train our children in all the perfections of humankind so that they will shine out as brilliant stars in the world of humanity.

PURITY AND NOBILITY: THE TRUE OBJECTIVES TO BE ACHIEVED

When the soul is conceived it enters the world pure and unblemished. The experiences of this world contribute blemishes and impurities. The purpose of life is to recognize and deal with these imperfections and to try to regain purity of motive and action. The purity of the infant is a bestowal of God. The imperfect purity we strive to regain becomes the conscious fruit of our lives. Our nobility comes from successful choice. Successful choice has only one criterion, alignment with the spiritual premises of the active Divine attributes. Bahá'ís call the process of aligning our choices with Divine Will, personal transformation.

COOPERATION AND COMPETITION

We often say that we are living in a competitive age. This word "Competition" is coined so much as a 'mantra' of today's success and survival that most schools are tending to be 'arenas' where students are trained and enabled to face various competitions. Thus, the focus shifts from "acquiring true knowledge" to gaining tips and tricks for defeating others. The Darwinian theory of the "survival of the fittest" gave this notion of competition a scientific basis. But even Darwin and his followers could not reply one thing. If men and animals are just designed to "survive" by increasing their 'fitness' anyhow, why we find the spirit of sacrifice and love working in this universe? Why a mother (even in animals) should sacrifice her life and put herself in trouble when she can easily choose her own survival in difficult conditions of life such as hunger, famine and other odd conditions? Why lovers stake their lives for protecting their beloveds when, according to Darwin, they should care for their own survival?

This question finds its answer in this basic belief that every human being is basically a spiritual creature and he is governed by such rules as love, care, sacrifice, help, co-living, etc. Vying for excellence is competition in its finest sense. It is competition which encourages cooperation, which seeks the elevation of all performance as an integral consequence of its practice

JUSTICE AND MERCY

A 'sense of justice' is perhaps the most powerful objective of all education. Bahá'u'llah states, 'Set your reliance on the army of justice, put on the armour of wisdom, let your adorning be forgiveness and mercy and that which cheereth the hearts of the well-favoured of God.' Our adolescents must be taught that in true spiritual sense this is a world of mercy but we mankind have made it cruel and unjust. Our purpose should be to equip them with a sound choice of just thought, just action, just purpose for life. It is this choice that sets man apart from animals. Nobility is derived from making the right choices in a world where wrong choices are possible.

CONSULTATION AND DECISION-MAKING

Bahá'í empowerment programs focuses our attention on new modes of decision-making, defined by Bahá'u'llah as the spiritual processes of consultation. There is a host of Bahá'í principles guiding the decision-making process. Consultation is a process, and the mastery of consultation an important objective of moral empowerment. The skills of decision-making are essential to success, in the family, in the workplace, in social institutions, and even in casual human interaction. One straight point is to understand the definition of an effective decision: a decision based upon analysis of facts and circumstances and of the principles which apply; a decision which has been informed by the opinion and perspective of all those concerned; and a decision which is conscientiously implemented by all.

Part of the decision-making process, whether by an individual or a group, is to explain the decision and assist with its implementation. Conscious understanding is essential in both making and implementing decisions. Roles must be clearly defined and understood. There is a time to offer advice and input to a decision. After a decision is made it is essential for everyone to be united in implementing it; otherwise it is impossible to make a good judgement about its effectiveness. Its failure may simply be a function of strife rather than of its own weakness.

CONCLUSIONS

A child's basic behavior patterns are established by the age of 6, so that what happens in the home and community and pre-primary school regarding sexual and reproductive behavior while the child is young can have a powerful positive or negative impact that could be life long.

Therefore, the challenge before us is to incorporate a systematic moral education in schools, families and communities from an early stage. We should remember that the World Health Organization has added "spiritual health" as a new dimension of Health, we can't take the risk of defining health just as physical wellness or mental alacrity.

It is at this point that we have to understand the value of "spirituality" which is the mother of all ethical values. Life should have a positive driving force. Intellect should have a motivation. Moral values serve as "positive driving force" without which children will never know to which direction they are going.

An effective adolescent empowerment programme may consider to incorporate the following elements in it:

- Provide opportunities for students to be responsible for each other by providing cross-age grouping and cross-age tutoring. The older will benefit by being a role model and by developing patience and tact, and the younger will benefit by being helped academically and witnessing a caring, helping relationship.
- Relate educational experiences to students' lives providing opportunities for students to share their points of view.
- Develop cooperative activities in the community with service projects to help students develop a sense of responsibility and connection to the community as a whole.
- Encourage discussions with and among students concerning aspects of school life and how to interact with other people in the appropriate manner.
- Guide children in playing a role in decision making in the classroom and school.
- Provide for forms of student self-government in public schools as a means of helping students contribute to others and develop critical thinking and interaction skills.
- Use day-to-day activities and what is happening in the students' lives as opportunities to deal with values and ethics.
- Encourage students to think in complex ways about moral issues in life as they appear in the curriculum.
- Use reading and writing activities to encourage moral and ethical thought.
- Structure the learning environment so that it models democratic values and provides a safe environment for learning, sharing, and cooperating.
- Encourage self-discipline through cooperative interaction between persons in the learning environment.
- Use discussion, role-playing, and analytical and creative projects as a basis for critical thinking about values, attitudes, character traits, and moral issues.
- Use cooperative learning activities to help students develop social interaction skills. Establish parent support groups to develop a moral consensus.

SUGGESTED READING

1. Baha'i International Community, www.news.bahai.org.
2. Baha'i Community of India (including youth desk), www.bahaindia.org.
3. Benson PL, Donahue MJ, Erickson JA. Adolescence and religion: A review of the literature from 1970 to 1986. Research in the Social Scientific Study of Religion 1989;1:153–81.
4. King PE, Furrow JL. Religion as a resource for positive youth development: Religion, social capital, and moral outcomes. Developmental Psychology 2004;40:703-13.
5. Lal S. Editorial: Reaching adolescents for health and development. Indian J. Community Medicine XXVI, 2001;4,167-72, Oct-Dec.
6. Roehlkepartain EC, et al (Eds.) Spiritual development in childhood and adolescence: Moving to the Scientific Mainstream, Handbook of spiritual development in childhood and adolescence.
7. Search Institute, Developmental Assets: An Overview, available from www.search-institute.org/assets, 1996.
8. Villarreal M. Adolescent Fertility: Socio-cultural Issues, FAO, Sustainable Development Department, FAO of the UN, 1998.
9. World Bank, Preventing HIV/AIDS in India, available from www.worldbank.org.in, 2004.
10. Wuthnow, R. Studying religion, making it sociological. In: M. Dillon (Ed.). Handbook of the sociology of religion (pp.17–30). Cambridge, UK: Cambridge University Press, 2003.

46 Statistical Review of ARSH: Indian Perspective

Kalpana Apte

INTRODUCTION

In a rapidly developing country like India, the dynamics of change affect many in myriad ways. Young people are the most caught and swept in this change. Therefore, any discussion on the sexual and reproductive health of young people can only indicate towards the multi-faceted, multi-layered situations shaping the lives of Indian young people.

Today, India remains a very young country, with only 4% people above the age of 65,[1] and over 30% population in the age group of 10 - 24.[2] Based on the population projections by the Registrar General of India (1996) this means that, (Table 46.1) over 90% people in India (age group 15-59) will require sexual and reproductive health services.

Table 46.1: Projected age structure of the population as on 1st March[3] (in million)

Year	*1997*	*2002*	*2007*	*2012*
Under 15	353.64	345.11	334.80	337.93
15-59	532.60	610.55	692.64	758.61
60+	63.64	71.94	84.01	98.50

Out of these, there are an estimated 300 million young people in the age—group 10-24, whose need for sexual and reproductive health information and services remains very high.[4] As like other groups, young people's SRH needs vary based on many factors like their literacy levels, socioeconomic situation, religion, gender, marital status and urbanization of their geographical locations. These factors play an important role in access to information and services. For example, a young married adolescent of age 16 can relatively easily access a contraceptive method, but an unmarried adolescent of the same age can not.

EDUCATION AND LITERACY LEVELS

There is a wide disparity among literacy levels across states. Although overall literacy rate in the country has increased to 65% which indicates an overall increase of 13% at highest decadal rate since independence (National Literacy Mission)[5] however, literacy level among young people still remains low and generally depend on their socioeconomic profile as well as gender. Far less young girls are likely to be literate as compared to young boys in the same age group. For example 72% of young men are literate as compared to only 44% young girls from the same age group. Similarly, 63% young people (age group 15-17) residing in urban areas attend school as compared to only 44% of the same group attending school in rural areas (NFHS—2).[6] However, the total proportion of literate young women in the age 20 - 24 is higher today with 34% reporting literacy as compared to only 18% literacy among older women aged 40-44 (Singh, 1998).[7]

SOCIOECONOMIC SITUATION AND URBANIZATION

As per the 1991 census, over 25% of India's population lived in urban areas. In 2001 census this increased to around 28%. That translates to about 285 million people living in urban areas and 742 million in rural areas out of a total population of 1027 million.[8]

The statistics show that a large number of young people are engaged in income generating activities. Over 44% boys (15-19 age) and 26% girls are economically active. The young people in rural areas are more likely to drop out from school to engage in income—generating activities (ILO, 1998).[9] However, these figures do not include the household work done by young people for which they do not receive wages. Therefore, access to information remains low as these young people can not be reached as a group like school or college going young people.

SEXUAL ACTIVITY AND AGE AT MARRIAGE

In spite of a legal provision against child marriage, almost 50% girls remain at a risk of getting married before 18.[10] Also, over 32% girls get married by age 15, however, as compared to this only 6% adolescent boys get married by that age (IIPS and ORC Macro, 2000).

However, there is increasing evidence that the onset of sexual activity before marriage is starting at a younger age amongst men. More young men (ranging from 15-26%) report premarital sexual activity as compared to only (3-6%) young women reporting premarital sexual activity.[11]

SEXUAL AND REPRODUCTIVE HEALTH CONCERNS

Young people are at high risk of negative sexual and reproductive health consequences like unwanted pregnancies, sexually transmitted infections and unsafe abortions. The access to services and information depends on their marital status and gender. Rapid urbanization and technological advances like internet and mobile phones have brought about a change in the way young people interact and share information. However, this remains available to very few. Also very few internet sites contain accurate, specific and reliable information.

In India, adolescent fertility remains critically high with 20% girls giving births by age 17. Also 19% of the total fertility rates in India are contributed by girls aged 15-19 years. This early childbearing age contributes to high maternal morbidity and mortality. Many studies have also indicated the risk of closely spaced births in young women.

It is estimated that between 1 and 10% of all abortion seekers are adolescents (Ganatra 2000).[12] Other studies have indicated varying proportions ranging from 10-30% abortion seekers being young women. Although most of these are married adolescents, at least 50% of unmarried women seeking abortions are adolescent[13] and amongst these a significant proportion are below 15 years of age.

The contraceptive use remains low among young married adolescent. Only 8% married adolescent (age 15-19) have reported using any method of contraception. The unmet need remains high in this age group with 27% reporting an unmet need for contraception. Women in the age 15 to 24 years are more likely to discontinue use of contraceptives because of method failure and due to difficulty in access.[14] This indicates a higher unmet need for contraception in young women as compared to older women.

Due to unequal power dynamics young people are at a higher risk of sexual violence as well as gender based violence. Unmarried adolescent and young girls are more vulnerable to violence in the form of eve teasing, sexual coercion, child abuse, physical and emotional violence. The outcomes are early marriage, unwanted pregnancy and abortion, unprotected sex, and related health problems. It affects their self-esteem and image, education; restricts mobility, limits expressions of opposite sex friendship. 'Culture of silence' inhibits them and their families from seeking support and services.

Married young girls face violence from husbands or other adults in the form of sexual coercion/nonconsensual sex, unprotected sex, physical and emotional violence. The outcomes of the violence are unwanted pregnancy, abortion, miscarriage, still birth, female feticide, sexual violence resulting in RTIs and STIs like HIV and related health problems. It affects day to day household work, results in loss of work and economy and an increase in health costs. Stigma inhibits them from seeking support, information and services.

FPAI EXPERIENCE

FPA India reaches out annually to over 100, 000 young people providing information and services.

FPA India reaches out to a large number of young people (age 10-19). As indicated in Table 46.2, over 20, 000 young people accessed various services. This included contraceptives, maternal care and also specialized services related to HIV/AIDS, and other reproductive health care. Over 300 adolescents sought safe-abortion services. Abortion services show an increase by 143% over the previous year (2004). Services related to maternal health care also increased by 15% over 2004. Data regarding the number of adolescent seeking counselling service, is shown in Table 46.3.

Table 46.2: Number of adolescents accessing services, 2004-05

ADOLESCENTS (10-19 yr)			
Services		*2005*	*2004*
FamilyPlanning -	Boys	0	
permanent	Girls	145	
Family Planning -spacing	Boys	3,288	
	Girls	2,344	
Total		5,777	6,791
Maternal Health	Girls	4,031	3,517
Abortion	Girls	343	141
HIV/AIDS	Boys	92	572 (Boys + Girls)
	Girls	282	
Other RH	Boys	1,051	2,941
	Girls	4,427	4,324
Total number of services		21,780	18,286

Table 46.3: Number of Adolescents Provided Counselling Services, 2005

ADOLESCENTS (10-19 yr)—COUNSELING		
FP-permanent	Boys	106
	Girls	601
FP-spacing	Boys	1,226
	Girls	2,440
	Total	4,373
Maternal Health Care	Boys	747
	Girls	3,181
Safe Abortion	Boys	207
	Girls	940
HIV/AIDS	Boys	1,809
	Girls	4,194
Other RH	Boys	8,297
	Girls	13,919
	Total counseled	42,040

The following figure clearly shows the age profile of clients seeking services. As can be seen in Figure 46.1, the majority of population accessing services from FPA India is between the ages of 20 to 44 years (86% in 2005 and 88% in 2004). A marginal decrease by 1% in 10 to 14-year-old and 3% in 15 to 19-year-old accessing services was noted. There was a 4% increase in clients in the age group of 25 to 29 years and 45 to 49 years, and 2% in 50+ year's age group, thus, indicating the life cycle approach to SRH services.

SUMMARY

As can be seen from the Table 46.4, FPA India reached out to over 70,000 young people providing high quality services backed up by counseling and follow-up services. Even though a large proportion of FPAI's clients are in the age group of 10-14 and 15-19, the largest percent is within the 19-24 age group. Significantly, even in the 10-14 age group, 11 girls have sought and received safe abortion services legally and safely. Ability to reach out to this very young and vulnerable group makes FPAI services very important and significant.

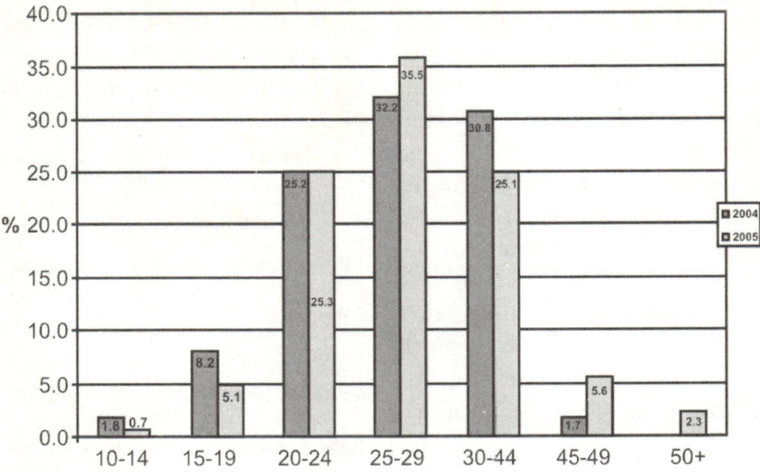

Fig. 46.1: Age of the clients, 2004-2005

Table 46.4: Counseling and SRH services provided to young people, 2005

		YOUNG PEOPLE (10-24 YEARS)		
COUNSELING		**10-14**	**15-19**	**20-24**
Abortion	Boys	34	173	632
	Girls	117	823	3,951
HIV/AIDS	Boys	462	1,347	2,317
	Girls	622	3,572	6,426
Other Rh	Boys	2,983	5,314	6,068
	Girls	4,572	9,347	15,220
Permanent methods	Boys	35	71	1,108
	Girls	59	542	8,632
Temporary methods	Boys	145	1,081	4,184
	Girls	302	2,138	9,783
Maternal health care	Boys	122	625	1,847
	Girls	399	2,782	14,114
	Total	**9,852**	**27,815**	**74,282**
	Total Boys	**3,781**	**8,611**	**16,156**
	Total Girls	**6,071**	**19,204**	**58,126**
Services				
Abortion	girls	11	332	2,914
HIV/AIDS	boys	15	77	406
	Girls	5	277	1,051
Other Rh	boys	234	817	2,548
	Girls	1,322	3,105	10,599
Male sterilisation	boys	0	0	42
Female sterilisation	girls	0	143	6,820
Temporary methods	boys	58	3,230	11,108
	Girls	144	2,200	11,710
Maternal health care	girls	71	3,960	23,197
	Total	**1,860**	**14,141**	**70,395**
	Total Boys	**307**	**4,124**	**14,104**
	Total Girls	**1,553**	**10,017**	**56,291**

RECOMMENDATIONS

FPA India works with parents/teachers and community leaders to ensure that appropriate sexuality education becomes accessible for young people. It is not only important to reach out to school and college going young people but programs need to reach out to the large contingent of out of school young people, in urban and rural areas.

Young people need to be more actively involved in developing programs and also implementing of such programs. The Peer educator model needs to be strengthened to ensure programmatic sustainability.

Specific training and sensitization programs need to be developed for teachers and parents to enable them to communicate with young people. The technologies like internet should be utilized appropriately and content monitoring of internet sites providing sexuality related information must be taken up.

The laws governing harmful practices like child marriage, sexual abuse should be strictly enforced through community sensitization and active involvement.

REFERENCES

1. Population Reference Bureau: 2000 World Population Data Sheet.
2. International Institute for Population Sciences (IIPS) and ORC Macro. 2000. National Family Health Survey (NFHS—2), 1998-1999; India. Mumbai: IIPS.
3. Report of the Technical Group on Population Projections constituted by Planning Commission, published as: Population Projections for India States 1996-2016, Registrar General, India 1996.
4. IIPS and ORC Macro, 2000; United Nations, 2001.
5. National Literacy Mission, Ministry of Human Resources, GOI.
6. National Family Health Survey-2, 1998-1999
7. Singh, S. Adolescent Childbearing in Developing Countries: A Global Review. Studies in Family Planning, 1998;29(2):117-63.
8. eCensus India: Issue 14:2003 (http://www.censusindia.net/results/eci14_page2.html).
9. International Labour Organization (ILO), 1998. Yearbook of Labour Statistics 1998. Geneva.
10. Santhya KG, Jejeebhoy SJ. 2003, Sexual and reproductive health needs of married adolescent girls, Economic and Political Weekly, 2003;38(41):4370-77.
11. Youth Sexuality 1993-94. A study of Knowledge, Attitudes, Beliefs and Practices among Urban Educated Indian Youth, FPAI 1994. And Abraham, L and K A Kumar. Sexual Experiences and their correlates among college Student in Mumbai, India International Family Planning Perspective 1999;25(3):139-46.
12. Ganatra, B.: What we know, and what we need to know. Women's Reproductive Health in India: 186-253. Rawat Publications.
13. Jejeebhoy S J. Adolescent Sexual and reproductive behaviour: A review of the evidence from India. Women's reproductive Health in India 2000;40-101.
14. Gandotra MM and Das N P: Factors influencing choice of a contraceptive and the reason for its discontinuation. Spacing as an Alternate Strategy: India's Family Welfare Programme: 1996;95-114. B R Publishing Corporation; Mari Bhat P N and Hasalkar J B. Factors influencing IUD retention in Northern Karnataka. Spacing as an Alternate Strategy: India's Family Welfare Programme:1996;63-94. B R Publishing Corporation.

47 Youth Friendly Health Services

Ashwini Bhalerao-Gandhi

INTRODUCTION

When young people are looking for urgent treatment for their own problems, public sector health services are often their last resort because there are many barriers in using existing health services.

BARRIERS

- Lack of knowledge on the part of the youth
- Legal or cultural restrictions
- Physical or logistical restrictions
- Poor quality of clinical services
- Unwelcoming services
- High cost
- Gender barriers
- Peer pressure.

HEALTH PROBLEMS FACED BY YOUNG PEOPLE

Young people come from different strata and communities—being not only of different ages and sexes but also of different cultures and life experiences. When in trouble, they usually do not know where to go and seek help. They often hesitate to visit any health care facility because they are afraid about the stigma and also wonder whether they will be treated well at a clinic. In addition to general health disorders, adolescent and young people face multiple specific problems.

Health problems faced by young people:

- General health problems
- Malnutrition/obesity/eating disorders
- Mental health problems
- Scholastic difficulties
- Addictive behaviors, accidents, violence
- Menstrual problems
- Early and unprotected sex
- Premarital sex, minimal use of contraceptives
- Unwanted pregnancies, abortions
- Prevalence of RTIS, STDS
- Female genital mutilation
- Sexual abuse.

NEWER CHALLENGES FACED BY YOUNG PEOPLE

- Early puberty
- Nuclear famililities
- Academic pressures
- Urbanization
- Industrialisation
- Effect of mass media
- Explosion of technology
- Globalization
- Experimentation (internet, mobile phones, etc).

ADOLESCENT AND YOUTH FRIENDLY HEALTH SERVICES (AFHS)

AFHS Represent an approach which brings together the qualities that young people demand, with the high standards that have to be achieved in public as well as private services. The characteristics of adolescent and youth friendly health services were discussed during the global consultation process initiated by WHO in 2000, and continued during the discussions by the expert group convened by WHO in Geneva in 2001.

CHARACTERISTICS OF ADOLESCENT FRIENDLY HEALTH SERVICES

Adolescent friendly health services need to be accessible, equitable, acceptable, appropriate, comprehensive, effective and efficient. They require:

Adolescent Friendly Policies that—

- Fulfil the rights of adolescents as stated in the UN Convention on the rights of the child and other declarations.
- Do not restrict providing health services on basis of sex, religion, age, disability, race, etc.
- Provide special attention to gender needs.
- Take into account needs of general population including vulnerable and under served groups.
- Ensure privacy and confidentiality, and promoting autonomy so that adolescents can consent to their own treatment and care.
- Make sure that services are provided free of cost or at affordable charges for adolescents.

Adolescent Friendly Procedures to Provide—

- Quick as well as confidential registration, storage and retrieval of records of patients.
- Minimal waiting time and prompt referral, if necessary.
- Flexibility of availing consultation with or without appointment welcoming walk-in clients.

Adolescent Friendly Health Care Providers who—

- Are trained to provide specific promotive, preventive and curative services tailor-made to each client's circumstances and maturity level.
- Are well motivated and supportive.
- Have non-judgmental attitude and are trustworthy.
- Have good communication skills.
- Can spare adequate amount of time for clients.
- Act in the best interest of their clients.
- Can respect as well as care for the clients irrespective of their gender, age, religion, culture, etc.
- Provide information enabling each adolescent to take a right decision out of their free will.

Adolescent Friendly Support Staff—

- Trained and motivated.
- Able to treat each adolescent client with equal care and respect.

Adolescent Friendly Health Facilities—

- Are located at a convenient place with an appealing ambience.
- Provide safe and clean environment.
- Have flexible and convenient hours of working.
- Offer privacy and are devoid of stigma.
- Provide IEC material.

Involvement and Participation of Adolescent and Youth, so that they are—

- Aware of their rights and services available.
- Encouraged to respect the rights of others and are involved in giving suggestions regarding variety of services provided.

To Solicit Involvement of Gatekeepers for example, Parents, Teachers, Social Workers, Politicians, etc.

- So that they develop trust in the health care system endorsing its utilization by the youngsters.
- To diffuse opposition by staunch religious, social and cultural authorities.

Provision of outreach, as well as Community based services involving peer educators.

Appropriate and Comprehensive Services that—

- Provide umbrella of services looking after physical, mental, social, sexual and spiritual needs of adolescents.
- Provide majority of services under one roof and referring to higher services only if required.
- Avoid unnecessary procedures, investigations, etc.

Effective Health Services for Adolescents

- Involving evidence-based protocols and guidelines.
- Having technical expertise, necessary equipments and supplies including medicines, vaccines, etc., necessary to deliver adequate health care.
- Having a process of quality improvement by on-going assessment and evaluation of existing facilities.

Efficient Services which have—

- A management information system including information on the cost of resources.
- Ability to foresee evolving issues and health problems and to adapt and incorporate changes to tackle them effectively in time to come.

LOCATIONS

Adolescent and youth friendly health services can be offered at various levels and centers. Making existing services more friendly is one option whereas establishing specific stand alone clinics is yet another option available.

- Services at health centres or hospitals—Existing services can definitely take care of the basic needs of young people provided medical and support staff are given proper training. There are also dedicated health centers which provide a full range of services especially for young people. Such services can provide training and inspiration for other health providers, but they usually only have an impact in that specific area, e.g. SHAHN at Safdarjang Hospital in New Delhi.
- Services located at other kinds of center—As same adolescents are reluctant to visit health facilities, services can also be taken to places where young people already go for example, Go for Health Youth Clubs of FPA India. Health services in Sweden reach large numbers of adolescents, including an increasing number of boys, through a network of youth centres nationwide.
- Out reach services—These are important to cater for the needs of young people who are unlikely to attend conventional health centres for example, Friend corners in Thailand were started in local shopping malls and community housing areas. The first point of contact is with adolescents trained as peer counsellors. Health staff are also on hand to provide counselling or to refer adolescents to specialized services as necessary.
- School/College health clinics—Schools and colleges are ideal places to screen for or treat a range of common illnesses, for health education and referral to a higher centre if required, e.g. Welingkar—FOGSI Growel centre at Welingkar College of Business Management, Mumbai. Services can be located anywhere where young people go—no single setting should become the only model.

A STRATEGY FOR PLANNING SERVICES

- Achieve a national consensus for action
- Decide on essential services to be provided
- Identify and set quality standards
- Link related services, networking, referrals
- Involve young people, parents and community leaders, professionals, teachers
- Political support

- Marketing, media, help-Lines
- Public private sector co-ordination
- Involvement of NGOs.

A VARIETY OF SERVICES CAN BE PROVIDED TO YOUNG PEOPLE

Specialized services concentrating on their Reproductive and sexual health include:

- Screening and advice on nutrition, self-care issues, body-image
- Counselling services
- Contraceptive services
- Pregnancy test, HIV testing, etc
- Safe Abortions
- Prenatal and postnatal care
- Mental health services
- Sexual and reproductive health education
- Space for youth groups to hold meetings
- Referral services.

These services can be provided by a team of professionals especially trained in ARSH.

GUIDELINES FOR STAFF

Staff—Gynecologists, pediatricians, physicians, psychologists, counselors, support staff, lab technicians.

Qualities and Skills

Non-judgmental and unbiased attitude, Ensure confidentiality, competence, warm and friendly approach, optimism and motivation, respect for clients irrespective of age, sex, socio-economic and marital status; adequate time for interaction, welcome drop-in clients, skills in record keeping, empathy, sensitivity.

Communicating with Young People

Good communication skills are very important to reach out to young people. They create trust and develop bonding.

- Take young people seriously
- Offer help quickly
- Give attention and encouragement
- Do not offer false assurance
- Encourage them to talk it out
- Help them to understand the cause of distress
- Maintain continued contact
- Focus on positive behavior
- Expect rebuffs.

Creating awareness and providing specific services catering to adolescent reproductive and sexual health in this manner is the need of the hour. It is essential in transforming today's adolescent boys and girls into tomorrow's responsible citizens, spouses and parents.

SUMMARY

We need to focus our attention towards the health needs of adolescents (a) to reduce mortality and morbidity now, and during their future lives (b) to respect their rights to health care, in general and reproductive health care, in particular (c) to enable them to pass on good health to their own children as they are the future parents.

Young people face dangers more complex than previous generations faced with less support and safety network.

SUGGESTED READING

1. Adolescent Friendly Health Services—An Agenda for change by Peter McInture, Oxford, UK with support from Department of Child and Adolescent Health and Development, WHO, Geneva in 2003.

48 Setting-up Adolescent Friendly Health Clinics in Private

Swati Y Bhave

INTRODUCTION

The Family welfare Dept. of Govt. of India is taking up the adolescent health delivery component in a very big way both in the RCH II and the NRHM (National Rural Health Mission) program, AFHS (Adolescent Friendly Health services) are going to be set up in district hospitals mainly to deliver ARSH services which will run on the standard for AFSH laid down by WHO.

Since adolescent medicine is not a post graduate specialty in India, there are very few special clinics geared to deliver adolescent services in the private sector.

Majority of the problems that are seen in the adolescents of today, both in the higher and lower socioeconomic groups in the urban setup, are mainly due to a high risk lifestyle and are potentially preventable. The incidence of lifestyle associated diseases like obesity, Type2 DM, hypertension and cardiovascular diseases are on the rise compounded by the physical and mental stress of today's competitive world. Premarital sex is here to stay. We should always try to emphasize the safety of abstinence and delaying initiation of sex. However one has to accept reality and empower the adolescents who are already indulging or plan to have premarital sex, to practice safe sex and prevent unwanted pregnancies and sexually transmitted diseases.

Adolescents do not belong to any specialized branch. They will approach a variety of specialists. They will continue going to their family physicians and pediatricians for day to day problems and immunizations, to an adult physician for diseases, to a gynecologist for menstruation and pregnancy related problems, to a mental health professional for their anxiety and depression and so on. Hence, managing an adolescent is a team work and hence the clinic also should have a team of specialists.

There are trained gynecologists available to look after adolescent girls but very few specialists for dealing with adolescent boys who are often neglected.

STARTING A CLINIC FOR ADOLESCENTS

The person in charge of an adolescent clinic can belong to any specialty, but should have undergone special training in adolescent health The entire staff including the receptionists, nurses and the peons, etc. have to be oriented towards the special issues of adolescent health to make the clinic *adolescent friendly* in the true sense.

The same principles outlined in Chapter 47 for youth friendly health services can be applied to a private set up also. Before starting an adolescent clinic in private practice, one has to do some basic homework. It is good to make a survey of the available adolescent services in the area and also survey if there are any area specific, specialized needs to be set up for adolescents. A referral system needs be set up with the community and nearby schools to get the adolescent clients. All specialists need to be available but specifically pediatrician, adult physician, gynecologists and mental health professionals should be available on routine basis. Dermatologists, orthopedic, ophthalmologists, ENT, etc should be as referrals.

BASIC PRINCIPLES

Hoffman established six basic principles for providing adolescent services which are as follows:

- Availability
- Accessibility
- Approachability
- Acceptability
- Appropriateness
- Affordability.

Availability

In a private set up, the best setting to establish such services is either in a corporate hospital or a polyclinic where all the required services are easily available under one roof. If an adolescent has to be sent elsewhere for a referral, there is a possibility that he/she may be lost to future follow-up.

However, this does not mean that adolescent services cannot be delivered in a small private clinic. A super specialty adolescent practice can be set up in an already existing clinic in a private set up. But the referral system has to be well established. This is not an easy task and one would need to put in diligent effort to do this in a private set up.

In Thailand, adolescent centers have been established in shopping malls. These centers have help lines, individualized counseling services and classes for training in dancing, public speaking and so on. Being in a mall many adolescents feel comfortable in accessing services.

Accessibility

The clinic timings should be suitable for the adolescents if one wants a good attendance.. Hence, weekdays during school or college hours should be avoided. The most convenient timing for adolescents are in the evening between 6 and 8 pm. These are generally after-school hours, and parents can also come if needed, as these are after office hours also. Saturday afternoons are another choice since many schools are closed or have half-day timings. Sunday mornings may be suitable for both adolescents and parents but due to many families wanting to have family time together this timing may not become very popular

The clinic should be at a location that is easily accessible by public transport, which is primarily used by unaccompanied adolescents.

Approachability

Adolescents are very sensitive to the atmosphere in a clinic and it needs to be welcoming and comfortable. The ambience has to be very sophisticated if it is for the affluent but this may be inhibitory to the middle and lower class. A clean and comfortable setting should be the minimum requirement.

Adolescents are unsure about the topics or the questions which can be answered in this clinic. A way to break this barrier is to keep pamphlets on various subjects in the waiting room. These should be on obesity, diet, exercise, stress management, sexually transmitted disorders, use of condom, menstrual hygiene, masturbation, etc. This serves a dual-purpose it educates them in a non-threatening manner and it also gives a signal to them that it is okay or 'done' to ask questions on these issues. Magazines or other reading material on these aspects also should be kept in the waiting room.

Acceptability

Adolescents will come back for follow-up to the clinic only if a good rapport is established with them. The staff should not be judgmental or moralistic. They should remember that they are in the clinic to help and to guide the adolescent through their problems, which could include delicate issues like sexuality and substance abuse.

The appointment should not be forced upon them but it should be set up with their consent and preferences so that it does not overlap with their important academic assignments and other activities such as hobbies, sports, etc.

An informatory notice could be put up in the clinic addressed to the adolescents and their parents explaining the rationale behind setting up the adolescent clinic.

Individual files of the patient's medical records should be maintained, but matters regarding ARSH and substance abuse should be kept confidential and not be accessible to everyone in the clinic.

Appropriateness

Teenagers are not the easiest to handle unless the clinician has the skills for it. Hence, it is not just enough to undergo training in adolescent care before venturing into starting a clinic but it is equally important that the service providers must genuinely like teenagers which many adults do not.

When advice is given for sensitive issues like sexuality, it is important to keep in mind the teen's upbringing, socio-cultural aspects, mental and emotional capacity.

Ideas about dating, premarital sex, contraception, abortion, etc in higher socioeconomic groups could be quite different from those of a conservative middle class ideology that emphasizes moral values.

The advice has to be based on individuals and generalized advice on these issues may not yield the desired results.

Affordability

As in other areas of medicine practice, the clinician needs to keep the fees flexible. A needy teenager should not be deprived of services just because she/he cannot afford the clinic fees. In case the adolescent cannot afford the clinic fees, they should be referred to centers which have free services, especially in cases of ASRH.

In a Western set up where teenagers start earning at an early age they pay for their consultations.

THE SETTING

The ambience should put the adolescent at ease so that they are comfortable discussing their problems especially sexually intimate issues. If space permits, the consultation and examination rooms should preferably be separate to allow for privacy. Minimal interruptions also contribute to an appropriate atmosphere.

It is important to do group counseling to both parents and adolescents for conveying preventive health messages. It is good to have an access to a seminar room with audiovisual facilities. It could be used to conduct health awareness programs and group discussions with the adolescents.

The services provided by the adolescent clinic should be holistic and should include annuual health check-ups, immunization, family life education and life skill classes, premarital counseling, etc.

COMMUNICATING SKILLS

Adolescents are very self-conscious, and have difficulty in discussing intimate issues specially related to sexuality. The clinician has to be very sensitive, patient, flexible and requires good communication skills specially orientated to the adolescent development. Open ended questions should be asked so that communication is bi-directional.

It is necessary to discuss ideas and thoughts clearly according to their chronological age and individual maturity. Physical appearance and chronological age may be misleading as measures of cognitive development

Early adolescence has concrete thinking and they can only relate to the present and immediate consequences whereas late adolescence develop abstract thinking and can project into the future. This understanding is very important when one gives health messages or anticipatory guidance and preventive counseling.

A non-judgmental attitude has to be adopted at all times. As a clinician, one may have strong personal moral values and ethics, but one has to be objective and help the adolescent with the problem on hand, be it the consequences of premarital unsafe sex or substance abuse.

The clinician should neither act like a figure of authority nor be too friendly as both will put off adolescents since they have come to a technically resourceful person with a potential to provide desired help. It is best to behave in the natural and appropriate manner of a physician.

It is important to assess the body language and non verbal cues while history taking and physical examination. An adolescent, who has an attitude or appears hostile is actually showing a defense mechanism to cover inner fear. A sullen, non-communicative adolescent is often hiding inner turmoil and will open up to a warm and caring attitude.

Adolescents often show a verbal-nonverbal mismatch. While the facial expression and body language conveys sadness verbally they will keep saying "everything is fine and there is no problem". They may react with anger if further pressed.

Sometimes the clinician may subconsciously emit negative vibrations if he or she is faced with an adolescent that indulges in premarital sex, substance abuse or has come to seek abortion. These non verbal cues will be picked up by the adolescent and cause barrier in communication A clinician has to have empathy to the adolescents's problems.

HISTORY TAKING AND EXAMINATION

History taking should achieve various objectives—determining health problems, motivating them to carry out the treatment plan and monitoring them. It is also very important for developing a rapport with them for ensuring a proper follow-up Assurance of confidentiality is a must but the limits should be clearly stated for, e.g. parental information and cooperation will be needed in cases of abortion, HIV testing, substance abuse, suicidal risk, etc. Parental involvement in the interview is a judgment that needs to be individualized in each case.

The first interview should be a detailed one and will take 30 to 45 minutes. Subsequent take less time depending upon the specific problem.

HISTORY TAKING

History taking in an adolescent needs a special approach.

Using the mnemonic HEADSS FIRST (Goldenring) approach for medico-social history.

H Home,
E Education,
A Abuse,
D Drugs,
S Safety practices,
S Sexuality,

F Friends,
I Image,
R Recreation,
S Spirituality
T Threats.

One can add to the above like Health in **H,** Activities (hobbies) in **A,** depression in **D,** family in **F,** Sexual orientation and sexual abuse, suicide in **S** and so on

A psychosocial assessment is as important as a physical assessment. Screening questionnaires aid in helping identify problems and high-risk situations. A questionnaire saves time and is good for keeping records, however, it is not a substitute for a personal interview.

Examination should be done for an adolescent boy in the presence of a male attendant and for a girl in the presence of a female attendant if the clinician is of the opposite sex.

This is also important for the protection of the physician from any false charges of molestation and also from problems of infatuation by the impressionable adolescents or temptation of flirting by the clinician.

While eliciting a history and performing a physical examination, the opportunity to provide anticipatory guidance should not be missed.

MONITORING THE ADOLESCENT

Adolescents need to be monitored on the lines of a "well baby clinic".

A chart for Tanner's classification to assess and monitor puberty should be placed in each file along with the growth and height charts for future follow up of the individual teen. A blood pressure measurement and BMI record also should be kept for follow-up.

Depending on the weight, appropriate advice needs to be given for obesity, eating disorders and malnutrition, etc.

While eliciting a history and doing an examination, *anticipatory guidance* should be given for high risk behavior, school performance, eating disorders, nutritional status, physical activity, high blood pressure and visual defects.

Adolescent clinics are good avenues to provide *preventive counseling* for individual or in groups on lifestyle modification, stress management, prevention of reproductive tract infections, teenage pregnancy, etc.

SUGGESTED READING

1. Bhave Swati Y, Galagali P. Setting up adolescent clinic in private practice, in Bhaves Textbook of adolescent medicine 1st ed 2006 Chief Ed Bhave Swati Y Jaypee publishers, New Delhi, 91-16.
2. Bhave Swati Y. Setting up adolescent clinic in private set up in Course Manual for Adolescent health. Part 2. IAP-ITPAH 2002 Chief Ed Swati Y Bhave Cambridge press, New Delhi.
3. Coupey SM. Interviewing Adolescents. Pediatr Cli of North Am 1997;44:1349-62.
4. Elster Arthur B, Kuznets Naomi J (Eds.) AMA Guidelines for Adolescent Preventive Services. USA. Williams and Wilikins: 1994.
5. Elster Arthur B, Levenberg Patricia. Integrating Comprehensive Adolescent Preventive Services into routine medical care. Pediatr Cli of North Am 1997;44:1365-78.
6. Felice M E, Friedman S B: Behavioral considerations in the health care of adolescents: PCNA 1982 vl.29, no.2: 399-413: Goldenring MN, Cohen E. Getting into adolescent heads. Contemp Pediatr 98;5:75-90.
7. Goldenring MN, Cohen E. Getting into adolescent heads. Contemp Pediatr 1998;5:75-90.
8. Hofmann AD (Ed). Adolescent Medicine. Menlo-Park, CA: Addison-Wesley, 1983.
9. Larsen K M, Smith C K. Assessment of non-verbal communication in the patient-physician interview: J Fam Pract. 1981:12:481-8
10. Mehta R. Approach to adolescent client in in Bhaves Textbook of adolescent medicine 1st ed 2006 Chief Ed Bhave Swati Y Jaypee Publishers New Delhi, 1.4; 16-21.
11. Neinstein Lawrence S. The office visit and interview technique. In: Lawrence S Neinstein, Urban and Schwarrzenberg (Eds.). Adolecent Health Care A Practical Guide. Baltimore-Munich 45-56.
12. Patel DR. Setting up adolescent services: office practice. In; Greydanus DE Chief Editor Part 2. IAP-ITPAH 2002 Chief Ed Swati Y Bhave New Delhi: Cambridge press, 9-13.
13. Schubiner H, Eggly S. Strategies for mental health education for adolescent patients: A preliminary investigation J Adolesc Health 1995;17:37-41.

Index